Ultra Medicine

**Essential Preparation
for Medical Finals**

Ultra Medicine

Essential Preparation for Medical Finals

David Cockshoot

MRCGP MRCP
Honorary Senior Lecturer
Department of Primary Care
University of Leeds

Oliver Monfredi

Bsc (Hons) MB ChB (Hons)
Senior House Officer
St James' Hospital, Leeds

www.ultramedicine.co.uk

Blackwell
Publishing

© 2005 David Cockshoot and Oliver Monfredi
Published by Blackwell Publishing Ltd
Blackwell Publishing, Inc., 350 Main Street, Malden, Massachusetts 02148-5020, USA
Blackwell Publishing Ltd, 9600 Garsington Road, Oxford OX4 2DQ, UK
Blackwell Publishing Asia Pty Ltd, 550 Swanston Street, Carlton, Victoria 3053, Australia

The right of the Authors to be identified as the Authors of this Work has been asserted in accordance with the Copyright, Designs and Patents Act 1988.

First published 2005

2   2009

Library of Congress Cataloging-in-Publication Data
Cockshoot, David.
   Ultra medicine : essential preparation for medical finals / David Cockshoot, Oliver Monfredi.
      p. ; cm.
   Includes index.
   ISBN 978-1-405-12403-4
   1. Medicine — Examinations, questions, etc.
   [DNLM: 1. Medicine — Examination Questions. W 18.2 C666u 2005]
I. Monfredi, Oliver.   II. Title.

R834.5.C63 2005
   610′.76 — dc22

2004020629

A catalogue record for this title is available from the British Library

Set in 8.75/11.5pt Minion by SNP Best-set Typesetter Ltd., Hong Kong
Printed and bound in Singapore by Ho Printing Singapore Pte Ltd

Commissioning Editor: Vicki Noyes
Development Editor: Karen Moore
Production Controller: Kate Charman

For further information on Blackwell Publishing, visit our website:
http://www.blackwellpublishing.com

The publisher's policy is to use permanent paper from mills that operate a sustainable forestry policy, and which has been manufactured from pulp processed using acid-free and elementary chlorine-free practices. Furthermore, the publisher ensures that the text paper and cover board used have met acceptable environmental accreditation standards.

Contents

Preface

This book is aimed primarily at the medical student preparing for finals, but will also be helpful in preparation for MRCP. The material was largely originally written to form the basis of a series of revision courses, and therefore has already been tried and tested. Our intention in writing this material was to take the student through all the 'core' subjects in medicine and some non-core but important 'chestnuts' that seem to feature regularly in examinations. By working through the material and reading around the subject matter, the candidate will be prepared to face most eventualities in medical finals. The book is divided into two main sections; four practice examinations (each of 24 MCQs and 5 or more EMQs) with expanded answers, and a section on the 50 commonest OSCE stations.

The difficulty in revising for medical examinations as an undergraduate (and frequently as a postgraduate) is attempting to cover a vast amount of factual information without having the clinical experience to 'hang' the knowledge on in order to make it stick. Although the ideal way to learn is to see a case and read around it, practical constraints will frequently prevent this being a feasible option. Challenging your knowledge using questions based on clinical cases is the next best option. To this end we hope we have achieved our aims.

Acknowledgements

Dr Sheila M. Clark FRCP, Department of Dermatology, Leeds General Infirmary. For help with the fine art of describing skin problems.

Dr Sally Nicholson MB ChB, Department of Surgery, St James' Hospital, Leeds.

Dr Bushera Choudry MB ChB.

Dr David Scullion, Consultant Radiologist, Harrogate District General Hospital. For contribution of the radiographs herein.

Normal Values

Haematology

Haemoglobin		
Male	13.5–18.0	g/dL
Female	11.5–16.5	g/dL
Mean corpuscular volume (MCV)	76–96	fL
White cell count	4–11	$\times10^9$/L
Neutrophils	2.0–7.7	$\times10^9$/L
Lymphocytes	1.6–4.0	$\times10^9$/L
Eosinophils	0.04–0.4	$\times10^9$/L
Monocytes	0.2–0.8	$\times10^9$/L
Basophils	0.01–0.1	$\times10^9$/L
Platelets	150–450	$\times10^9$/L
PT	10–14	seconds
APTT	35–45	seconds
D-dimer	<500	ng/mL

Blood gases

PaO_2	>10.6	kPa
$PaCO_2$	4.8–6.1	kPa
HCO_3^-	20–28	kPa
pH	7.35–7.45	
Anion gap	12–20	mmol/L

Biochemistry

Albumin	35–50	g/L
Amylase	25–125	U/L
Alkaline phosphatase	30–150	U/L
Bilirubin	3–17	µmol/L
Calcium (total)	2.12–2.65	mmol/L
Creatinine	80–120	µmol/L
CRP	<10	mg/L
Phosphate	0.8–1.45	mmol/L
Potassium	3.5–5.0	mmol/L
Sodium	135–145	mmol/L
Protein (total)	60–85	mmol/L
Urate	0.18–0.46	mmol/L
Urea	2.5–6.7	mmol/L

Part 1 Practice Papers

Introduction

Ideally, it is best to take each paper as a practice examination of 24 MCQs and 5 (or more) EMQs, completed without interruption in one sitting. Allow yourself 2 hours. For EMQs, attempt to reach the answer first without recourse to scanning the picking list, as these will have been constructed deliberately to throw you off the scent. For MCQs we recommend you go through them rapidly, writing down the answers for the ones you are sure about on the first run through, leaving the rest. Go through the questions a second time, concentrating on the questions you did not know the answers for the first time through. Go with your first instinct, don't be tempted into indecision unless your original answer is clearly incorrect — the questions are written to tempt you into indecision. Then go through the MCQs a third and final time, checking all your answers carefully, being sure you have read the question in full.

Good luck!

Paper 1 Questions

MCQs

[1] Concerning cardiac failure . . .
(a) valvular disease is the most common cause in the UK
(b) raised levels of atrial natriuretic peptide (ANP) are thought to be beneficial in heart failure
(c) a third heart sound is a common finding on ausculation
(d) the heart looks small on plain postero-anterior chest radiograph
(e) all diuretics used in treatment of cardiac failure potentially cause hypokalaemia

[2] Concerning hypertension . . .
(a) approximately 50% of all cases of hypertension are caused by renal dysfunction
(b) patients with Conn's syndrome usually have a raised serum potassium level
(c) hypothyroidism does not cause hypertension
(d) the 'Cushing reflex' is an increase in systolic blood pressure that occurs secondary to Cushing's syndrome
(e) malignant hypertension can be diagnosed on fundoscopy alone

[3] Acute myocardial infarction . . .
(a) causes chest pain not relieved by glyceryl trinitrate (GTN)
(b) can be entirely painless in elderly diabetic patients
(c) should prompt administration of intramuscular morphine to relieve pain
(d) can be diagnosed on the history alone
(e) first shows on ECG in the form of 'Q' waves

[4] The following are recognized complications of acute MI . . .
(a) Sheehan's syndrome
(b) acute aortic regurgitation

(c) Dressler's syndrome
(d) electromechanical disociation
(e) left ventricular aneurysm

[5] The following cardiac events are matched correctly to the corresponding ECG changes . . .
(a) inferior infarct → ST-segment depression in leads II, III and aVF
(b) pericarditis → downward-sloping ST-segment depression in all anterior chest leads
(c) atrial fibrillation → irregularly irregular P-waves
(d) first degree heart block → broad QRS complexes
(e) ventricular aneurysm → persistent ST-segment elevation in chest leads

[6] In peripheral arterial occlusive disease . . .
(a) the relationship between radius of artery and flow within it is described by the Fick principle
(b) claudication means 'cramping' in Latin
(c) Leriche syndrome is arterial occlusive disease below the popliteal trifurcation
(d) 'rest pain' commonly occurs in the feet and metatarsal heads
(e) arterial ulcers are usually painless

[7] Concerning aortic stenosis . . .
(a) all aortic valve murmurs are heard best with the patient on their left side with breath held in end-expiration
(b) it causes hypertrophy of only the left ventricle
(c) it causes a 'Waterhammer' character in the radial pulse
(d) it causes an 'ejection systolic' murmur
(e) it is a common cause of atrial fibrillation

[8] Concerning atrial fibrillation (AF) . . .
(a) it is commonly caused by dehydration

(b) when caused by high levels of circulating thyroid hormone, it is always accompanied by thyroid eye signs
(c) no P waves are present on the ECG
(d) the QRS complex is broad
(e) class Ic antidysrhythmics (e.g. flecainide) are safe to give to most patients with atrial tachyarrhythmias

[9] Concerning the respiratory organs of the body . . .
(a) the right main bronchus lies more vertically than the left
(b) the lung is an organ with a single blood supply (i.e. the pulmonary artery)
(c) the alveolar lining of the lungs comprises mainly type I pneumocytes
(d) only the right lung has an oblique fissure
(e) in healthy subjects, the strongest stimulator of ventilation is an increase in the arterial partial pressure of CO_2 ($PaCO_2$)

[10] On examination of the chest of a patient with a unilateral tension pneumothorax . . .
(a) chest wall movements are decreased on both sides
(b) the mediastinum is pulled towards the affected side
(c) the percussion note may be hyperresonant
(d) breath sounds may be decreased or absent on the affected side
(e) tactile vocal resonance will be increased on the affected side

[11] Concerning chronic obstructive pulmonary disease (COPD) . . .
(a) the airway obstruction is entirely irreversible
(b) chronic bronchitis is believed to be due mainly to mucous gland hypertrophy
(c) patients commonly demonstrate asterixis
(d) 'cor pulmonale' is defined as lung disease secondary to ventricular hypertrophy
(e) it mainly leads to type II respiratory failure

[12] Concerning respiratory failure . . .
(a) $PaCO_2$ is, by definition, elevated in all types of respiratory failure
(b) the commonest cause of type II respiratory failure is pneumonia
(c) pulsus paradoxus is a sign commonly associated with respiratory failure
(d) it always presents with dyspnoea

(e) it causes 'bat's wing' pulmonary oedema, upper lobe diversion and Kerley-B lines on chest radiograph

[13] Concerning asthma . . .
(a) airway limitation is uniformly reversible in asthma
(b) typical asthma attacks occur during exercise
(c) ACE inhibitors should not be given to asthmatic subjects
(d) symptoms of asthma are usually worse at night
(e) β_2 adrenoceptor antagonists are commonly used in treatment of asthma

[14] Tuberculosis . . .
(a) is caused by the Gram-negative bacillus *M. tuberculosis*
(b) is a recognized cause of apical lung fibrosis
(c) is classically associated with the presence of non-caseating granulomas
(d) is diagnosed using one test with two different names: Heaf and Mantoux
(e) is a recognized cause of erythema nodosum

[15] Concerning palpation of the abdomen . . .
(a) in healthy, slim individuals, the liver is normally palpable in the right upper quadrant in deep inspiration
(b) the normal liver extends superiorly to the 3rd intercostal space
(c) hepatic enlargement usually proceeds toward the left iliac fossa
(d) in healthy, slim individuals, the spleen is normally palpable on deep inspiration in the left hypochondrium
(e) splenic enlargement occurs obliquely, toward the right iliac fossa

[16] The following are recognized gastrointestinal causes of finger clubbing . . .
(a) fibrosis
(b) coeliac disease
(c) Plummer–Vinson syndrome
(d) gastrointestinal lymphoma
(e) cystic fibrosis

[17] The following are recognized medical causes of abdominal pain . . .
(a) diabetic ketoacidosis
(b) myocardial infarction
(c) Addison's disease

(d) hypercalcaemia
(e) lead poisoning

[18] The oesophagus . . .
(a) lies anterior to the trachea
(b) lies entirely within the thorax
(c) has no serosal layer
(d) is composed entirely of smooth muscle
(e) disorder oesophageal achalasia is caused by pathological spasm of the lower oesophageal sphincter

[19] Concerning gastrointestinal (GI) bleeding . . .
(a) melaena is loss of fresh blood per rectum
(b) blood from an upper GI bleed always arrives at the rectum in the form of melaena
(c) the commonest cause of upper GI bleeding is oesophageal varices
(d) octreotide infusion is useful in the acute management of upper GI bleed
(e) melaena is typically described to have a 'coffee ground' character

[20] Concerning gastric ulcers (GUs) . . .
(a) they are usually caused by acid hypersecretion
(b) they cause pain that is exacerbated by fasting
(c) they are not associated with malignant transformation
(d) medical therapy is better at healing GUs than duodenal ulcers
(e) Curling's and Cushing's ulcers are subtypes of gastric ulcer disease

[21] Concerning gallstones . . .
(a) the most common type of gallstone is the pigment type
(b) 90–95% of gallstones are visible on plain abdominal radiograph if the patient is fasted
(c) the term 'choledocholithiasis' literally means 'stones within the cystic duct'

(d) gallstones are commoner in females
(e) rapid weight loss is a known risk factor for biliary lithogenesis

[22] Concerning self poisoning . . .
(a) a cherry red colour to the skin indicates carbon dioxide poisoning
(b) opiates cause miosis
(c) ventricular tachycardia is common in significant benzodiazepine poisoning
(d) carbon monoxide poisoning is treated by flumazenil infusion
(e) flumazenil is given to treat suspected benzodiazepine overdose

[23] Concerning acute pancreatitis . . .
(a) it is most commonly caused by pancreatic trauma
(b) it causes hypogastric abdominal pain
(c) higher levels of amylase are seen in patients with gallstone pancreatitis compared with alcoholic pancreatitis
(d) the severity of an attack of pancreatitis is indicated by Ranson's score
(e) treatment includes administration of large quantities of intravenous fluids

[24] Concerning small bowel obstruction . . .
(a) it is most commonly caused by tumours in the UK
(b) a volvulus is where a more proximal region of bowel telescopes through the lumen of adjacent distal bowel
(c) gallstone ileus occurs when a gallstone passes down the common bile duct into the bowel to obstruct the lumen
(d) typically, bowel sounds are absent
(e) paralytic ileus is caused by mechanical malignant obstruction of the bowel lumen

EMQs

Question 1

Match the following examination findings to the most accurate diagnosis:

(1)

JVP	Normal
Apex	'Tapping' in character, not displaced laterally
Auscultation	Grade 3 mid-diastolic murmur at apex, no pre-systolic accentuation
Chest	Clear
BP	155/82 mmHg

(2)

JVP	Elevated
Apex	Displaced laterally, and 'thrusting' in character
Auscultation	Pan-systolic murmur at apex
Chest	Bi-basal end expiratory crepitations
BP	143/65 mmHg

(3)

JVP	Normal
Apex	'Tapping' in character, not displaced
Auscultation	Grade 3 mid-diastolic murmur at apex, pre-systolic accentuation
Chest	Clear
BP	162/73 mmHg

(4)

JVP	8 cm
Apex	Displaced, thrusting in character
Auscultation	Short early diastolic murmur
Chest	Few bi-basal crepitations
BP	180/62 mmHg

(5)

JVP	Normal
Apex	'Heaving' in character and displaced laterally
Auscultation	Grade 3 crescendo-decrescendo systolic murmur over whole precordium, not heard in carotid area
Chest	Few bi-basal crepitations
BP	110/93 mmHg

(a) Mitral stenosis
(b) Mitral regurgitation
(c) Aortic regurgitation
(d) Aortic sclerosis with atrial fibrillation
(e) Aortic regurgitation with left ventricular failure
(f) Mitral stenosis with atrial fibrillation
(g) Mitral regurgitation and stenosis
(h) Aortic stenosis
(i) Aortic sclerosis
(j) Mitral regurgitation with diastolic flow murmur
(k) None of these

Question 2

Match the following case histories to the best diagnosis given in the list below.

(1) A 47-year-old woman presents with a history of recurrent headaches over 5 years. The pain is described as unilateral, behind the eye and severe. She is well between episodes. There is no vomiting although she feels nauseated and has abdominal discomfort. The onset is typically sudden. She occasionally has 'hazy' disturbance of her vision. There are no abnormal features on systemic review. In the past she has had hypertension, but is currently not taking treatment. She has three children. There are no regular medications. On examination she has a BMI of 29 and a BP recording of 170/95 mmHg. Otherwise a full neurological examination was normal, including fundoscopy.

(2) A 15-year-old girl presents with a 5-week history of persistent headaches. These are described as 'all over the head'. There is associated episodic blurring of vision and dizziness. There is no history of head injury. These headaches occur throughout the day. There have been several episodes of vomiting. In the past she has been fit and well. Her mother and sister have both suffered episodes of migraine since childhood. She takes the oral contraceptive pill as her only medication. On examination she is obese and has a BMI of 32. She is normotensive. Cranial nerve examination is normal. Fundoscopy reveals bilateral blurring of the optic disc margins. There are no abnormal findings in the peripheral nervous system.

(3) A 52-year-old patient attends complaining of episodic bouts of headache. He has no previous history of headaches. The pain is described as burning and severe. The pain occurs behind the right eye, and is associated with lacrimation, and running of the nostril on the same side. Each episode lasts approximately 1 h and then subsides. In the past he has suffered from diabetes and angina. He smokes 20 cigarettes per day. His current medication includes metfomin and GTN spray for occasional use. You happen to see him during an acute episode. He has conjunctival injection on the side of the pain. Cranial nerve examination and fundoscopy findings are normal.

(4) A 58-year-old female patient presents with her relatives with a history of increasing headaches. The pain is felt worse at the top of the head. These occur every day and improve towards the end of the day. In addition there have been several reported episodes of irregular 'jerking' of the left arm, each lasting around 5 min. There is no history of head injury. There is a 10-year history of excessive alcohol consumption, 30 units per day. She takes no regular medication. On examination she is apyrexial. There is a bilateral coarse tremor. There is a single spider naevus on the upper chest wall, but no jaundice or hepatomegaly. Cranial nerve examination reveals a right-sided homonymous inferior quadrantanopia.

(5) A 19-year-old university student presents acutely with a headache, vomiting and photophobia. He had been found confused, wandering around his hall of residence looking for his room. He had been fit and well until a few hours ago. Prior to admission, in the ambulance, he had been observed to have a grand mal fit, which has responded to rectal diazepam. Past medical history includes an admission for observation 6 months previously following a minor head injury after falling off his bike. He had received the meningitis C vaccine before going to university. On examination he was pyrexial at 38.7°C. Confused and GCS 10/15. There was obvious neck stiffness and photophobia. There was no rash. Cranial nerve examination was normal. The pupil size was 3 mm bilaterally and reactive and the optic discs were thought to be normal.

(a) Trigeminal neuralgia
(b) Migraine
(c) Acute bacterial meningitis
(d) Tension headache

(e) Giant cell arteritis
(f) Space occupying lesion
(g) Chronic subdural haematoma
(h) Epilepsy
(i) Cavernous sinus thrombosis
(j) Viral meningitis
(k) Benign intracranial hypertension
(l) Cluster headache
(m) Referred pain
(n) Hypertensive encephalopathy
(o) Acute encephalitis
(p) None of these

Question 3

Match the following chest examination findings to the most likely diagnosis:

(1)
Respiratory rate	36 b.p.m.
Central cyanosis	Present
Trachea	Central
Chest shape	Normal
Expansion	Equal
Percussion note	Resonant bilaterally
Auscultation	Normal breath sounds

(2)
Respiratory rate	32 b.p.m.
Central cyanosis	Present
Trachea	Deviated to the right
Chest shape	Normal
Expansion	Reduced on left
Percussion note	Hyperresonant on left
Auscultation	Reduced breath sounds on left

(3)
Respiratory rate	16 b.p.m.
Central cyanosis	Absent
Trachea	Deviated to left side
Chest shape	Depressed chest wall at left apex
Expansion	Reduced in left upper zone
Percussion note	Dull over left clavicle
Auscultation	Normal

(4) Respiratory rate — 20 b.p.m.
Central cyanosis — Absent
Trachea — Deviated to the right
Chest shape — Normal
Expansion — Reduced at right base
Percussion note — Stony dull at right base
Auscultation — Reduced breath sounds at right base

(5) Respiratory rate — 28 b.p.m.
Central cyanosis — Present
Trachea — Central
Chest shape — Normal
Expansion — Normal
Percussion note — Dull at right base
Auscultation — Bronchial area at right base

(6) Respiratory rate — 28 b.p.m.
Central cyanosis — Present
Trachea — Central
Chest shape — Hyperinflated bilateral
Expansion — Equal
Percussion note — Resonant equally left and right sides
Auscultation — Diffuse polyphonic expiratory wheezing

(a) Lung abscess
(b) Right lower lobe pneumonia
(c) Right sided pleural effusion
(d) Old tuberculosis at right apex
(e) Acute pulmonary oedema
(f) Asthma
(g) Tension pneumothorax on the right
(h) Left ventricular failure
(i) Left apical lung fibrosis
(j) Right ventricular failure
(k) Pulmonary embolism
(l) Inhaled foreign body in right main bronchus
(m) None of these

Question 4

From the following questions, choose the best diagnosis from the list below.

(1) A 7-year-old boy presents with spontaneous onset of swelling and pain, in his right knee. The previous day he had run a cross-country race at school without problems. There is no family history of haemophilia or other bleeding disorder. On examination he was mildly pyrexial at 37.5°C and he appeared in pain. The right knee was hot, swollen and locally tender. The following investigations were obtained:

Hb — 12.3 g/dL
WCC — 5.6×10^9/L
Platelets — 354×10^9/L
PT — 12 s (NR 10–15 s)
APPT — 72 s (NR 25–35 s)
Bleeding time — Normal
Factor VIII:C — 5% of normal

(2) A 34-year-old man presents with a swollen and painful right knee. There is no preceeding history of trauma. His brother had had similar problems in the past. The following investigations were obtained:

Hb — 14.7 g/dL
WCC — 10.6×10^9/L
Platelets — 373×10^9/L
PT — 14 s (NR 10–15 s)
APPT — 79 s (NR 25–35 s)
Bleeding time — Normal
Factor VIII:C — Normal

(3) A 27-year-old female is investigated for heavy periods. Her mother had similar problems. She had also noticed prolonged bleeding from simple cuts and after blood taking. She was on no medication. The following investigations were obtained:

Hb — 10.2 g/dL
WCC — 9.6×10^9/L
Platelets — 175×10^9/L
PT — 11 s (NR 10–15 s)
APPT — 79 s (NR 25–35 s)
Bleeding time — 18 min (normal <10 min)
Factor VIII:C — 20% of normal

(4) A confused 78-year-old patient is admitted and noted to have numerous bruises. Her relatives say she takes a range of medications, but the details are not known and no reliable history can be obtained from the patient. In her bag is found a cardiology outpatients appointment card. On examination she is confused and drowsy with a GCS of 9/15. There are multiple large bruises of the skin. She has an enlarged right pupil that reacts poorly to light. Her pulse is 52/min and irregularly irregular and blood pressure is 200/110. The following investigations were obtained:

Hb	14.3 g/dL
WCC	7.5×10^9/L
Platelets	415×10^9/L
PT	31 s (NR 10–15 s)
APPT	82 s (NR 25–35 s)
Bleeding time	5 min (normal <10 min)
Factor VIII:C	Normal

(5) An asymptomatic 54-year-old female consults her GP because of concern over frequent bruising episodes. She complains of bleeding when brushing her teeth. On examination she has numerous old and new bruises, particularly on her lower legs. The following investigations were obtained;

Hb	14.7 g/dL
WCC	10.6×10^9/L
Platelets	405×10^9/L
PT	11 s (NR 10–15 s)
APPT	25 s (NR 25–35 s)
Bleeding time	7 min (normal <10 min)
Factor VIII:C	Normal

(a) Haemophilia A
(b) Vitamin K deficiency
(c) Von Willebrand's disease
(d) Liver disease
(e) Haemophilia B
(f) Treatment with unfractionated heparin
(g) Thrombocytopenia
(h) Treatment with warfarin
(i) Treatment with low molecular weight heparin
(j) Disseminated intravascular coagulation
(k) Easy bruising syndrome
(l) Vitamin K deficiency
(m) Henoch–Schönlein purpura

Question 5

In the diagnosis of chest pain, match the following clinical scenarios to the most likely diagnosis in the list below.

(1) A 35-year-old male patient presents with a history of chest pain for several days. The pain is localized over the anterior aspect of the chest. It does not radiate. Although the patient does not have a cough, coughing exacerbates the pain. In the past he has been fit and well. He plays Sun-day league football regularly and has not had to miss any games recently. He takes no medication. On examination he is slim, athletic and not in distress. Examination of the cardiovascular system and chest are unremarkable. There is, however, tenderness over a number of sterno-costal joints with associated swelling.

(2) A 19-year-old previously healthy female presents with a short history of right-sided chest pain and gradually increasing shortness of breath. Coughing exacerbates the pain. She has had a non-productive cough for 2 days prior to the onset of the pain and intermittent fever. There has been no haemoptysis. She is pregnant at 32 weeks gestation. She smokes 15 cigarettes per day. On examination she is unwell. Her body mass index is raised at 29 kg/m². Her temperature is recorded at 39.5°C. The respiratory rate is 30 b.p.m. and the pulse is 110/min and regular. Her JVP is measured at 4 cm above the angle of Louis. The blood pressure is recorded at 80/48 mmHg and the heart sounds are normal. Chest expansion is equal. There is no abnormality on percussion. On auscultation there is a pleural rub at the right base.

(3) A 20-year-old male patient returns from his summer holiday in Devon complaining of a constant bilateral lower anterior chest pain. He has been unwell whilst away with a dry cough, sore throat and sweating. He is otherwise usually well, with no significant past medical history. On examination there is tenderness of the lower anterior chest wall and epigastria. Otherwise the cardiovascular system and respiratory system are unremarkable. ECG and chest radiograph are reported as normal.

(4) A 54-year-old male was admitted to casualty with severe chest pain by emergency ambulance. The pain occurred suddenly at work when he was lifting a heavy steel plate into a rolling machine. He described the pain as a 'pulling sensation' in his chest. The pain was located in the centre of the chest and did not radiate. He felt sick but did not vomit. The pain was not improved by position. There were no respiratory symptoms. In the past he had been treated with ACE inhibitors for essential hypertension. He did not smoke. On examination he appeared pale, sweaty and unwell. Intravenous morphine was required for the pain. Examination of the cardiovascular and respiratory systems were unremarkable. In particular there were no cardiac murmurs or central cyanosis, all peripheral pulses were present and the respiratory rate was 20/min. The abdomen was soft without any masses and there was no evidence of a neurological deficit. An initial ECG was normal apart from a sinus tachycardia of 115/min. This remained unchanged when repeated at 15 and 30 min. A chest radiograph revealed fluffy shadows in the left upper and right lower zones. Subsequent cardiac enzymes were normal.

(5) A 55-year-old man is recovering in hospital 3 days following an acute anterior myocardial infarction. His initial ECG showed Q waves and ST elevation in the anterior chest leads. He had not been given thrombolysis on arrival in the A&E department because he did not give consent. You are called to the ward because he has developed a dull central chest pain, which is relieved by leaning forward. He is not nauseated but feels short of breath. On examination he is in atrial fibrillation at a rate of 110/min. The blood pressure is 140/78 mmHg. His JVP is elevated to 8 cm, with elevation during inspiration. The heart sounds are faint and there are no added sounds.

(a) Angina pectoris
(b) Prolapsing mitral valve
(c) Musculoskeletal chest pain
(d) Tietze's syndrome
(e) Acute pericarditis
(f) Myocarditis
(g) Pulmonary embolism
(h) Constrictive pericarditis
(i) Herpes zoster
(j) Neuralgic amyotrophy
(k) Dressler's syndrome
(l) Hiatus hernia
(m) Restrictive cardiomyopathy
(n) Aortic dissection
(o) Epidemic myalgia (Bornholm disease)
(p) Lobar pneumonia
(q) Gastro-oesophageal reflux disease
(r) Acute myocardial infarction

Question 6

Match the following scenarios to the best diagnosis from the list given below.

(1) A 38-year-old female developed gradually increasing shortness of breath on exercise. There was no associated cough, wheeze or sputum production. She had in addition suffered several recent episodes of what were described by her husband as fainting episodes. There had been no chest pain, but she did report occasional episodes of palpitations that were associated with increased breathlessness. In the past she had been entirely fit and well apart from mild asthma treated with occasional β_2 agonists. Six months previously she had given birth to her third baby following an uneventful pregnancy and delivery. She did not smoke or take any regular medications. On examination she became breathless getting undressed and getting onto the examination couch. She had central cyanosis. There were no splinter haemorrhages or other stigmata of infective endocarditis. The JVP was measured at 10 cm above the angle of Louis with prominent V waves. She was normotensive. There was a left parasternal heave but the apex beat was normal in character and not displaced. Auscultation of the heart revealed a loud second sound in the pulmonary area and a pansystolic murmur at the left sternal edge. The lung fields were clear on auscultation. In the abdomen the liver was palpable 4 cm below the costal margin and thought to be pulsatile. An ECG showed right axis deviation and a chest radiograph showed cardiomegaly, and dilatation of the proximal pulmonary with peripheral arterial 'pruning'.

(2) A 27-year-old man attends the A&E department complaining of recurrent episodes of anterior chest pain and episodes of fainting. The pain was described as a 'heavy' feeling and radiated to the neck. It occurred both at rest and variably during exercise, relieved by resting. These episodes had been getting worse over several months but he was vague about the details. He was known to abuse amphetamines (which exacerbated the symptoms) and alcohol, according to a friend who accompanied him. There is no history of cough, haemoptysis or wheeze. He smoked 20 cigarettes per day. In the past he had visited the doctor infrequently. There was a variety of social problems and he had lived in hostel accommodation on-and-off since the age of 20. On examination he was thin and unkempt. There was no lymphadenopathy. There was no evidence of central cyanosis, clubbing or stigmata of infective endocarditis. The pulse was regular but 'jerking' in character. He was normotensive. The JVP was not elevated but there was a prominent 'a' wave. The apex beat was not displaced although thought to be 'heaving' in character with a double impulse beat. There was a harsh ejection systolic murmur with a thrill in the aortic area. In addition there was a fourth heart sound. An ECG showed voltage criteria for left ventricular hypertrophy and ST segment depression in the lateral leads.

(3) A 39-year-old female presents to her GP with gradually increasing symptoms of shortness of breath on exercise. She has had no chest pain or cough, but has had several episodes of palpitations when she has felt dizzy. She has had several recent episodes of 'fainting'. In the past she had been entirely well apart from rheumatic fever in childhood. She did not smoke or take any regular medications. On examination she appeared cyanosed at rest. There was evidence of clubbing, but no stigmata of infective endocarditis. The JVP was raised at 12 cm above the angle of Louis. There was a left parasternal heave. Auscultation of the heart revealed a diastolic murmur over the tricuspid area and wide fixed splitting of the second heart sound.

(4) A 29-year-old man presents in the A&E department with a history of gradually increasing shortness of breath over several days. There has been no cough, haemoptysis or fever. He has smoked 15 cigarettes per day since the age of 17 but has not seen a doctor since he was at school. He is rather evasive when more closely questioned, however. On examination he is cyanosed and short of breath on minimal exertion. There are numerous healing papules along the veins in both forearms. There is no evidence of clubbing or stigmata of bacterial endocarditis or chronic liver disease. His JVP is elevated to 8 cm and there is a parasternal heave. There is an early decrescendo murmur in the pulmonary area. The lung fields are clear on auscultation. There is mild pitting oedema of the ankles. An ECG shows right axis deviation and right bundle branch block. A chest radiograph shows clear lung fields and a suggestion of right ventricular enlargement. Oxygen saturation is recorded at 86%.

(5) A 45-year-old female patient presents with tiredness, weight loss and joint pains over several weeks.

She has also been experiencing increasing breathlessness and describes feeling short of breath when climbing stairs. She has previously been fit and well, although had recently received treatment for her acne with minocycline. On examination she is mildly obese. There is facial erythema in the malar region with fine scaling. There is no clubbing or cyanosis. Her temperature is 38.2°C. The pulse is 100/min and regular and the JVP is not elevated. The cardiac apex is not displaced and there are no abnormal heart sounds. Her respiratory rate is 24 b.p.m. and she has stony dullness at the right base with an area of bronchial breathing immediately above this. Examination of the abdomen and nervous system are unremarkable.

(a) Aortic stenosis
(b) Asthma
(c) Chronic pulmonary embolism
(d) Atypical pneumonia
(e) Pleural effusion
(f) Cardiac tamponade
(g) *Pneumocystis carinii* infection
(h) Pneumothorax
(i) Bacterial endocarditis
(j) Anxiety symptoms
(k) Tricuspid regurgitation
(l) Systemic lupus erythematosus
(m) Fibrotic lung disease
(n) Tricuspid stenosis
(o) Tetralogy of Fallot
(p) Atrial septal defect
(q) Angina pectoris
(r) Hypertrophic obstructive cardiomyopathy
(s) Anaemia
(t) Ventricular septal defect
(u) Myocardial infarction
(v) Primary pulmonary hypertension
(w) Pulmonary stenosis

Paper 2 Questions

MCQs

[1] Concerning cardiac failure . . .
(a) the prevalence is decreasing in British females
(b) 'high output' cardiac failure is less common than 'low output' cardiac failure
(c) if it is due to mitral regurgitation, the liver will likely be pulsatile on palpation
(d) left heart failure is the most common cause of right heart failure
(e) treatment in heart failure aims to increase both preload and afterload

[2] Concerning hypertension . . .
(a) a single blood pressure recording >160/90 is sufficient cause to instigate antihypertensive medication
(b) Caucasian populations have a higher mean blood pressure than do Afro-Caribbean populations
(c) headache is a common symptom of hypertension
(d) radio-femoral delay is diagnostic of renal artery stenosis
(e) the ECG in a hypertensive patient usually shows smaller than expected QRS complexes in the anterior chest leads

[3] Concerning ischaemic heart disease . . .
(a) myocardial ischaemia results from excessive CO_2 in the blood
(b) hyperthyroidism is a recognized cause of angina
(c) coronary artery disease is the single most common cause of death in the UK
(d) a 'foam cell' is a type of neutrophil involved in atherogenesis
(e) a high level of high-density lipoprotein (HDL) is considered detrimental to health

[4] In the management of acute myocardial infarction (MI) . . .

(a) aspirin should be given stat in a dose of up to 75 mg
(b) a chest radiograph should be obtained before treatment is commenced
(c) thrombolysis causes 10% of those receiving it to have a stroke
(d) clopidogrel should never be given to a patient who is also receiving aspirin due to the risk of upper gastrointestinal bleeding
(e) thrombolysing agent should be administered within 30 min of the initial cardiac event, otherwise the risks outweighs the potential benefits

[5] Concerning the diagnosis of acute MI . . .
(a) T-wave inversion is always followed by the appearance of Q-waves
(b) Q-waves on the ECG are always pathological
(c) a shift in the axis of the ECG may indicate evolution of a myocardial infarct
(d) a rise in serum levels of creatine kinase MM isoform is pathognomonic for acute MI
(e) increased troponin T isoform is pathognomonic for MI

[6] The following cardiac events are matched correctly to the corresponding ECG changes . . .
(a) lateral infarct → ST-segment elevation in leads I and aVL
(b) septal infarct → ST-segment elevation in leads V1 and V2
(c) occlusion of the right coronary artery → ST-segment elevation in leads II, III and aVF
(d) old septal infarct → Q-waves in V3 and V4
(e) ventricular tachycardia → saddle-shaped ST-segment elevation

[7] Infective endocarditis . . .
(a) most commonly occurs in the acute, fulminant form
(b) is more common in developing countries
(c) is commoner in patients with a history of rheumatic fever
(d) is most commonly caused by *Streptococcus pyogenes*
(e) typically affects the right-sided heart valves

[8] Concerning syncope . . .
(a) it is defined as 'permanent global cerebral hypoperfusion'
(b) onset is classically instantaneous, with no pre-warning
(c) jerking movements rule out syncope as a cause of collapse
(d) when due to arrhythmias, is usually due to tachyarrhythmia rather than bradyarrhythmia
(e) it can lead to a cerebral infarction

[9] Mitral stenosis . . .
(a) is most commonly caused by rheumatic heart disease
(b) causes enlargement of both the left atrium and the left ventricle
(c) may lead to development of non-cardiogenic pulmonary oedema
(d) rarely causes AF
(e) causes a 'tapping' apex beat

[10] Concerning the respiratory organs of the body . . .
(a) the pleural space between visceral and parietal layers of pleura is approximately 1 mm in healthy individuals
(b) the diaphragm is innervated by the vagus nerve
(c) stretching of the visceral pleura causes pleuritic chest pain
(d) normal expiration at rest is a passive process
(e) doxapram is used in the treatment of hyperventilation

[11] On examination of the chest of a patient with unilateral consolidation . . .
(a) chest wall movements are increased on the affected side
(b) the mediastinum is not displaced
(c) the percussion note is described correctly as 'stony dull'
(d) breath sounds will be absent over the affected area

(e) vocal resonance will be increased over the affected area

[12] Concerning upper respiratory tract infections . . .
(a) viruses causing the common cold are mainly togaviruses
(b) sinusitis is usually caused by *Staphylococcus aureus*
(c) perennial allergic rhinitis is usually caused by pollens
(d) pharyngitis is usually viral in aetiology
(e) tonsillitis should always be treated by antibiotics

[13] Concerning chronic obstructive pulmonary disease (COPD) . . .
(a) it is common in non-smokers
(b) 'blue bloaters' are believed to be suffering predominantly from emphysema
(c) people in type I respiratory failure should not routinely be given 100% O_2 to breathe
(d) it is a recognized cause of cor pulmonale
(e) COPD is commonly accompanied by appropriate polycythaemia

[14] Concerning pleural effusions . . .
(a) they are clinically detectable when their volume approaches 200 mL
(b) they demonstrate bronchial breathing upon auscultation of the affected area
(c) during aspiration, the needle should be introduced at the lower border of the appropriate rib
(d) transudates are usually unilateral
(e) transudates contain a higher protein concentration than do exudates

[15] Concerning asthma . . .
(a) increased IgE-producing ability is believed crucial in the pathogenesis of asthma
(b) eosinophils release histamine during asthma attack
(c) expectoration of yellow sputum in an asthmatic indicates respiratory tract infection, and should prompt rapid commencement of broad-spectrum antibiotics
(d) the wheeze associated with asthma is monophonic
(e) salbutamol can be used in a hyperkalaemic patient to lower potassium levels

[16] The following signs would suggest that a left-sided abdominal mass was a kidney and not a spleen . . .
(a) presence of a notch
(b) resonance to percussion

(c) ability to bimanually palpate

(d) enlargement toward the left iliac fossa

(e) inability to palpate superiorly

[17] The following are recognized causes of a mass in the right iliac fossa . . .

(a) acute appendicitis

(b) myelofibrosis

(c) Crohn's disease

(d) tuberculosis

(e) Sister Mary Joseph's nodule

[18] Concerning infection in surgical patients . . .

(a) corticosteroids enhance wound healing

(b) haemoglobin potentiates bacterial virulence

(c) reducing length of operation is demonstrably effective in reducing infection rates after surgery

(d) an early postoperative fever is usually caused by abscess formation at the site of the operative wound

(e) an infected operative wound that contains pus can be effectively treated with systemic antibiotics

[19] Concerning gastro-oesophageal reflux disease (GORD) . . .

(a) a 'sliding' hiatus hernia is much more likely to cause symptomatic acid reflux than a 'rolling' one

(b) most hiatus herniae are of the sliding type

(c) all hiatus herniae should be repaired surgically upon discovery

(d) the symptoms of GORD are due to acid of an unusually low pH being refluxed into the oesophagus from the stomach

(e) the pain of GORD may be partially relieved by sublingual GTN spray

[20] Concerning gastroduodenal anatomy and physiology . . .

(a) the stomach has two anatomical sphincters

(b) the branch of the aorta that supplies blood to the stomach is the superior mesenteric artery

(c) the stomach receives sympathetic nervous supply from the vagus nerve

(d) parietal cells, chief cells and goblet cells are found diffusely throughout the stomach

(e) the duodenum is anatomically split into five parts

[21] Gastric carcinoma . . .

(a) is more common in the UK than in Japan

(b) is an almost inevitable development in the polyps of patients with Peutz-Jehgers syndrome

(c) is more common in patients with blood group A

(d) pernicious anaemia is considered a premalignant condition for gastric carcinoma

(e) is associated with Krukenberg's tumour

[22] Concerning the diagnostic evaluation of the patient with gallstones . . .

(a) biliary 'colic' is paradoxically a constant pain

(b) pruritis is caused by deposition of unconjugated bile acids within the tissues

(c) biliary colic is caused by gallbladder inflammation

(d) Murphy's sign is positive in patients with gallstones

(e) a jaundiced patient who has an enlarged gall bladder is more likely to have cancer of the head of the pancreas than a stone in the common bile duct

[23] Concerning hepatitis . . .

(a) it is only caused by either viruses or alcohol

(b) all hepatitis-causing viruses are RNA-viruses

(c) hepatitis A is spread mainly by the faeco-oral route

(d) hepatitis B is mainly spread by the faeco-oral route

(e) less than 10% of patients infected with hepatitis C go on to develop chronic liver disease

[24] Concerning the rarer causes of cirrhosis . . .

(a) primary biliary cirrhosis (PBC) mainly affects male patients

(b) painless jaundice is usually the first symptom in PBC

(c) hereditary haemochromotosis (HH) is caused by excessive deposition of copper within the various organs and tissues of the body

(d) Wilson's disease solely affects the liver

(e) α_1-antitrypsin deficiency solely affects the liver

EMQs

Question 7

From the following case histories, choose the most likely diagnosis from the list below.

(1) A 38-year-old farmer presents to his GP with a history of weakness in his legs progressing over several weeks. He first became aware that he might have a problem when he found he was unable to whistle his dog when at work. He then noticed that he had developed weakness of the hands such that he was having difficulty inserting keys into locks. There had been no sensory symptoms of paraesthesiae or numbness. He had noticed some cramp-like pains in the legs. The symptoms did not fluctuate in their severity. He had not lost weight and a review of systems history was otherwise unremarkable. In the past he had been fit and well. On examination there is wasting of the lower limb muscles with occasional fasciculation. Tone however is increased in the quadriceps and there are brisk knee reflexes. The plantar reflex is up going. There is wasting and fasciculation of the tongue. Sensory testing is normal.

(2) A 23-year-old male presents to his GP with a history of episodic double vision. His girlfriend confirms this and also reports associated slurred incoherent speech. In addition he had had to stop playing five-a-side football due to increasing shortness of breath. He was previously fit and well apart from mild asthma for which he took occasional salbutamol. His mother and sister had rheumatoid arthritis. On examination the cranial nerves were intact with no evidence of abnormality. Peripheral neurological examination also revealed no abnormality. His chest and cardiovascular system were unremarkable.

(3) A 34-year-old female patient presents with a 48-h history of weak legs. There was associated 'pins and needles' in both legs for the same period. In addition she complained of difficulty voiding urine. There is no history of back pain, rigors or trauma. She had previously been well, with no hospital admissions. She had, however, consulted her GP 3 years previously complaining of 'pins and needles' in the left hand. This had resolved spontaneously. She took no regular medications, but smoked 20 cigarettes per day. On examination she was thin, not clinically anaemic and there was no evidence of finger clubbing. Lower limb tone was symmetrically increased. Power was reduced in both lower limbs to grade 3/5 symmetrically, and there was generalized lower limb hyper-reflexia. Sensory testing revealed reduced sensation to the T4 level. Palpation of the bladder revealed a full bladder.

(4) A 54-year-old male smoker is admitted from work with sudden onset of severe occipital headache and vomiting. Little other history is available. His wife on arrival reported that he had been well on leaving the house that morning and previously well apart from mild hypertension treated with bendroflurazide. Three days prior to the event he had consulted his GP regarding a severe headache, which had resolved after 24 hours using simple analgesics. Following admission his condition deteriorated with a decline in the GCS from 13 to 6 and a fixed dilated pupil on the left side. He was severely photophobic and there was obvious neck stiffness. There was no evidence of trauma. A left-sided hemiparesis was recorded, with increased tone and hyperreflexia. He was apyrexial, and there was no skin rash. Blood pressure is recorded at 230/130, pulse rate at 50/min. and respiratory rate at 12 b.p.m.

(5) A 65-year-old female attends her GP with increasing weakness in the upper and lower limbs. She is otherwise fit and well and systemic review is unremarkable. On examination she has weak legs with increased tone and hyper-reflexia. There is in the upper limbs wasting of the biceps with reduced power and absent biceps and supinator tendon reflex. The triceps reflex is brisk and power is reduced. Sensory testing is normal in the upper limbs but shows diminished position and vibration in the lower limbs. There is no skin change or evidence of fasciculation.

(a) Guillain–Barré syndrome
(b) Multiple sclerosis
(c) Friedreich's ataxia
(d) Vasculitis
(e) Acute subdural haematoma
(f) Tabes dorsalis
(g) Motor neurone disease
(h) Porphyria
(i) Myasthenia gravis
(j) Brown Séquard syndrome

(k) Acute poliomyelitis
(l) Migrane
(m) Subarachnoid haemorrhage
(n) Cerebrovascular accident
(o) Pott's disease
(p) Cervical spondylosis with myelopathy
(q) Cluster headache
(r) Syringomyelia
(s) Subacute combined degeneration of the cord
(t) Acute bacterial meningitis

Question 8

From the following clinical information choose the most likely diagnosis from the list provided below.

(1) A 73-year-old man presents with back pain and tiredness for several weeks. On examination you find bruising on the lower limbs. Investigations were as follows:

Hb	8.2 g/dL
WBC	3.2×10^9/L
Platelets	97×10^9/L
ESR	150 mm/h
Na$^+$	138 mmol/L
K$^+$	4.5 mmol/L
Ur	20 mmol/L
Cr	235 mmol/L
Ca^{2+}	3.2 mmol/L
Phosphate	0.98 mmol/L (NR 0.8–1.6)
Alkaline phosphatase	75 U/L

(2) A 78-year-old man presents with a several month history of lower limb and pelvic pain. He has lost no weight and does not smoke. On examination he is wearing a hearing aid. His lower limb examination is normal with normal pulses and normal neurological examination. Investigations were as follows:

Hb	15.3 g/dL
WBC	5.6×10^9/L
Platelets	442×10^9/L
ESR	30 mm/h
Na$^+$	143 mmol/L
K$^+$	3.5 mmol/L
Ur	7.8 mmol/L
Cr	98 mmol/L
Ca^{2+}	2.52 mmol/L
Phosphate	1.20 mmol/L (NR 0.8–1.4)
Alkaline phosphatase	823 U/L

(3) A 56-year-old Asian woman complains of increasing buttock and quadriceps pain on movement. She has noticed difficulty in climbing stairs and getting out of a chair. Investigations reveal:

Hb	12.4 g/dL
WBC	7.6×10^9/L
Platelets	432×10^9/L
ESR	45 mm/h
Na$^+$	138 mmol/L
K$^+$	3.8 mmol/L
Ur	8.2 mmol/L
Cr	97 mmol/L
Ca^{2+}	2.10 mmol/L
Phosphate	0.69 mmol/L (NR 0.8–1.4)
Alkaline phosphatase	498 U/L

(4) A 65-year-old man presents with increasing confusion, abdominal pain and polyuria. Investigations were as follows:

Hb	15.3 g/dL
WBC	6.7×10^9/L
Platelets	352×10^9/L
ESR	28 mm/h
Na$^+$	139 mmol/L
K$^+$	3.5 mmol/L
Ur	8.8 mmol/L
Cr	92 mmol/L
Ca^{2+}	3.68 mmol/L
Phosphate	0.68 mmol/L (NR 0.8–1.4)
Alkaline phosphatase	482 U/L

(5) A 78-year-old female patient presents with spontaneous onset of localized lower back pain. The pain is worse with movement exercise and improved by rest. There is no radiation. There has been no weight change or fever. Examination reveals normal hands and peripheral joints, mild central obesity and a restricted range of movement in the lumbar spine. There is local tenderness over the second lumbar vertebra. Investigations reveal:

Hb	14.7 g/dL
WBC	8.8×10^9/L
Platelets	222×10^9/L
ESR	48 mm/h
Na$^+$	140 mmol/L
K$^+$	4.2 mmol/L
Ur	7.8 mmol/L
Cr	100 mmol/L
Ca^{2+}	2.35 mmol/L

Phosphate	1.15 mmol/L (NR 0.8–1.4)
Alkaline phosphatase	42 U/L

(a) Monclonal gammopathy of uncertain significance (MGUS)
(b) Waldenstrom's macroglobulinaemia
(c) Primary hyperparathyroidism
(d) Metastatic bone disease
(e) Mechanical back pain
(f) Osteomalacia
(g) Amyloidosis
(h) Multiple myeloma
(i) Secondary hyperparathyroidism
(j) Sciatica
(k) Osteoporosis with pathological fracture
(l) Secondary hyperparathyroidism
(m) Tertiary hyperparathyroidism
(n) Polymyalgia rheumatica
(o) Paget's disease

Question 9

Match the following blood gas results to the most accurate description in the list below.

(1)	PaO_2	23.46 kPa
	$PaCO_2$	4.69 kPa
	pH	7.29
	HCO_3	16.7 mmol/L

(2)	PaO_2	8.92 kPa
	$PaCO_2$	3.71 kPa
	pH	7.47
	HCO_3	19.9 mmol/L

(3)	PaO_2	5.74 kPa
	$PaCO_2$	7.78 kPa
	pH	7.36
	HCO_3	32.4 kPa

(4)	PaO_2	17.03 kPa
	$PaCO_2$	1.94 kPa
	pH	7.685
	HCO_3	17.03 mmol/L

(5)	PaO_2	12.5 KPa
	$PaCO_2$	6.8 KPa
	pH	7.65
	HCO_3	34.3 mmol/L

(6)	PaO_2	7.8 KPa
	$PaCO_2$	7.2 KPa
	pH	7.32
	HCO_3	28.24 mmol/L

(7)	PaO_2	20.2 KPa
	$PaCO_2$	4.0 KPa
	pH	7.23
	HCO_3	29 mmol/L

(a) None of these
(b) Respiratory alkalosis
(c) Type II respiratory failure with compensated respiratory acidosis
(d) Compensated respiratory acidosis
(e) Metabolic alkalosis
(f) Metabolic acidosis
(g) Type I respiratory failure with respiratory alkalosis
(h) Compensated respiratory alkalosis
(i) Type II respiratory failure with uncompensated respiratory alkalosis
(j) Metabolic alkalosis with partial compensation

Question 10

From the following clinical information choose the best diagnosis from the list below.

(1) A 35-year-old male patient presents with a 4-day history of dry cough and increasing shortness of breath. There has been no chest pain or haemoptysis. He is a non-smoker and was previously healthy. He works as a dentist. On examination he looks unwell. There is a rash consisting of 'target' shaped erythematous lesions on the trunk and face. His pulse is 120/min. The JVP is elevated at 6 cm with paradoxical movement. The apex beat cannot be palpated. The heart sounds are quiet. There was no cyanosis or anaemia. Examination of the chest revealed inspiratory crepitations in left basal zone. Investigations reveal:

FBC	Hb	14.2 g/dL
	WCC	8.7×10^9/L
	Platelets	102×10^9/L
Cold agglutinins		Positive
ECG		Sinus tachycardia, widespread T wave inversion
Echocardiogram		'Significant pericardial effusion with reduced left ventricular ejection fraction'

(2) A 56-year-old male is being treated for right lower lobe pneumonia and is admitted to hospital. Despite 10 days of intravenous antibiotics (erythromycin, cefotaxime and flucloxacillin) he continues to be very unwell with a high swinging temperature and productive cough. Until this current illness he had been entirely fit and well and was a non-smoker on no medication. Ten days before admission to hospital he had had a retirement party at home, during which he had a bout of coughing from which he initially recovered. He then started to feel unwell 3 days later. There were no atypical features to the illness and systemic review was normal, apart from the respiratory system. On examination he was pyrexial with clinical and radiological evidence of right lower lobe consolidation.

(3) A 42-year-old male presents with increasing shortness of breath over 6 weeks, but without productive cough or sputum. He has noticed a recent weight loss of 5 kg. He feels lethargic and has been experiencing excessive sweating particularly at night. There has been no chest pain or haemoptysis. He is a non-smoker and was without previous lung disease. As a child he had had mild asthma that resolved. He takes mesalazine for mild distil ulcerative colitis, which is under control. Two years previously he received chemotherapy for stage III Hodgkin's disease. On examination he is pyrexial at 38.6°C, thin, pale and weak. Examination of the chest revealed stony dullness at the left base. Examination of the abdomen suggested hepatomegaly to 5 cm below the right costal margin. A chest X-ray showed numerous round opacities in both lung fields and a significant left-sided pleural effusion.

(4) A 19-year-old female is referred with a history of productive cough failing to respond to antibiotics over several weeks. She is producing half a cup full of thick green sputum per day, occasionally flecked with blood. There has been no chest pain. She complains of breathlessness on walking short distances. She has not lost any weight but has 'always been thin' according to her mother. She is a non-smoker and works as a cashier in a bank. In the past she has had frequent chest infections during the winter and occasionally the summer months. She did report occasional bulky and loose stools. Otherwise a review of systems was normal. On examination she is pale and thin with a BMI of 17.3 kg/m^2. There was evidence of clubbing. Pulse is 60/min. The JVP is elevated and there is a loud second sound over the pulmonary area. There is

mild cyanosis. There is no lymphadenopathy. The respiratory rate is 24 cycles per minute. In the chest there are diffuse wheezes and coarse inspiratory crepitations in all areas.

Peak flow rate	220 L/min (predicted 510 L/min)
Chest radiograph	'Hyper-inflation with apical bronchiectasis in both lungs'

(5) A 58-year-old man attends the A&E department. He is a regular patient and known to abuse alcohol and sleep rough on most nights. As usual he is drunk and aggressive. He complains, however, of difficulty breathing and a persistent cough. He is a known heavy smoker. He appears to have lost some weight. On examination he is unkempt and smells of alcohol. He is thin. There are several enlarged lymph nodes in the cervical area, which are firm but not tender. Examination of the chest reveals stony dullness at the left base. A chest radiograph reveals left upper lobe fibrosis and a left-sided pleural effusion. On the ward a subsequent pleural aspirate produced a straw-coloured fluid with a protein content of 52 g/L and abundant lymphocytes. No malignant cells were seen. Culture of the aspirate produced no growth at 1 week.

(a) Chronic obstructive airways disease
(b) Bronchiectasis
(c) Cystic fibrosis
(d) Pneumocysitis pneumonia
(e) Pulmonary tuberculosis
(f) Coxsackie virus infection
(g) Legionnaire's disease
(h) Atypical pneumonia
(i) Systemic lupus erythematosus
(j) Mesothelioma
(k) Bronchogenic carcinoma
(l) Aspiration causing pneumonia
(m) Sarcoidosis
(n) Mycoplasma pneumonia
(o) Underlying HIV infection
(p) Asthma
(q) Pulmonary embolism
(r) Lymphoma
(s) None of these

Question 11

Match the following haematology results to the condition(s) in the list given below, which may take these patterns:

(1) Hb   10.6 g/dL
     WCC 7.6×10^9/L
     Platelets 342×10^9/L
     MCV   78 fL

(2) Hb   7.8 g/dL
     WCC 2.8×10^9/L
     Platelets 145×10^9/L
     MCV   108 fL

(3) Hb   12.8 g/dL
     WCC 9.8×10^9/L
     Platelets 350×10^9/L
     MCV   102 fL

(4) Hb   18.2 g/dL
     WCC 15.6×10^9/L
     Platelets 653×10^9/L
     MCV   95 fL

(5) Hb   9.8 g/dL
     WCC 6.8×10^9/L
     Platelets 345×10^9/L
     MCV   88 fL

(6) Hb   13.8 g/dL
     WCC 1.5×10^9/L
     Platelets 342×10^9/L
     MCV   92 fL

(a) Hypothyroidism
(b) Idiopathic
(c) Pregnancy
(d) Folate deficiency
(e) Myelofibrosis
(f) Primary polycythemia (polycythemia vera)
(g) Alcoholism
(h) Methotrexate treatment
(i) Iron deficiency
(j) Tuberculosis
(k) Renal failure
(l) Vitamin B12 deficiency
(m) Gaisbock's syndrome
(n) Septicaemia
(o) High altitude training

Question 12

From the following cases choose the most likely diagnosis from the list below.

(1) A 76-year-old lady presents with a 6-week history of progressive swallowing difficulties, particularly of solids. She has lost 6 kg in weight. There has been no pain associated with the dysphagia. She is able to drink normally. She occasionally reports regurgitation of solids. In the past she has had a myocardial infarction 10 years ago. She takes prophylactic aspirin therapy and oral sustained release nitrates for occasional angina. She has regularly consumed 30 units of alcohol per week for many years. She smokes 20 cigarettes per day. On examination she is jaundiced. Examination of the neck reveals no abnormality. There is no lymphadenopathy. Her cardiovascular system and chest are normal. Examination of the abdomen reveals a hard irregular hepatomegaly to 3 cm below the left costal margin.

(2) A 35-year-old male smoker presents with a history of pain in the chest developing over several months. This is located behind the sternum and occurs at rest. There is some radiation to the neck. There is no precipitation by exercise and he has normal exercise tolerance. He occasionally experiences a bitter taste in his mouth. The pain can be precipitated by alcohol or a large meal. The pain is worse at night. There have been no swallowing difficulties and he has not lost any weight. On examination he has a BMI of 32.2. Otherwise there are no abnormal clinical findings.

(3) A 76-year-old male who lives alone is referred to outpatient's clinic with a 2-month history of epigastric pain and occasional vomiting. There has been no haematemesis or dysphagia. He has lost 5 kg in weight over the period and admits to a reduced appetite. He has consumed 40 units of alcohol per week for many years, but denies smoking. In the past he has taken antacids for 'indigestion' and was recently prescribed a proton pump inhibitor by his GP. This, however, failed to provide any symptom relief. On examination he is thin and has nicotine staining of the fingers. There is no jaundice clinically. There is a palpable lymph node behind the head of the left sterno-clavicular junction. There is no evidence of hepatomegaly. There is a rash consisting of a pigmented velvet like lesion on the back of the neck and in the axillae.

(4) A 38-year-old male complains of intermittent swallowing difficulties for both liquids and solids over many months. He occasionally experiences severe retro-sternal pain, particularly after drinking hot liquids. There has been no weight loss. His wife reports choking episodes occurring at night. On examination he appears well with no anaemia or jaundice. There are no skin abnormalities and he has no findings on examination of the gastrointestinal tract. A chest radiograph reveals a dilated oesophagus with a fluid level within it.

(5) A 45-year-old female is investigated for weight loss and epigastric pain over several months. Her appetite is good and there has been no dysphagia or vomiting. The pain occurs after meals and is felt in the epigastrium and radiates to the back. There has been no alteration of the bowel habit. On examination she is thin and pale. There is no clubbing or lymphadenopathy. The chest and cardiovascular system are unremarkable. Examination of the abdomen reveals mild epigastric discomfort but no overt mass. There is no evidence of organomegaly. She has pitting oedema of both ankles. A dip test of the urine is clear for blood, protein and leucocytes. Subsequent upper gastrointestinal endoscopy revealed abnormal thickening and enlargement of the gastric mucosal folds.

(6) A 24-year-old single mother attends with a complaint of intermittent difficulty in swallowing with asso-

ciated pain and a feeling of a lump in the throat. She has not lost weight and has had no reduction in her appetite. She is a smoker. In the past she has been fit and well apart from an episode of postnatal depression treated with antidepressants by her GP. On examination she appears anxious and thin. There is no lymphadenopathy. There is no abnormality in the oropharynx. Abdominal examination is unremarkable. A subsequent upper GI endoscopy is reported as normal.

(a) Systemic sclerosis
(b) Bulbar palsy
(c) Achalasia of the oesophagus
(d) Gastro-oesophageal reflux disease (GORD)
(e) Oesophageal candidiasis
(f) Pseudobulbar palsy
(g) Peptic stricture
(h) Schatzki ring
(i) Gastric carcinoma
(j) Foreign body
(k) Oesophageal carcinoma
(l) Myasthenia gravis
(m) Menetrier's disease
(n) Diffuse oesophageal stricture
(o) Globus hystericus
(p) Pharyngeal pouch
(q) Plummer–Vinson syndrome
(r) Hiatus hernia
(s) Oesophageal varices
(t) Gastric ulcer

Paper 3 Questions

MCQs

[1] Concerning pulmonary oedema . . .
(a) paroxysmal nocturnal dyspnoea (PND) is an early form of pulmonary oedema
(b) it classically causes rusty sputum
(c) chest radiograph typically shows Kerley-C lines
(d) first-line treatment is with nebulisers and steroids
(e) it is typically treated with both arterial and venous vasodilators

[2] Concerning aneurysms . . .
(a) 'true' aneurysms involve all three layers of the arterial wall
(b) 'saccular' aneurysms involve the artery symmetrically
(c) they most commonly involve the infrarenal aorta
(d) the 'Venturi' effect explains how tangential wall stress within an artery increases with increasing diameter of the vessel
(e) aneurysms of the abdominal aorta should only be repaired when their diameter exceeds 10 cm

[3] Raynaud's . . .
(a) disease is when the symptoms of Raynaud's phenomenon occur without any other disorder
(b) disease usually affects elderly men
(c) phenomenon is usually unilateral
(d) phenomenon typically affects fingers worse than toes
(e) phenomenon can be caused by ingestion of calcium channel antagonists

[4] Concerning venous thromboembolism . . .
(a) in health, perforating veins of the leg carry blood from deep → superficial veins
(b) treatment of choice for superficial thrombosis is with NSAIDs and warm compress

(c) the major risk factors for deep venous thrombosis (DVT) are described by Beck's triad
(d) calf pain on dorsiflexion of the foot is known as Lasegue's sign
(e) initially, warfarin treatment makes the patient's blood hypercoagulable

[5] Rheumatic fever . . .
(a) is due to infection with Lancefield group A streptococci
(b) has its effects by direct bacterial infection of the involved parts of the body
(c) is associated with formation of Aschoff nodules within the heart
(d) may be diagnosed using the Keith–Wagener criteria
(e) causes characteristic dermatological manifestations

[6] Mitral regurgitation . . .
(a) can develop acutely
(b) causes the apex beat to be 'heaving' on palpation
(c) typically causes an 'early systolic' murmur
(d) causes the cardiac shadow to be enlarged on plain AP chest radiograph
(e) is associated with malar flushing of the face

[7] Atrial myxoma . . .
(a) is a complication of hypothyroidism
(b) usually develops in the left atrium
(c) can cause systemic symptoms
(g) is a malignant tumour
(h) should be treated by surgical removal

[8] The following are recognized causes of sinus bradycardia . . .
(a) athletic training

QUESTIONS 3

23

(b) old age

(c) subarachnoid haemorrhage

(d) Addison's disease

(e) atropine

[9] Concerning bradycardias . . .

(a) in sick sinus syndrome, the PR interval is longer than normal

(b) in first degree AV block, frequency of P waves is vastly decreased

(c) in first degree AV block, P:QRS ratio is greater than or equal to 2

(d) in second degree AV block, some P waves conduct to the ventricles whilst others do not

(e) in Wenkebach heart block, PR interval is constant

[10] T-cells . . .

(a) comprise 70–80% of normal circulating lymphocytes

(b) secrete IgG

(c) are the primary defence against bacterial infection

(d) are infected with Epstein–Barr virus in glandular fever

(e) indicate good prognosis when they are the predominant cells in acute lymphatic leukaemia

[11] Concerning asthma . . .

(a) it can be diagnosed by a >15% improvement in lung function following inhalation of bronchodilator

(b) clumps of eosinophils on sputum microscopy suggest a diagnosis of asthma

(c) asthma retards growth in children

(d) inhaled corticosteroids do not retard growth in children

(e) status asthmaticus should be initially treated with saline nebulisers

[12] Pneumonia . . .

(a) is caused by 'atypical' infective organisms in approximately 50% of cases

(b) is always due to infective causes

(c) community-acquired pneumonia usually causes more florid symptoms in elderly people

(d) showing large cavities with air-fluid levels on chest radiograph suggests *Mycobacterium tuberculosis* as the cause

(e) caused by aspiration is usually due to anaerobic organisms

[13] Bronchiectasis . . .

(a) involves permanent thickening and dilatation of the airways

(b) is the most common cause of 'massive' haemoptysis in the UK

(c) is caused most commonly by cystic fibrosis in the UK

(d) may be associated with Kartagener's syndrome

(e) may be associated with Eisenmenger's syndrome

[14] Concerning cryptogenic fibrosing alveolitis (CFA) . . .

(a) it causes localized fibrosis in the lung

(b) it typically affects teenagers

(c) it eventually leads to type I respiratory failure

(d) it typically causes fine, end-inspiratory crepitations on auscultation of the chest

(e) it can be cured using high-dose corticosteroid and immunosuppressant treatment

[15] Small cell bronchial carcinoma . . .

(a) is more common in males than females

(b) is the most aggressive form of bronchial carcinoma

(c) is less common than non-small cell bronchial carcinoma

(d) is also known as 'oat-cell carcinoma'

(e) arises from endocrine cells

[16] Concerning oesophageal carcinomas . . .

(a) they are 4× more common in females

(b) their incidence varies little throughout the world

(c) invasion of local structures is rare

(d) dysphagia is the most common symptom at presentation

(e) they generally have a good prognosis

[17] Concerning gastroenteritis . . .

(a) most cases of gastroenteritis should be effectively treated with antibiotics

(b) it can be caused by *Staphylococcus aureus*

(c) that caused by *E. coli* is uniformly associated with bloody diarrhoea

(d) a member of the Salmonella family of bacteria causes typhoid fever

(e) *Campylobacter jejuni* is a relatively rare cause of gastroenteritis in the UK

[18] Concerning the diagnostic evaluation of the patient with gallstones . . .
(a) levels of serum amylase do not increase in acute cholecystitis/cholangitis
(b) a patient with long-standing obstructive jaundice would be expected to have normal clotting parameters (i.e. normal INR, PT, APTT, and TT)
(c) ERCP is the first-line investigation of choice
(d) HIDA scans may be used
(e) the finding of a raised alkaline phosphatase is diagnostic of bile duct obstruction

[19] Concerning cirrhosis . . .
(a) it may be caused by cystic fibrosis
(b) it may be caused by the Budd–Chiari syndrome
(c) patients should have regular measures of their β-hCG levels
(d) liver function may be estimated using Child's grading
(e) cirrhotics with concomitant hepatocellular carcinoma (HCC) should not receive a liver transplantation

[20] Concerning paracetamol poisoning . . .
(a) it occurs because the glutathione-mediated inactivation of toxic metabolites becomes saturated
(b) the antidote to paracetamol overdose is Pabrinex
(c) threshold for treatment of high-risk patients with N-acetylcysteine is higher levels of blood paracetamol than for patients who are at normal risk
(d) plasma paracetamol levels are reliable in the first 4 h following ingestion
(e) it is an absolute contraindication to liver transplantation

[21] Pseudocysts . . .
(a) are defined as 'abnormal sacs containing gas, fluid or semi-solid material, with a membranous or epithelial lining'
(b) are a rare complication of pancreatitis
(c) rarely cause pain
(d) are suggested by persistent elevation of serum amylase
(e) resolve spontaneously in 95% of cases

[22] Concerning herniae . . .
(a) an indirect inguinal hernia occurs when bowel protrudes directly through a defect in the anterior abdominal wall
(b) indirect inguinal herniae are the commonest type of hernia in males, but not in females
(c) indirect inguinal herniae protrude initially laterally to the inferior epigastric vessels
(d) the internal/deep inguinal ring is located at the mid-inguinal point
(e) femoral herniae arise below and medial to the pubic tubercle

[23] Concerning appendicitis . . .
(a) it occurs due to obstruction of the appendiceal lumen
(b) the pain of acute appendicitis classically begins in the right iliac fossa
(c) patients with acute appendicitis classically have a positive Murphy's sign
(d) the pain eventually becomes localized to McBurney's point
(e) patients with appendicitis classically have a positive Rovsing's sign

[24] Concerning Crohn's disease (CD) . . .
(a) it is curable by surgical resection of the diseased portion of the intestine
(b) development of fissures and fistulae is common
(c) perianal complications are relatively common
(d) smoking increases the likelihood of developing CD
(e) corticosteroids are rarely indicated in the treatment of CD

QUESTIONS 3

EMQs

Question 13

From the following case histories choose the most likely diagnosis from the list below.

(1) A 45-year-old female presented to her GP with a 6-week history of abdominal discomfort and bloating. She had not lost any weight but felt lethargic. There had been no alteration of the bowel habit. She has previously been fit and well. She worked in a bar and admitted to an alcohol intake of 40 units per week. On examination there were no stigmata of chronic liver disease. Her chest and cardiovascular system were unremarkable. Her abdomen was soft, non-distended and not tender. The liver and spleen were not palpable. Six weeks later following a trial of symptomatic treatment for presumed irritable bowel syndrome she returned with continued symptoms. She had also developed unsteadiness at work. This time her abdomen was distended with a mass arising centrally out of the pelvis. There was some shifting dullness on percussion of the abdomen. Examination of the nervous system revealed nystagmus and an ataxic gait with staggering to the right on walking. An urgent abdominal ultrasound showed: a small amount of ascites; normal liver, kidneys and spleen; left ovary containing several cysts, but right ovary could not be seen owing to a large omental mass. Urinalysis showed no abnormality.

(2) A 35-year-old female attends outpatients with a 4-month history of abdominal pain and altered bowel habit. She describes intermittent loose motions with occasional mucus. During an episode she can pass up to six loose motions per day. The pain is central and in the left iliac fossa. It is relieved by defecating or passing wind. Her appetite has been normal and she has not lost any weight. There has been no vomiting. There have been no urinary and/or gynaecological symptoms. In the past she had had similar symptoms 18 months previously, which had been investigated with flexible colonoscopy, but this did not show any abnormality. She had also suffered from recurrent tension headaches and had been previously referred by her GP for a neurology opinion. She smokes 20 cigarettes per day and takes occasional ibuprofen for her headaches. On examination she is slim with a BMI of 19.2. She is clinically euthyroid. There is nicotine staining of the fingers but no clubbing. There is

no lymphadenopathy in the cervical region. Examination of the abdomen reveals mild tenderness in the left iliac fossa. There is no organomegaly. A PR examination is refused by the patient. A full blood count, urea and electrolytes and CRP are all normal. Urinalysis is normal.

(3) A 54-year-old male attends with a 3-week history of bloody diarrhoea, reduced appetite and weight loss. He has also been experiencing pain in the left iliac fossa. His bowel habit has altered such that he has been opening his bowels up to six times per day. His appetite is reduced. In the past he had received 'white tablets' for a duodenal ulcer, but had been otherwise fit and well. There is no history of recent travel or contact with other cases of diarrhoea. On examination he is not clubbed, there is evidence of weight loss and his conjunctiva appears pale. His temperature is 37.8°C. There is no lymphadenopathy. Examination of the abdomen reveals mild tenderness in the left iliac fossa. There is no enlargement of the spleen or liver. A PR examination reveals blood and mucus, but no mass. Investigations reveal:

Hb	10.1 g/dL
WCC	15.2×10^9/L
Platelets	808×10^9/L
MCV	80 fL
CRP	262 (reference range <10)

(4) A 70-year-old female is admitted to hospital with suspected pneumonia by her GP. The diagnosis is confirmed and she is treated on the ward for 1 week, during which she makes a steady improvement. Following a successful home visit, she is discharged home for her GP to follow up. The following week her GP is called to see her, as she has become unwell with profuse watery diarrhoea. On examination the temperature is 37.8°C. The patient is drowsy and lethargic. Pulse 110/min, blood pressure 100/60 lying and 82/52 standing. There is generalized abdominal tenderness.

(5) A 50-year-old female is referred for investigation of diarrhoea and weight loss over several months. The diarrhoea is described as 'loose stools' without blood or mucus. There has been no reduction in appetite; in fact, she claims to be eating well. In the past she has been fit and well apart from hypothyroidism diagnosed ten years previously. She smokes 20 cigarettes per day. On examination she looks anxious and thin. Her pulse is 120/min and irregularly irregular. There is no clubbing or conjunctival pallor. Otherwise examination of the chest, cardiovascular system and abdomen are unremarkable.

(a) Irritable bowel syndrome
(b) Tropical sprue
(c) Alcoholic liver disease
(d) Right ventricular failure
(e) Ovarian carcinoma
(f) Coeliac disease
(g) Thyrotoxicosis
(h) Laxative abuse
(i) Small bowel Crohn's disease
(j) Pancreatic insufficiency
(k) Inflammatory bowel disease
(l) Small bowel lymphoma
(m) Hypothyroidism
(n) Enteric fever
(o) Whipple's disease
(p) Sigmoid colon carcinoma
(q) Diverticulitis
(r) Anxiety
(s) Pseudomembranous colitis

Question 14

From the following case histories choose the most accurate diagnosis from the list below.

(1) A 26-year-old male patient presents to the A&E department with a 4-day history of feeling unwell. He is anorexic but has had no vomiting. He complains of itching. He has had a productive cough that more latterly has contained significant amounts of fresh blood. He is complaining of breathlessness. He smokes 20 cigarettes per day and drinks 20 units of alcohol per week. In the past he has been well, but had complained of a sore throat 2 weeks previously. He works as a journalist and has had no dust or pet exposure. On examination he is thin and pale. There is no lymphadenopathy. There is mild cyanosis. The JVP is not elevated. There are scratch marks on the chest and thighs. He has a pulse of 96 BMP and regular. His heart sounds are normal and there was no peripheral oedema. Examination of the chest reveals a respiratory rate of 24 b.p.m. Otherwise breath sounds are clear. Investigations reveal the following results:

Na$^+$	138 mmol/L
K$^+$	6.8 mmol/L

Ur	52 mmol/L
Cr	1045 mmol/L
CXR	Diffuse alveolar shadowing in both bases

(2) A 78-year-old man with ischaemic heart disease attends casualty complaining of lethargy, nausea and itching increasing in severity over the preceding week. In the past he had suffered from three previous myocardial infarctions. He was known to have hypertension and had recently been reviewed by his GP who had altered his medications. On examination he was drowsy, his skin showed evidence of excoriation. Pulse 60/min, JVP elevated at 6 cm. Heart sounds revealed a quiet pan-systolic murmur at the apex radiating to the left axilla. His respiratory rate was 20 cycles per minute. There were fine end inspiratory bi-basal crepitations at both bases. Examination of the abdomen revealed no evidence of organomegaly. There was a murmur heard over the umbilicus. Initial blood tests revealed:

Ur	32.3 mmol/L
Cr	432 mmol/L
Na$^+$	132 mmol/L
K$^+$	7.9 mmol/L
ECG	'Tented T waves'

(3) A 25-year-old male patient presents with a 2-week history of tiredness, exertional dyspnoea and ankle swelling. He has been previously well, although had been prescribed a course of ibuprofen recently following an ankle sprain playing rugby. On examination his pulse was 90/min and regular, blood pressure 178/100 mmHg and JVP 3 cm. Normal heart sounds. There is dullness to percussion at the right lung base. He has bilateral oedema of the legs to below the knee. Examination of the abdomen reveals hepatomegaly to 3 cm below the right costal margin, and shifting dullness. Investigations revealed:

Hb	10.3 g/dL
WCC	6.7 × 10^9/L
Pl	236 × 10^9/L
MCV	88 fL
Ur	24.6 mmol/L
Cr	254 mmol/L
Na$^+$	135 mmol/L
K$^+$	5.6 mmol/L
Albumin	27 g/L
CXR report	'Right-sided pleural effusion. Normal cardiac size and outline'

(4) A 24-year-old female presents with an acute illness consisting of vomiting, a high temperature, rigors and left-sided loin pain. The pain was severe and continuous. It had gradually become worse during the previous 3 days. There was no history of trauma. She is ordinarily fit and well. There were no respiratory symptoms. There was no frequency of micturition or pain on passing urine. She had not noticed any haematuria. On examination she appeared unwell. Temperature 39.2°C, pulse 106/min and blood pressure 90/60 mmHg. The heart sounds were normal, there were no murmurs and examination of the respiratory system was unremarkable. Her abdomen revealed tenderness in the left renal angle. Investigations revealed:

Pregnancy test: Positive
Urine: Blood, non haemolysed +++
                   WBC ++
                   Protein ++

(5) A 25-year-old male patient presents with a short history of illness. He feels unwell with nausea and vomiting. He has been experiencing diffuse abdominal pain and painful swelling of his right knee joint. On examination there is a rash consisting of pupuric spots over the abdomen and lower limbs. His pulse is 70/min sinus rhythm. Blood pressure 170/110 mmHg. His cardiovascular system was otherwise clear, but he had bilateral pitting oedema of both ankles. There are fine bi-basal inspiratory crepitations. There are no specific tender areas in the abdomen. Investigations reveal:

Na$^+$	131 mmol/L
K$^+$	5.4 mmol/L
Ur	126 mmol/L
Cr	502 mmol/L
Hb	14.6 g/dL
WCC	8.6 × 10^9/L
Platelets	243 × 10^9/L
Urine	Protein++
	RBCs++
	WBCs ++ (granular casts noted)

(a) Wegener's granulomatosis
(b) Renal infarction
(c) Acute pyelonephritis
(d) Renal tuberculosis
(e) Nephrotic syndrome
(f) Acute renal failure
(g) Pulmonary embolism

(h) Acute renal failure due to angiotensin converting enzyme inhibitors
(i) Lymphoma
(j) Physiological symptoms of pregnancy
(k) Nephritic syndrome
(l) Acute ureteric colic
(m) Systemic lupus erythematosus
(n) Henoch–Schönlein syndrome
(o) Renal artery thrombosis
(p) Meningococcal infection
(q) Renal artery stenosis
(r) Goodpasture's syndrome

Question 15

Match the following case synopses to the most likely diagnosis from the list below.

(1) A 28-year-old female presents with an acute left-sided weakness. She is admitted to hospital where an urgent MRI scan confirms a thrombotic cerebrovascular accident affecting the right middle cerebral artery territory. She is a non-smoker and does not take oral contraception. In the past she had been on warfarin for two previous deep vein thrombosis events, which were presumed to be secondary to taking long-haul flights. One year ago after getting married she had two miscarriages close together. She is currently on no medication. On examination she had typical features of a left hemiplegia. She was in sinus rhythm, was normotensive and there was no evidence of a carotid bruit. She had a patchy, lace-like, dusky-coloured rash over the buttocks and thighs.

(2) A 56-year-old Turkish male patient presents with a purpuric rash on the lower limbs. This has been present for a number of weeks. In addition he gives a history of recurrent mouth ulcers. On the morning of admission his doctor had become concerned that he had become unsteady on his feet and was having difficulty standing and walking. On examination he was confused with an abbreviated mental test score of 6 out of 10. There were several large ulcers on the buccal mucosa. He had injection of the cornea, with pupil irregularity and mild photophobia in the left eye. There was a vasculitic rash on the lower limbs. Examination of the central nervous system revealed nystagmus to the right, an intension tremor and past pointing worse on the right side. There was no defect in tone, power, sensation or reflexes. He walked with a broad based gait. The left knee appeared swollen, mildly tender on palpation of the joint line, with a small effusion.

(3) A 35-year-old female patient attends complaining of pain in the left arm and hand of gradually worsening severity over several months. The pain is made worse by exercise of the affected limb. She complains that the arm and hand feel cold and occasionally experience 'pins and needles'. She obtains some relief by dangling the arm over the side of the bed at night. She has also experienced some blurring of vision affecting both eyes. She has lost 4 kg in weight during the period. In the past she has been fit and well. She is a non-smoker. On examination she is thin. There is no palpable pulse in either the left brachial or radial arteries. The left external carotid artery cannot be palpated either and there is a prominent bruit over the right external carotid artery.

(4) A 56-year-old male attends A&E with increasing symptoms of abdominal pain and passing offensive, dark-coloured stools. This had commenced 3 days previously and is described as a central colicky pain radiating to the back. He has vomited several times and has a reduced appetite. Prior to the onset of the abdominal pain he has consulted his general practitioner with symptoms of tiredness, weight loss and night sweats over several weeks. He is a smoker, but does not drink alcohol. In the past he has been investigated for weight loss with upper and lower gastrointestinal endoscopy, but no obvious cause was found. He takes no regular medications. On examination he appears unwell. He has a temperature of 37.8°C. There is no evidence of peripheral lymphadenopathy, anaemia or jaundice, but there is a dusky-coloured, lace-like rash over the upper and lower limbs. His pulse is 110/min and his blood pressure is 200/110 mmHg. The remainder of the cardiovascular system and respiratory system were unremarkable. Examination of the abdomen revealed central abdominal tenderness, but no masses or enlargement of the internal organs. The following results were obtained:

Hb	8.9 g/dL
WCC	15.9×10^9/L
Pl	234×10^9/L
ESR	121 mm/h
Na$^+$	132 mmol/L
K$^+$	5.6 mmol/L
Ur	14.6 mmol/L
Cr	235 mmol/L

Urine dip	Blood +++
	Protein ++
Amylase	56 U/L

Colonoscopy: normal

Hepatitis B surface antigen: positive

Arteriography of mesenteric vessels: 'numerous 0.5–1.0 cm aneurisms within the superior and inferior mesenteric arterial tree'

(5) A 73-year-old female presents with a history of weight loss and weakness over several months. She has noted a particular difficulty in swallowing for both solids and liquids over this period. She also reports pain around the hip and shoulder areas. In the past she has had a myocardial infarction at the age of 52. She takes enalapril, aspirin and atenolol as part of her regular medications. Although she does not drink alcohol she smokes five cigarettes per day. On examination there is wasting of the deltoid, gluteal and quadriceps muscle groups. In addition there is tenderness of these muscles to palpation. It is also noted than there is a purple discolouration around the eyes and raised, scaly purple lesions over the knuckles bilaterally.

(a) Behçet's syndrome
(b) Polyarteritis nodosa
(c) Giant cell arteritis
(d) Systemic lupus erythematosus
(e) Polymyositis
(f) Systemic sclerosis
(g) Dermatomyositis
(h) Cervical rib
(i) Neuralgic amyotrophy
(j) Wegener's granulomatosis
(k) Sjögren's syndrome
(l) Carcinomatosis
(m) Mycoplasma pneumonia
(n) Amyotrophic lateral sclerosis
(o) Muscular dystrophy Becker type
(p) Oesophageal carcinoma
(q) Takayasu's arteritis
(r) Dissection of the aorta
(s) Antiphospholipid syndrome
(t) Upper limb arterial embolism
(u) Subclavian steal syndrome
(v) Acute viral hepatitis
(w) Typhoid fever

Question 16

Match the following case histories to the most likely diagnosis from the list below.

(1) A 20-year-old West Indian female presents with increasing shortness of breath over a 10-week period. She has noticed increasing difficulty in climbing stairs and carrying her shopping home. She has also developed a dry, persistent cough, and has lost 5 kg in weight. There has been no chest pain. She is a non-smoker, but has lived in a city all her adult life. In the past she had been fit and well apart from occasional upper respiratory tract infections over the winter periods. She takes no regular medications. She works in an air-conditioned building as a receptionist. She has not had contact with birds. On examination she is thin and pale. There is no evidence of central cyanosis. There is no finger clubbing or flap of CO_2 retention. There are several enlarged lymph nodes in the anterior cervical area bilaterally, which are rubbery and non-tender. The trachea is central, and the cardiac apex undisplaced. Chest expansion is symmetrical but reduced bilaterally. Percussion is normal. Auscultation reveals fine end inspiratory crepitations at both lung bases. There was a rash on both shins consisting of dusky red lesions, which were tender to palpation.

(2) A 43-year-old male presents with a 6-week history of a persistent non-productive cough and increasing shortness of breath. There has been no haemoptysis. He is a lifelong smoker. His wife reports that he has lost approximately half a stone (3.5 kg) in weight and has also had weakness in his legs with resulting difficulty in getting in and out of a chair. He is normally active and can walk any distance. In the past he has received salbutamol for mild asthma. The GP he saw recently about his new symptoms added an additional inhaled corticosteroid and prescribed a course of amoxycillin. He takes no other regular medication. On examination he is thin, and tanned following a recent holiday. There is an early increase in fluctuance of his nail beds bilaterally. There are no abnormal findings in the head and neck, and in particular there is no evidence of lymphadenopathy. On examination of the chest he has reduced expansion in the left lower zone, with associated reduced air entry and local stony dullness also on the left. Examination of the cardiovascular system and abdomen are unremarkable. Neurologically he has reduced power in the proximal muscles of his upper and lower limbs to grade 4 out of 5.

(3) A 25-year-old male patient attends complaining of episodic episodes of shortness of breath. He has noticed these particularly in the morning after walking upstairs to his office in the city. He takes regular exercise and has noticed a reduction in his recent performance. In addition he has developed persistent rhinorrhoea with associated nasal itching for the last 2 months. The past medical history includes asthma, chicken pox as a child and an episode of hepatitis A after returning from Tunisia 1 year previously. His regular medications include twice a day beclomethazone and four times a day salbutamol. On examination he is slim and athletic in build. There are no findings in the periphery. There is no clinical evidence of anaemia, central cyanosis or lymphadenopathy. His respiratory rate is 16 b.p.m. Examination of the chest reveals widespread polyphonic wheezing. There are a few purpuric lesions on the lower shins bilaterally. His peak flow is 335 L/min (predicted 510 L/min), and FBC reveals a relative eosinophilia.

(4) A 65-year-old female presents with gradually increasing shortness of breath over several months with an associated non-productive cough. She has also lost 5 kg in weight. She has noticed the shortness of breath with modest exercise such as walking on the flat. She has been an occasional smoker for most of her adult life. Past medical history includes Raynaud's disease, for which she is prescribed nifedipine. Three years ago she had been investigated for altered bowel habit. A lower GI endoscopy had revealed a small area of ulcerative colitis, which had resolved with mesalazine treatment. She had had no relapse of the condition. On examination there was obvious clubbing and central cyanosis. There was no clinical anaemia. The JVP was elevated and a third heart sound was present. The trachea was central. Expansion was symmetrical and percussion was normal all round. Auscultation revealed bi-basal fine end inspiratory crepitations. Examination of the abdomen was normal. There was pitting oedema of the ankles. Spirometry was performed and gave the following results: FEV1 2.9 L, FVC 3.1 L.

(5) A 19-year-old female medical student presents to A&E with an acute illness. She has developed a right-sided chest pain for 36 h that is gradually getting worse, and is exacerbated by coughing and moving. In addition she has developed a productive cough with brown-coloured sputum. She had recently returned from her elective in Nepal and was recovering from a diarrhoeal illness. There is no history of any respiratory problems in the past, but she had not been given the BCG vaccination as an adolescent as she had developed a vigorous reaction to the Heaf test. A chest radiograph taken before entry to medical school, however, was reported as being normal. She has never smoked. Her only medication was the oral contraceptive pill. On examination she is slim. There is pyrexia of 39.2°C. The respiratory rate is 40 b.p.m. There is no evidence of clubbing. Her pulse is 105/min and regular. The heart sounds were normal without any added sounds or murmurs. There is a cold sore on the upper lip. There is no clinical evidence of lymphadenopathy. There is, however, evidence of central cyanosis. The trachea is central, but expansion reduced on the right side. The percussion note was dull at the right base. The breath sounds were bronchial at the right base with an associated pleural rub throughout the respiratory cycle.

(a) Mycoplasma pneumonia
(b) Empyema
(c) Sarcoidosis
(d) Congestive cardiac failure
(e) Cryptogenic fibrosing alveolitis
(f) Histiocytosis
(g) Pulmonary TB
(h) Miliary tuberculosis
(i) Churgg–Strauss syndrome
(j) Simple pulmonary eosinophilia
(k) Asthma
(l) Systemic sclerosis
(m) Pulmonary embolism
(n) Pneumothorax
(o) Legionnaire's disease
(p) Staphylococcal pneumonia
(q) Pneumococcal pneumonia
(r) Bronchogenic carcinoma
(s) Lymphoma
(t) Systemic lupus erythematosus

Question 17

Match the following case histories to the best underlying diagnosis in the list given below.

(1) A 65-year-old female attends the A&E department having developed gradually increasing shortness of breath over several days She has no past history of breathing difficulties. There is no history of chest pain or cough. She has noticed increased shortness of breath is made worse when lying flat and has taken to using several pillows at night. Her past medical history includes long-standing type II diabetes complicated by peripheral neuropathy and background retinopathy. She is a non-smoker. There is no past history of thromboembolic disease. On examination her pulse is 105/min and regular and her blood pressure is 134/68 mmHg. She is apyrexial. She appears short of breath, her JVP is elevated to 7 cm above the angle of Louis. The first and second heart sounds are normal, but she has an additional third and fourth heart sound. There are no murmurs. There is mild ankle oedema, but no clinical evidence of deep vein thrombosis. A chest radiograph shows an increased cardiothoracic ratio, pulmonary plethora and small bilateral pleural effusions.

(2) A previously healthy 72-year-old male patient is recovering on the ward following a transurethral resection of the prostate operation. The operation was technically difficult and took longer than usual, owing to the large size of the prostate gland. You are asked to see him 3 h after the procedure because of increasing shortness of breath. There has been no chest pain. On examination he has an intravenous infusion running. He is distressed. The pulse is 102/min and regular and the blood pressure is 180/90 mmHg. The JVP cannot be seen because of obesity. There is an ejection systolic murmur in the aortic area, which was noted before the operation. There is a third heart sound. Chest reveals coarse crepitations in both lower zones. There is no oedema of the ankles. An urgent chest radiograph shows diffuse, fluffy pulmonary shadowing with a normal heart size. An ECG shows a pattern of left ventricular strain but without any acute features of myocardial infarction.

(3) A 55-year-old businessman is brought into casualty with a headache and visual disturbance. A prescription for atenolol is found in his jacket pocket. On examination he is confused and there is no available history. There is no evidence of trauma. His wife later reports that he had seen his GP 1 week previously with increasing headaches, and that he had seemed 'vague' before setting off for work that morning. His pulse is 70/min and blood pressure 220/134 mmHg. He has had several retinal haemorrhages and shows evidence of bilateral papilloedema. He has a loud second sound. Examination of the chest reveals coarse bi-basal crepitations. Examination of the abdomen is difficult owing to obesity, but there is no evidence of tenderness or a mass. Auscultation of the abdomen reveals a bruit in the central area. There is no focal abnormality on neurological examination. Dip test of the urine reveals haematuria. An ECG shows left ventricular hypertrophy with ST segment depression in the lateral chest leads. A random blood glucose is measured at 6.7 mmol/L.

(4) A 48-year-old female patient presents to the A&E department with anterior chest pain. The pain had commenced after an argument with her husband's mistress. It was described as 'heavy' and radiated to the neck area. It had continued for 15–20 min after stopping the exertion. There had been no cough or haemoptysis. She is a non-smoker. Her records showed six recent previous attendances with similar symptoms, following which she had been admitted for observation and subsequently discharged. In addition, she had presented on numerous occasions to several different GPs with less severe episodes. On every occasion that she had been admitted to hospital, she had had a normal ECG on arrival in casualty. She had also not had any rise in the troponin I value during any admission. A subsequent exercise ECG had shown ST segment depression on reaching stage III of the standard Bruce Protocol, but subsequent coronary artery angiography had shown entirely normal coronary arteries. She had also had a normal upper gastrointestinal endoscopy. On examination she appeared tanned and fit and not in pain. Her pulse was regular and 80/min. The JVP was unremarkable. Her blood pressure was 132/68 mmHg. The apex beat was normal as were the heart sounds. There were no cardiac murmurs. The chest was clear.

(5) A 65-year-old man presents with several days of intermittent central chest pain. The pain is scored '5 out of 10' on a pain rating scale. It is described as a 'heavy ache' that radiated to the left shoulder area. There is associated mild shortness of breath. He has had a dry cough for the previous 2 weeks following return from holiday in Spain. He smokes 10 cigarettes per day. He takes no regular exercise and there is no history of exercise precipitating the pain. In the past he has been investigated for altered bowel habit but with no abnormality having been found. He has type II diabetes that is treated by diet alone. On examination he has a BMI of 31.6. His pulse is regular at 70/min and blood pressure is recorded at 178/94 mmHg. The JVP is 4 cm above the angle of Louis. There are no murmurs or bruits, but the second heart sound is loud and there is thought to be a fourth heart sound. Exami-

nation of the respiratory system is unremarkable. His ECG shows lateral ST segment depression greater than 1 mm in three adjacent leads. Cardiac troponin levels are not raised. His chest radiograph is unremarkable.

(a) Acute cardiogenic pulmonary oedema
(b) Silent myocardial infarction
(c) Syndrome X
(d) Unstable angina
(e) Dissection of the aorta
(f) Acute rheumatic fever
(g) Acute non-cardiogenic pulmonary oedema
(h) Temporal arteritis
(i) Pleuritic chest pain
(j) Intracranial haemorrhage
(k) Drug overdose
(l) Cardiac neurosis
(m) Abdominal aortic aneurysm
(n) Acute pericarditis
(o) Acute bacterial meningitis
(p) Migraine
(q) Acute pulmonary embolism
(r) Cavernous sinus thrombosis
(s) Acute myocardial infarction
(t) Chronic LVF
(u) Accelerated hypertension

Question 18

From the following case descriptions choose the most likely diagnosis from the list given below.

(1) A 48-year-old female patient experiences an acute onset of lumbar back pain on bending to pick up shopping bags. The pain is severe and radiates to the sole of the left foot. She has no history of back problems in the past, but does have type II diabetes for which she takes metformin therapy. On examination she is in distress if she attempts to move. There is limitation of straight leg raise on the left to 30 degrees caused by a 'shooting pain down the leg'. The quadriceps reflexes were bilaterally symmetrical and normal. The ankle reflexes were asymmetrical with a reduced left response. In addition there was a relative defect in sensation over the left sole.

(2) A 32-year-old female patient develops acute onset of lumbar back pain in the puerperal period after bending over to pick up her baby. The pain is described as severe and exacerbated by movement. The pain is located in the perineum and anterior thighs. She has also developed weakness getting out of a chair. She has previously been fit and well but has had occasional bouts of anxiety for which she took propranolol. On examination she was slim, there was loss of the lumbar lordosis and straight leg raise was equal on the left and right sides to 80 degrees. There was some patchy loss of sensation over the anterior thighs and perineum. There was evidence of wasting of the quadriceps and the knee and ankle reflexes were bilaterally absent. The plantar reflexes were down going. In addition, a full bladder was palpated, of which the patient was unaware, and following the passage of a urinary catheter 300 mL of urine is drained.

(3) A 62-year-old male patient presents with increasing lumbar and thoracic back pain for 2 months. The pain is constant and has occurred at night. It is unaffected by position. There is no history of trauma or unaccustomed exercise. In addition he has lost his appetite and felt generally weak and unwell. He complains of dizziness and increasing shortness of breath on taking minimal exercise. There has been neither chest pain nor cough. He is an ex-smoker having quit 10 years previously. On examination he is thin and pale, with evidence of marked bruising over the arms and legs. There is no clubbing. The chest and cardiovascular system are unremarkable. The abdomen is soft without discernable hepatomegaly. Some routine investigations were as follows:

Hb	9.2 g/dL
WCC	2.1×10^9/L
Platelets	42×10^9/L
Ur	23 mmol/L
Cr	322 mmol/L
K^+	4.9 mmol/L
Na^+	135 mmol/L

(4) A 45-year-old alcoholic vagrant complains of constant pain in the mid-thoracic area increasing in severity over recent months. In addition he has lost a significant amount of weight and has developed severe episodes of night sweating. Over the past week he had developed difficulty in climbing stairs. He had had a chronic cough for 'many years' and had been a lifelong smoker. On examination he is thin and without evidence of clubbing. There is a palpable firm lymph node in the left anterior cervical triangle of the neck. Examination of the chest was

unremarkable. Lower limb neurological examination revealed bilaterally increased tone and weakness in all muscle groups tested. An abnormal sensory testing result was found in the lower limbs extending up to around the area of the lower chest. A chest radiograph shows apical fibrosis, fluffy shadowing, a cavitating lesion in the left lung and a bulky hilar region with evidence of calcification. A radiograph of the lateral thoracic spine reveals irregular destruction of the body of T5 with early collapse.

(5) A 22-year-old university student has a history of chronic intermittent lower back pain with stiffness of the back in the mornings lasting up to an hour after getting out of bed. Over recent months he had developed increasing shortness of breath on exertion. On examination there was a reduction in the forward flexion of the spine and an increase in the kyphosis of the thoracic spinal region. Examination of the cardiovascular system revealed an early de-crescendo diastolic murmur down the left sternal edge.

(a) Spinal stenosis
(b) Intervertebral disc prolapse with compression of the S1 root
(c) Tuberculosis of the spine
(d) Postural or mechanical back pain
(e) Ankylosing spondylitis
(f) Inflammatory arthritis
(g) Rheumatic fever
(h) Spinal stenosis with myelopathy
(i) Conus medullaris compression due to central disc prolapse
(j) Leaking abdominal aortic aneurysm
(k) Metastasic pyogenic bone infection
(l) Multiple myeloma
(m) Cauda equina syndrome due to central disc prolapse
(n) Intervertebral disc prolapse with compression of the L4 root
(o) Rheumatoid arthritis
(p) Lymphoma
(q) Metastatic disease
(r) Intervertebral disc prolapse with compression of the L5 root
(s) Central lumbar disc prolapse above the T8 level

Paper 4 Questions

MCQs

[1] Concerning heart failure . . .
(a) it causes the patient to be both centrally and peripherally cyanosed
(b) it can cause the patient to be jaundiced
(c) β-blockers are contraindicated in the management of acute heart failure
(d) chronic lung disease is a common cause of left-sided heart failure
(e) cachexia can occur in severe long-standing heart failure

[2] Concerning hypertension . . .
(a) rib-notching on the chest radiograph of a hypertensive patient suggests renal artery stenosis
(b) thiazide diuretics are recognized to cause hypercholesterolaemia as a side effect
(c) ACE inhibitors cause a dry cough because they prevent formation of bradykinin
(d) doxazosin is an example of a non-dihydropyridine calcium-channel antagonist
(e) benign intracranial hypertension is commonest in young males

[3] Concerning cholesterol . . .
(a) myocardial infarction disrupts accurate reading of plasma cholesterol levels for up to 3 days
(b) cholestyramine is found in high concentrations in the blood of patients with hypercholesterolaemia
(c) 'statin' drugs work by direct inhibition of the enzyme cholesterol synthetase
(d) high levels of chylomicrons in a single blood sample indicate significant cardiovascular risk
(e) 'statin' drugs are potentially hepatotoxic

[4] Concerning angina . . .
(a) 'classical' angina typically occurs at night

(b) 'variant' or 'Prinzmetal's' angina typically comes on during exercise
(c) a 'myoscan' demonstrates perfusion of the heart
(d) GTN spray used in angina commonly causes headache
(e) β-blockers should not be given to asthmatics because they cause bronchodilation

[5] Concerning the management of ischaemic heart disease (IHD) . . .
(a) percutaneous transluminal coronary angioplasty (PTCA) has no effect on the prognosis of a patient with IHD, even though it may improve symptoms
(b) PTCA can precipitate acute coronary occlusion and myocardial infarction
(c) the mortality of PTCA is 1/10 000
(d) the left internal mammary artery is currently the vessel of choice for coronary artery bypass grafts (CABGs)
(e) long-term patency of venous grafts is superior to that of arterial grafts

[6] The following are recognized causes of acute pericarditis . . .
(a) hyperbilirubinaemia
(b) uraemia
(c) MI
(d) restrictive cardiomyopathy
(e) Coxsackie virus

[7] Concerning subarachnoid haemorrhage (SAH) . . .
(a) bleeding is usually secondary to trauma
(b) the diagnosis can be confirmed 3 weeks after the acute episode by examination of cerebrospinal fluid
(c) a sixth nerve palsy is a valuable localizing sign

(d) a third nerve palsy is a valuable localizing sign
(e) berry aneurysms are the commonest cause of SAH

[8] Recognized causes of pancytopenia include . . .
(a) folic acid deficiency
(b) paroxysmal nocturnal haemoglobinuria
(c) tuberculosis
(d) acute leukaemia
(e) myelofibrosis

[9] Concerning aortic stenosis . . .
(a) 'aortic sclerosis' is aortic stenosis caused by rheumatic carditis
(b) it causes symptoms predominantly attributable to increased left atrial pressure
(c) it causes the apex beat to be displaced downwards and outwards
(d) it causes an 'opening snap' on auscultation of the chest
(e) it causes a murmur best heard at the apex of the heart

[10] Concerning bradycardias . . .
(a) in AV node blockade, the QRS complexes have a bizarre morphology
(b) in Mobitz type II heart block, PR interval is constant
(c) Wenkebach is the most malignant form of second-degree heart block
(d) first-degree heart block necessitates treatment by permanent pacing
(e) in third-degree heart block, conduction of P waves to the ventricles is variable

[11] Concerning the respiratory organs of the body . . .
(a) the epithelial lining cells of the upper respiratory tract each have a single cilium
(b) type I pneumocytes are derived from type II pneumocytes in the lung
(c) in the terminal airways of the lungs, gas flow occurs solely by diffusion
(d) airway tone is normally constant throughout the day in a non-asthmatic patient
(e) 'dead space' describes a situation where an area of lung is being ventilated but not perfused with blood

[12] Concerning upper respiratory tract infections . . .
(a) sinusitis is common in infants under 5 years
(b) croup is caused by parainfluenza virus

(c) epiglottitis is caused by *Streptococcus pneumoniae*
(d) epiglottitis should be diagnosed under direct vision using a tongue depressor
(e) croup can be prevented by immunization

[13] Acute intermittent porphyria . . .
(a) is recognized to be precipitated by barbiturates
(b) is an autosomal dominant disorder
(c) is recognized to be precipitated by tetracycline
(d) affects more women than men
(e) is recognized to be precipitated by chlordiazepoxide

[14] Cystic fibrosis . . .
(a) commonly causes symptomatic steatorrhoea
(b) causes infertility in both males and females
(c) viscosity of secretions may be decreased using intravenous recombinant human DNAse
(d) is an absolute contraindication to lung transplantation
(e) necessitates a diet high in calories

[15] Eosinophils . . .
(a) in healthy individuals comprise 20% of white blood cell numbers
(b) are present in large numbers in the allergic response to penicillin
(c) are present in large numbers in rheumatic fever
(d) contain many large cytotoxic granules
(e) are present in large numbers in ulcerative colitis

[16] Tuberculosis . . .
(a) is caused solely by *Mycobacterium tuberculosis*
(b) is classically associated with the presence of 'cold abscesses'
(c) is associated with Pott's disease
(d) immunization using BCG is >95% effective
(e) is a recognized cause of lupus pernio

[17] Concerning non-small cell bronchial carcinoma . . .
(a) it is 3× more common than small cell bronchial carcinoma
(b) the 'squamous' type commonly causes cavitation in the lungs
(c) 'large cell' carcinoma is the type most likely to arise from occupational asbestos exposure
(d) 'alveolar cell' carcinoma is frequently associated with expectoration of large volumes of mucoid sputum

(e) the mean time from diagnosis to death is shorter than in small cell lung carcinoma

[18] The following are recognized causes of a mass in the right iliac fossa . . .
(a) sigmoid diverticulitis
(b) caecal carcinoma
(c) volvulus
(d) ovarian cyst
(e) Meckel's diverticulum

[19] The following are recognized risk-factors for the development of oesophageal carcinoma . . .
(a) alcohol
(b) tobacco
(c) oesophageal achalasia
(d) Barratt's oesophagus
(e) Plummer–Vinson syndrome

[20] Recognized signs of an acute occlusion of the left middle cerebral artery include . . .
(a) flaccidity of the limbs of the right side of the body
(b) left facial paralysis
(c) dysphasia
(d) headache
(e) visual field defect

[21] Concerning portal hypertension and variceal bleeding . . .
(a) the pressure in the hepatic portal vein in health is the same as in the hepatic artery
(b) patients with portal hypertension in general have a slow, sluggish circulation

(c) Sengstaken–Blakemore tubes should never be used to control bleeding from varices
(d) 'TIPS' is an effective procedure in reducing bleeding from oesophageal varices
(e) β-blockers are an effective choice for prophylaxis of recurrent variceal bleeding

[22] Marked vitamin B12 deficiency is recognized to occur with . . .
(a) chronic pancreatitis
(b) jejunal diverticulosis
(c) pernicious anaemia
(d) tropical sprue
(e) Osler–Weber–Rendu syndrome

[23] Concerning ulcerative colitis (UC) . . .
(a) 'skip lesions' are characteristic
(b) micro-abscesses do not occur
(c) sulphonylurea drugs are important in the management of UC
(d) it is curable
(e) it is more common than Crohn's disease

[24] Concerning Crohn's disease (CD) . . .
(a) it involves the mucosal and submucosal layers of the gut only, sparing the serosa
(b) it is characterized by the presence of non-caseating granulomas
(c) it is characterized by 'skip lesions'
(d) bloody diarrhoea usually predominates
(e) intestinal malabsorption is common

QUESTIONS 4

EMQs

Question 19

From the following case descriptions choose the most likely diagnosis from the list below.

(1) A 78-year-old female patient presents to her GP with increasing fatigue and listlessness over a period of 4 months. There are no other specific features in the history. In the past she had been troubled by osteoarthritis of the knees and hips and had taken Ibuprofen periodi-

cally for a number of years. On initial examination there were no significant findings other than she was significantly overweight and she appeared pale. Initial investigations revealed an Hb of 7.8 g/dL with an MCV of 92 fL. The urea and electrolytes were unremarkable and the urine was free from blood, protein, bilirubin and glucose. Upper and lower gastrointestinal endoscopies were reported as normal. Following a blood transfusion she was followed up and 3 months later she was found to have a similar recurrent picture of fatigue and anaemia. This time on examination of the abdomen, however, there is a mass in the left hypochondrium and loin. It is firm, 15–20 cm in size and the superior border can be palpated. In addition it moves with respiration and is resonant to percussion.

(2) A 34-year-old male patient presents to A&E with recurrent headaches and visual obscurations. The headaches were described as 'all over and made worse by coughing and bending down'. There had been no vomiting. On examination fundoscopy revealed several flame-shaped haemorrhages in the retina. There was no papilloedema. His blood pressure was checked several times and found to average 225/134 mmHg. On examination of his abdomen there were found to be irregular, bilateral 20-cm masses in each loin, that could be palpated above and which were resonant to percussion.

(3) A 66-year-old male patient presents with increasing listlessness and fatigue symptoms over a period of several months. He had enjoyed good health up until this point. He had noticed increasing shortness of breath and dizziness on climbing stairs. Occasional episodes of anterior chest pain were brought on by such exertion, radiating to the left shoulder. In addition he reported episodes of sweating at night. His wife had made him attend the doctors when he had seemed reluctant to attend a golf tournament. On examination he was slim and there was no clubbing. He appeared pale, but there was no evidence of angular stomatitis or glossitis. His chest and cardiovascular system were unremarkable. There were several firm lymph nodes in the axillae and groin. Examination of the abdomen revealed smooth hepatomegaly to 5 cm. In addition, a mass was found in the left hypochondrium, which was firm, extended across to the umbilicus and was dull to percussion. The superior border of the mass could not be palpated. The following results were obtained:

Hb	9.8 g/dL
WCC	122 × 10⁹/L
Platelets	146 × 10⁹/L

(4) A 55-year-old male presents to A&E with acute back pain radiating into the legs. He had been well earlier that morning, the pain starting on arrival at work. He had visited his GP 2 weeks before following a similar but milder episode of back pain which had subsided spontaneously. The current pain was constant and not relieved either by position or rest. He was normally well but took atenolol

for hypertension and atorvastatin for raised cholesterol. On examination he was an obese patient. He appeared unwell and distressed. He had a sinus tachycardia of 130/min and his blood pressure was recorded at 80/48 mmHg. His chest and cardiovascular system were clear but examination of the abdomen revealed central tenderness with some evidence of abdominal distension. There were no palpable pulses in the lower limbs.

(5) A 17-year-old male patient is investigated for tiredness and episodes of dizziness over several months. He had been adopted in early childhood and had previously been well and asymptomatic. On examination he appeared pale and jaundiced. Examination of the abdomen revealed a mass in the left hypochondrium that could just be palpated by the tip of the finger, but the superior border could not be felt. It was dull to percussion. The following results were obtained:

Hb	8.8 g/dL
WCC	5.6 × 10⁹/L
Platelets	178 × 10⁹/L
MCV	102 fL
Reticulocytes	4%
Bilirubin	34 mmol/L (unconjugated)

(6) A 20-year-old university student returns home for the Christmas vacation and shortly becomes unwell with a high temperature, rigors, headache and a sore throat. On examination she is unwell. The temperature was recorded at 40°C. She has yellow conjunctiva. The throat examination showed inflamed tonsils with a purulent exudates and petechiae on the hard palate. There was no generalized rash or evidence of meningism. The pupils were equal and reactive and there was no evidence of papilloedema. She was alert and not confused. Her GP visited her at home and prescribed Penicillin V. Two days later she developed acute abdominal pain and is found to have generalized abdominal tenderness and the suggestion of a mass in the left upper quadrant which is dull to percussion and no palpable upper border.

(a) Autosomal recessive polycystic kidney disease
(b) Acute myeloid leukaemia
(c) Acute lymphocytic leukaemia
(d) Abdominal aortic aneurysm
(e) Chronic myeloid leukaemia
(f) Renal artery stenosis
(g) Renal cell carcinoma
(h) Acute hepatitis A infection

(i)   Acute streptococcal infection
(j)   Chronic alcohol abuse
(k) Saddle embolism
(l)   Dissection of the aorta
(m) Meningococcal meningitis
(n) Leptospirosis
(o) Autosomal dominant polycystic kidney disease
(p) Hereditary spherocytosis
(q) Infectious mononucleosis
(r)   Bilateral hydronephrosis
(s)   Bilateral chronic pyelonephritis

Question 20

From the following clinical cases choose the most representative diagnosis from the list below.

(1) A 28-year-old type I diabetic who has poor glycaemic control develops increasing shortness of breath over several months. He last attended the diabetic clinic two years ago where he had an HbA1C of 10.6%. At that time his urea and electrolytes were measured as follows:

Ur   8.9 mmol/L
Cr   123 mmol/L
K$^+$ 4.6 mmol/L
Na$^+$ 132 mmol/L

  On arrival in A&E he is distressed and clinically cyanosed. He has several vomiting episodes in the waiting room before seeing the doctor. He appears pale and there are numerous scratch marks over the abdomen and arms. His JVP is estimated at 6 cm and rises with inspiration. The apex beat is displaced. The heart sounds were thought to be normal with no added sounds. His pulse was recorded at 130/min and his blood pressure was 80/52 mmHg. His respiratory rate was 36 b.p.m. The abdomen was soft with a palpable liver to 3 cm below the right costal margin. The kidneys and spleen were not palpable. There was ankle oedema extending to the mid-calf region. The urine was dipped and found to contain protein.

(2) A 48-year-old female type I diabetic, who was diagnosed at the age of 17 years, is referred by her GP to the diabetic clinic because of increasing difficulty in controlling her blood glucose, despite increasing her insulin dosage. In addition, she has refractory hypertension which is proving difficult to manage. In the past she had been treated for cervical cancer at the age of 42 years, and had undergone a hysterectomy and had received radiotherapy. Her current insulin regimen consisted of mixed human insulin, 52 units in the morning and 46 units in the evening. She also takes enalapril 20 mg once a day, atorvastatin 10 mg once a day and low-dose aspirin. On examination she is obese with a BMI of 38. Her adipose tissue is mainly distributed around hips and thighs. There were no skin abnormalities. Examination of the cardiovascular system is unremarkable apart from the blood pressure, which was measured at 192/105 mmHg. The urine is dip tested and found to contain one plus of protein.

(3) A 45-year-old diabetic patient was referred to the skin department in the local hospital after noticing a brown velvet-like skin lesion which had developed in both axillae.

(4) A 56-year-old patient with long-standing type I diabetes is referred for investigation of altered bowel habit to the gastroenterology clinic. This consists of diarrhoea that started several months previously. The symptoms are particularly troublesome at night. There is no history of blood or mucus in the stool. His appetite has remained unchanged and he had not altered his diet recently. There is no history of weight loss or vomiting. He had, however, experienced several recent episodes of palpitations and had had two episodes of 'fainting' when standing from a sitting position. Apart from twice-daily insulin, which has not recently altered in dose, and an angiotensin converting enzyme inhibitor, he takes no other medication. On examination he appeared well. His pulse was regular. His blood pressure was recorded at 134/76 mmHg. The heart sounds were normal and there were no abnormal findings in the respiratory system. Examination of the abdomen was unremarkable without any tenderness, masses or enlargement of the internal organs. Fundoscopy revealed early background retinopathy. The urine was sent for microalbumin testing which was positive. A resting ECG was performed which was reported as being within normal limits. Subsequent colonoscopy of the large bowel found several small polyps, which were removed but proved to be benign, but no other pathology.

(5) A 75-year-old female type II diabetic patient is sent to A&E after having been visited at home by her doctor. She lives alone and is known to have suffered from self-neglect in the past. She has no social support and no relatives living close to her. On arrival in hospital she was found to be drowsy and confused. She was noted to request a drink frequently. Her temperature was 37.8°C. She had poor skin turgor and dry mucous membranes. Her pulse was 110/min and regular. Her blood pressure was recorded at 100/60 mmHg with a significant drop to 80/52 on standing. The cardiovascular system was otherwise unremarkable on examination. Her respiratory rate was 28 cycles per minute and there were crepitations at the left base. The following blood results were obtained:

Random glucose	52.3 mmol/L
Ur	23.6 mmol/L
Cr	156 mmol/L
Na^+	158 mmol/L
K^+	5.5 mmol/L

Arterial blood gas analysis:

PaO_2	8.7 kPa
$PaCO_2$	4.5 kPa
pH	7.38
HCO_3	22.1 mmol/L

A chest radiograph reported a left basal pneumonia.

(6) A 56-year-old male patient reports symptoms of thirst and passing excessive amounts of urine to his GP. There has been no weight loss. He is concerned because his best friend who had long-standing diabetes recently died from a myocardial infarction. He is otherwise fit and well apart from essential hypertension, which he has had for a number of years and which is well-controlled on a thiazide diuretic. On examination he appears well. He is mildly obese with a central distribution of the adipose tissue. There are no abnormalities on examination of the skin. The blood pressure is recorded at 165/88 mmHg. The rest of the examination including fundoscopy and neurological examination is normal. His random blood glucose is measured at 11.5 mmol/L by his GP using a reliable assay

(7) A 78-year-old non-insulin diabetic attends the diabetic clinic. His visual acuity was measured and was found to be reduced substantially in the left eye: 18 over 60 m compared to 6 over 60 m at his last check 6 months previously. His HbA1C was 8.1%. There was no evidence of microalbuminuria or peripheral neuropathy. There was a normal red reflex. The retinas were thought to be normal on inspection with no evidence of retinopathy.

(a) The patient can be diagnosed as having diabetes
(b) Diabetes cannot be diagnosed from the information given

(c) The patient has impaired glucose tolerance
(d) The patient does not have diabetes
(e) (Diabetic) Syndrome X
(f) Hypoglycaemia
(g) Diabetic ketoacidosis
(h) Granuloma annulare
(i) Hyperosmolar non-ketotic coma
(j) CMV retinitis
(k) Diabetic dermopathy
(l) Cushing's disease
(m) Acute renal failure
(n) Ischemic heart disease
(o) Medication side effect
(p) Retinal artery occlusion
(q) Diabetic amyotrophy
(r) Cardiomyopathy
(s) Acanthosis nigricans
(t) Irritable bowel syndrome
(u) Diabetic maculopathy
(v) Autonomic neuropathy
(w) Cataract
(x) Uraemic pericarditis

Question 21

From the following case histories choose the correct diagnosis.

(1) A 78-year-old female patient is referred by her GP for general weight loss, diarrhoea and increasing lethargy. She lives alone, and her relatives report several recent falls and occasional episodes of vomiting. Past medical history includes treatment for tuberculosis in young adult life. You find a pale, slightly confused woman. Examinations of the cardiovascular system, respiratory system and abdomen are all normal. Blood pressure was 150/80 mmHg lying and 130/60 on standing. There is increased pigmentation within a previous appendectomy scar. Investigation results are as follows:

Na^+	130 mmol/L
K^+	5.6 mmol/L
Ur	10.6 mmol/L
Cr	156 mmol/L
Ca	2.8 mmol/L
Hb	10.2 g
WCC	5.2
Urine	NAD
CXR	Opacification of L apex

(2) A 37-year-old female patient presents with symptoms of polyuria and thirst over a period of several weeks. She has also complained of frequent headaches occurring all over the head, not exacerbated by coughing and without any diurnal variation in severity. There have been no visual disturbances associated with the headaches. There has been no weight loss and her menstrual cycle is regular. On examination she appears well although she is on the 2nd centile for height and weight. There is normal secondary sexual development and there is a normal distribution of body hair. There is no clinical evidence of thyroid under- or overactivity. The following results are obtained:

Baseline:

Fasting blood glucose	4.1 mmol/L
Plasma Ca	2.15 mmol/L
Plasma K	4.2 mmol/L
Plasma osmolality	272 mOsm/kg (normal 275–295)
Urine osmolality	50 mOsm/kg

After 8 hours of water deprivation:

Plasma osmolality	293 mOsm/kg
Urine osmolality	619 mOsm/kg

(3) A 45-year-old female presents with weakness and weight loss over a period of several weeks. In addition, she has noticed increased acne over her face and upper chest. Her husband has noticed a change in her facial appearance, which has become 'rounded'. Three days prior to admission she developed severe back pain whilst bending to lift a washing basket. She has previously been fit and well apart from several recent bouts of acute bronchitis. In the past she has had an anaphylactic reaction when given penicillin and was admitted to the intensive care unit. She takes no regular medication. She smokes 20 cigarettes per day. On examination she has a moon face with increased pigmentation. There are striae over the abdomen and around the axillae. There is no evidence of facial hair. Her cardiovascular and respiratory systems are unremarkable. There is some focal bony tenderness over the first lumbar vertebra. Her blood pressure is recorded at 210/98 mmHg. The following results are obtained:

Low dose dexamethazone suppression test:

Plasma cortisol at 48 h	235 nmol/L (normal <50 nmol/L)

High dose dexamethazone suppression test:

Pre-test cortisol	242 nmol/L
Day 2 post-high dose dexamethazone	245 nmol/L

(4) A 56-year-old female patient complains of muscle weakness, with increasing difficulty in getting out of a chair and ascending stairs. This has been gradually getting worse over a period of several months. She has also noticed decreased exercise tolerance and has not been sleeping well due to episodes of shortness of breath during the night. She has had no chest pain or palpitations. There has been no cough, but she has noticed herself wheezing occasionally. There is no history of altered gastrointestinal function or of weight loss. She does not smoke and does not take any regular medications. On examination she is apyrexial, her skin is dry, her pulse is 58/min and regular. She appears pale, but there is no evidence of pigmentation. Her blood pressure is 188/98 mmHg. Her JVP is elevated at 7 cm but has a normal waveform. The apex beat cannot be palpated. There is a third heart sound and stony dullness at the left base. Examination of the abdomen and nervous system was unremarkable. There is no evidence of muscle wasting. The following results were obtained:

Hb	10.8 g/dL
MCV	103 fL
Platelets	341×10^9/L
WCC	7.8×10^9/L
Ca	2.34 mmol/L
Alkaline phosphatase	98 U/L
Na$^+$	126 mmol/L
K$^+$	4.3 mmol/L
Ur	7.8 mmol/L
Cr	120 mmol/L
Chest radiograph	'Cardiomegaly, upper lobe venous diversion, bilateral pleural effusions more pronounced on the left side'

(5) A 42-year-old female patient complains of frequent and persistent headaches over several months along with muscular weakness and joint pains. There has been no vomiting or reported visual disturbance. She has noticed that her periods have become infrequent over the previous six months. In the past she had been fit and well although has recently been referred to an orthodontist for dental malocclusion and pain in both her temporomandibular joints. She takes no regular medications. On examination she is on the 50th centile for both height and weight and there is normal secondary sexual development. The JVP is elevated at 7 cm and there is a prominent third heart sound with mild pitting oedema of the ankles. On examination of her cranial nerves there is evidence of bitemporal hemianopia. Her blood pressure is measured at 178/100 mmHg and her urine contains glucose 3+.

(a) Addison's disease
(b) Cranial diabetes insipidus
(c) Nephrogenic diabetes insipidus
(d) Primary polydipsia
(e) Acromegaly
(f) Osteomalacia
(g) Diabetes mellitus
(h) Congestive cardiac failure
(i) Cushing's disease
(j) Graves' disease
(k) Ectopic adrenocorticotrophic hormone (ACTH) production
(l) Adrenal tumour producing cortisol
(m) Hypothyroidism
(n) Normal
(o) Growth hormone deficiency
(p) Hyperprolactinaemia
(q) Hypopituitarism
(r) None of these

Question 22

From the following case descriptions choose the most likely diagnosis.

(1) A 24-year-old female consults you with a 6-month history of progressive tiredness and weight loss. She has lost her appetite, but has had no alteration in bowel habit. She has reduced exercise tolerance such that she has to stop half-way up one flight of domestic stairs. She has had several episodes of a painful swollen knee joint over the previous two months. She is normally well apart from pneumonia as a child that required admission to hospital.

On examination she is thin and has early fluctuance of the nail bed. Her temperature is 38.5°C, pulse 110/min sinus rhythm and blood pressure is 110/60 mmHg. There is a quiet systolic murmur at the apex radiating to the left axilla. Examination of the chest reveals fine bi-basal crackles, but is otherwise clear. Examination of the abdomen reveals mild splenomegaly. Investigations reveal:

Hb	9.8 g/dL
MCV	90 fL

WCC	5.6×10^9/L
Platelets	600×10^9/L
Ur	6.5 mmol/L
Cr	96 mmol/L
Na$^+$	137 mmol/L
K$^+$	4.5 mmol/L
Urine	Non-haemolysed blood on dip test 2+
CXR	Reported as 'normal'

(2) A 48-year-old female patient reports episodes of short-duration chest pain which have developed over several months. The pain is described as 'sharp' in character and localized in the left infra-mammary area. She has also experienced increasing shortness of breath on moderate exertion and additionally has had several bouts of dizziness. On one occasion she reports collapsing during such an episode of dizziness, after carrying heavy bags of shopping back to her car. In the past she has been fit and well without any previous cardiac events. There is no history of rheumatic fever. She does not smoke or drink alcohol and is on no regular medications. She does take 'herbal' medicines for migraine episodes. On examination she appears slim and sun-tanned. There is no clubbing. The pulse rate is 84/min, essentially regular but with an occasional ectopic beat. The blood pressure is recorded at 140/62 mmHg and equal in each arm. All peripheral pulses are present. There is no cyanosis and the JVP is not elevated. The apex beat in normal in position and character. On auscultation there is a mid-systolic 'click' followed by a murmur that radiates to the left axilla.

(3) A 36-year-old Asian female mature student returns from India and becomes unwell with a short history of increasing breathlessness and palpitations. There has been no chest pain. She did not have a cough or wheeze and she is a lifelong non-smoker. She had also developed pain and swelling of the left knee over the last week. Her past medical history is unremarkable, and she took no regular medications. She had been unwell whilst away with a pharyngitis for which she took paracetamol. On examination she was mildly obese. Her temperature was recorded at 38.4°C with no lymphadenopathy. The pulse was regular with a rate of 120/min. The JVP was elevated but with a normal waveform. On auscultation there is a pan-systolic murmur radiating to the left axilla, with an additional short diastolic murmur radiating towards the apex area. A pink rash was noted on the anterior thighs.

(4) A 29-year-old male patient develops shortness of breath gradually increasing in severity over several weeks. In addition, he has had several episodes of collapse after standing from a sitting position. He has not experienced any chest pain but has experienced occasional palpitations. He is now breathless on minimal exertion and is sleeping with four pillows at night. There is neither a cough nor sputum production. He is a non-smoker, takes no regular medications and reports drinking only 6 units of alcohol per week. The past medical history includes chronic osteomyelitis for several years following a fractured tibia sustained in a motorbike accident. On examination his respiratory rate is 28 b.p.m. His pulse is irregularly irregular and is recorded at 120/min. The JVP is elevated at 7 cm. The apex cannot be palpated, but the heart sounds were normal. In the abdomen there was non-tender enlargement of the liver and the spleen. There was pitting oedema to the mid-thigh bilaterally. The urine contained three pluses of protein but was otherwise clear.

(5) A 42-year-old female presents with several necrotic areas in the toes of both feet. In addition, she has experienced periodic bouts of sweating and fever over several months. She has had no weight loss. On examination the patient has a pyrexia of 37.8°C. There are no splinter haemorrhages or Osler's nodes. The apex beat is not displaced and is normal in character; there is a mid-diastolic murmur at the apex followed by a loud first heart sound and a prominent third heart sound. The chest is clear and examination of the abdomen is normal.

(a) Atrial myxoma
(b) Subacute bacterial endocarditis
(c) Mitral valve prolapse
(d) Mitral stenosis
(e) Tuberculosis
(f) Streptococcal infection
(g) Aortic stenosis
(h) Systemic amyloidosis
(i) Ventricular septal defect
(j) Constrictive pericarditis
(k) Coarctation of the aorta
(l) Sarcoidosis
(m) Abdominal aortic aneurysm
(n) Rheumatic fever
(o) Lymphoma
(p) Syndrome X
(q) Hypertrophic obstructive cardiomyopathy

(r) Cardiac neurosis
(s) Mitral regurgitation

Question 23

Match the following case scenarios to the diagnoses listed below.

(1) A 67-year-old Jewish female presents with a short history of gradually progressive weight loss, lethargy and pain in the hips and shoulder. She has noticed a reduction in her appetite, but there has been no vomiting, abdominal pain, or alteration in bowel habit. Systemic review was otherwise normal. She is normally well, but has had several recent visits to the dentist for suspected dental pain on eating. On examination she is pale and there is no clubbing or rash. There is no evidence of lymphadenopathy. Examinations of the cardiovascular and respiratory systems are unremarkable. She has a reduction in power in all limbs to grade 4 out of 5, but otherwise normal peripheral and central neurological examination findings. There was no muscle swelling or tenderness. Investigations revealed:

Hb	8.9 g/dL
WCC	7.4×10^9/L
Pl	679×10^9/L
MCV	91.9 fL
Na$^+$	132 mmol/L
K$^+$	5.1 mmol/L
Ur	12.4 mmol/L
Cr	144 mmol/L
CRP	43 mg/L (normal <10)
Urinary Bence Jones protein	Negative

(2) A 38-year-old female who has rheumatoid arthritis is referred to outpatients for suspected pneumonia. She complains of a productive cough and left-sided pleuritic chest pain. She is concerned because she has had three similar episodes in the previous two years. She is a non-smoker with no history of previous chest problems. She has also been experiencing painful ankles and wrists intermittently over the same period. She is on no regular medications.

On examination she is thin and tanned. Her respiratory rate is 40 b.p.m. and there is evidence of consolidation at the left base. She has symmetrical swelling and tenderness of the wrists and metacarpal phalangeal joints (MCPJs). The following investigations were performed:

Hb	9.5 g/dL
WCC	2.8×10^9/L (neutrophils 15%)
Pl	52×10^9/L
Na$^+$	120 mmol/L
K$^+$	4.5 mmol/L
Ur	8.2 mmol/L
Cr	100 mmol/L
CXR	Left lower lobe shadowing

(3) A 23-year-old male complains of frequent bouts of acute pain and swelling in the left knee. This had been recurrent over the last three years since returning from Ibiza following a holiday. When seen in outpatients he appeared well and was apyrexial. There was a moderate effusion of the left knee with local warmth and some diffuse tenderness over the joint. The range of movement in the joint was limited to 40 degrees flexion from full extension. The knee was aspirated under aseptic conditions and 40 mL of straw-coloured fluid was obtained. Microscopy and culture of this was unremarkable and there was no evidence of crystals under polarized light. It was also noted that he had a skin lesion consisting of what was recorded in the notes as 'pustular psoriasis' on the right foot plantar area.

(4) A 36-year-old male patient attends A&E complaining of pain, swelling and morning stiffness in the right wrist and first metacarpophalangeal joints. He had been experiencing these symptoms for 9 months. He had recently had the thenar eminence of the hand explored by the orthopaedic team for a suspected foreign body, as he worked manually in the forestry industry, and there was suspicion of a forgotten injury. However, despite this the pain and swelling had continued. There is no previous history of joint, skin or eye problems. He had previously been well and was on no medications. On examination the wrist area was moderately swollen with boggy tissue. The temperature of the joint was increased. There was limited hand function. There was some pitting noted in several fingernails. Otherwise physical examination was normal including inspection of the skin.

(5) A 56-year-old male is found at a routine insurance medical to have hypertension. He is commenced on some medication and it is arranged for him to attend his GP for review. On attendance 1 week later he had developed severe pain and swelling of the left knee. Plasma uric acid levels were measured at 445 µmol/L (normal range <448 µmol/L).

(6) A well 78-year-old female attends the diabetic clinic for routine testing and is found to have raised calcium (3.03 mmol/L) incidentally. A subsequent parathormone assay is raised and primary hyperparathyroidism is diagnosed. Several weeks later, whilst waiting for a subsequently arranged out patient appointment, she develops an excruciatingly painful and swollen right knee joint. A joint radiograph shows calcification of the medial meniscus.

(a) Systemic lupus erythematosus
(b) Palindromic rheumatoid arthritis
(c) Drug side effect
(d) Acute gout
(e) Pseudogout
(f) Sarcoidosis
(g) Chronic renal failure
(h) Behçet's syndrome
(i) Polymyalgia rheumatica
(j) Polmymyositis
(k) Carcinomatosis
(l) Felty's syndrome
(m) Dermatomyositis
(n) Osteoarthritis
(o) Reactive arthritis
(p) Haemarthrosis
(q) Psoriatic arthritis
(r) None of these

Question 24

From the following information choose the next most appropriate steps as indicated in the list below.

(1) A 45-year-old patient is admitted to A&E having collapsed at home. On examination he is pale, sweaty and unconscious. A cuffed endotracheal tube has been inserted and intravenous access has been established by the paramedic ambulance crew, and the patient is being ventilated by hand. He had no pulse when collected and external cardiac massage was commenced at that time. On your initial assessment he still does not have a cardiac output. **(Give the next two steps.)**

(2) A 22-year-old man is brought into the Emergency Room accompanied by several friends, having been found on a park bench unconscious. He arrives in the department with an airway and intravenous access established by the paramedic crew. You find the patient has a cardiac output with a pulse of 60/min and a blood pressure of 120/80 mmHg. He has bilateral pin-point pupils. (**Give the next step.**)

(**3**) You are a GP called to the home of a 34-year-old well-controlled type I diabetic patient. His wife has found him unconscious prior to lunchtime. He appears pale and sweaty. He is breathing spontaneously and has a cardiac output on brief examination. (**Give the next two steps.**)

(**4**) A 24-year-old known asthmatic patient attends the A&E department with shortness of breath and wheeze. He is unable to complete sentences in one breath, his pulse is 120/min and his peak flow is un-recordable. His oxygen saturation on air is recorded at 89%. He is centrally cyanosed and examination of the chest reveals heavy use of accessory muscles for ventilation and quiet breath sounds without audible wheezes. (**Give the next three steps.**)

(**5**) A 56-year-old patient who was recently discharged from the hospital oncology ward is admitted to A&E in a collapsed state. His wife states that he has become increasingly unwell and confused during the course of that day. On examination you find the patient has a temperature of 39.4°C. The pulse is 114/min and blood pressure is 78/36 mmHg. He is maintaining his airway and has spontaneous respirations. (**Give the next two steps.**)

(a) Establish an airway
(b) Give intravenous fluids
(c) Give salbutamol nebulized on air
(d) Give intravenous naloxone
(e) Arrange urgent transfer to hospital
(f) Assess the patient's cardiac rhythm
(g) Check the position of the endotracheal tube
(h) Arrange an urgent chest radiograph
(i) Question a relative or friend about the circumstances of the event
(j) Give intravenous hydrocortisone 100 mg
(k) Commence intravenous insulin using a sliding scale
(l) Take blood for blood cultures
(m) Give high-dose oral prednisolone
(n) Check the peak flow rate
(o) Call for senior/ITU help
(p) Give salbutamol nebulized on high flow oxygen
(q) Give salbutamol and ipratropium nebulized on high flow oxygen
(r) Give intravenous epinephrine
(s) Give IM glucagon
(t) Commence an intravenous infusion of aminophylline
(u) Commence DC cardioversion if in ventricular fibrillation or ventricular tachycardia
(v) Check blood glucose with bedside test
(w) Perform Heimlich manoeuvre
(x) Give intravenous calcium gluconate
(y) Give intravenous dextrose and insulin
(z) Perform an urgent lumbar puncture

Part 2 Answers

Paper 1 Answers

MCQs

[1]	(a) F	(b) F	(c) T	(d) F	(e) F
[2]	(a) F	(b) F	(c) F	(d) F	(e) F
[3]	(a) F	(b) T	(c) F	(d) F	(e) F
[4]	(a) F	(b) F	(c) T	(d) T	(e) T
[5]	(a) F	(b) F	(c) F	(d) F	(e) T
[6]	(a) F	(b) F	(c) F	(d) T	(e) F
[7]	(a) F	(b) T	(c) F	(d) T	(e) F
[8]	(a) T	(b) F	(c) T	(d) F	(e) F
[9]	(a) T	(b) F	(c) T	(d) F	(e) T
[10]	(a) F	(b) F	(c) T	(d) T	(e) F
[11]	(a) F	(b) T	(c) T	(d) F	(e) T
[12]	(a) F	(b) F	(c) T	(d) F	(e) F
[13]	(a) F	(b) F	(c) F	(d) T	(e) F
[14]	(a) F	(b) T	(c) F	(d) F	(e) T
[15]	(a) T	(b) F	(c) F	(d) F	(e) T
[16]	(a) F	(b) T	(c) F	(d) T	(e) T
[17]	(a) T	(b) T	(c) T	(d) T	(e) T
[18]	(a) F	(b) F	(c) T	(d) F	(e) F
[19]	(a) F	(b) F	(c) F	(d) T	(e) F
[20]	(a) F	(b) F	(c) F	(d) F	(e) F
[21]	(a) F	(b) F	(c) F	(d) T	(e) T
[22]	(a) F	(b) T	(c) F	(d) F	(e) F
[23]	(a) F	(b) F	(c) T	(d) T	(e) T
[24]	(a) F	(b) F	(c) F	(d) F	(e) F

---

[1] (a) F (b) T (c) T (d) F (e) F

(a) Valvular disease only causes **7%** of cases of heart failure in the UK. The commonest cause of heart failure in the UK is **atherosclerotic ischaemic heart disease**. In general, the causes of *low-output* cardiac failure can be split up depending on whether they cause predominantly systolic, predominantly diastolic or acute failure of the myocardium . . .

- **Dominant systolic heart failure**
  - Ischaemic myocardial disease, coronary artery disease
  - Cardiomyopathy (alcoholic, diabetic, drug-induced, idiopathic)
  - Myocarditis
  - Valvular heart disease
  - Congenital heart disease with severe pulmonary hypertension
  - Terminal ventricular septal defect or atrial septal defect
- **Dominant diastolic heart failure**
  - Hypertension
  - Severe aortic stenosis
  - Hypertrophic cardiomyopathy
  - Restrictive cardiomyopathy
  - Ischemic myocardial disease, coronary artery disease
- **Acute heart failure**
  - Acute mitral or aortic regurgitation
  - Rupture of valve leaflets or supporting structures
  - Infective endocarditis with acute valve incompetence
  - Myocardial infarction

(b) Atrial cells store and release the 28-amino-acid **atrial natriuretic peptide** (ANP) in response to **stretch of the right atrium** by increased central venous pressure. The relative volume overload of the atria that occurs in heart failure causes levels of ANP to be high, leading to a variety of beneficial effects in heart failure, including . . .

- Increased sodium and water excretion by the kidney (**natriuresis and diuresis**)
- Increased glomerular filtration, hence increased sodium excretion (by selective vasodilatation of renal glomerular afferents, and vasoconstriction of renal glomerular efferents)

49

- Relaxation of vascular smooth muscle (vasorelaxation of capacitance vessels)
- Increased vascular permeability
- Inhibition of release/action of several undesirable hormones which exacerbate heart failure (e.g. aldosterone, angiotensin II, endothelin, ADH)

When it was first discovered, ANP was cast as the cardiovascular hero, standing opposed to the villainous intents of vasoconstrictors such as angiotensin, ADH and endothelin in heart failure. Unfortunately, its potential therapeutic use foundered with the discovery of its short plasma half-life. Subsequent attempts to devise ANP agonists or agents to block clearance of the endogenous peptide have been thus far unsuccessful.

(c) The third heart sound (S3) occurs in **early** diastole due to **rapid ventricular filling** as soon as the mitral and tricuspid valves open. It can be normal in children and young adults, but is abnormal in others and represents **heart failure or volume overload of the heart** (e.g. mitral or aortic regurgitation). It is commonly referred to as a 'distressed' sound.

The fourth heart sound (S4) occurs in **late** diastole in association with ventricular filling due to atrial systole, and is related to **reduced ventricular compliance**. It is a low-frequency oscillation that can be normal at older ages owing to a physiological decline in ventricular compliance, but is nearly always abnormal at younger ages especially if it is of high intensity or is palpable. It is **common in ventricular hypertrophy**, particularly with hypertension and aortic stenosis, and is almost invariable in acute myocardial infarction. S4 may arise from the right ventricle, the left ventricle or both. It is commonly referred to as a 'stressed' sound.

(d) The chest X-ray in a patient with heart failure has a classical pattern, comprising . . .

- Cardiomegaly (greater than the width of one hemithorax)
- Upper lobe venous diversion
- Kerley-B lines (fine peripheral septal lines; named after Peter J. Kerley, an English radiologist who also described Kerley-A and Kerley-C lines on chest radiographs)
- 'Bat's wing' hilar oedema
- Bilateral effusions

(e) Diuretics commonly used in the treatment of heart failure include . . .

- **Thiazide diuretics** (e.g. bendrofluazide, metolazone): decrease active reabsorption of Na^+ and Cl^- in the distal convoluted tubule by binding to the chloride site of the electroneutral Na^+/Cl^- co-transport system and inhibiting its action. Potassium loss with these drugs is significant and can be serious. Excretion of uric acid ($\rightarrow$ gout) and calcium is decreased, whereas that of magnesium is increased.
- **Loop diuretics** (e.g. furosemide, bumetanide): inhibit transport of NaCl out of the lumen of the thick segment of the ascending limb of the loop of Henle. These are the most powerful of all currently used diuretics, potentially causing loss of up to 25% of the Na^+ in the filtrate by direct inhibition of the $Na^+/K^+/2Cl^-$ carrier in the luminal membrane. Again, these drugs cause significant K^+ loss. There is an increase in the excretion of calcium and magnesium, and a decrease in the excretion of uric acid ($\rightarrow$ gout).
- **Potassium-sparing diuretics** (e.g. spironolactone, amiloride): Spironolactone has a limited diuretic action. By acting as an **aldosterone antagonist** it inhibits Na^+ retention and decreases K^+ excretion. Similarly, amiloride has limited diuretic efficacy. By blocking Na^+ reabsorption in the collecting tubules and ducts, it concomitantly decreases K^+ excretion. Importantly, drugs in this class are the only diuretics that **do not cause hypokalaemia**.

[2] (a) F (b) F (c) F (d) F (e) F

(a) Over 90% of all cases of hypertension arise due to **no known cause**, referred to as **'essential'** hypertension. The remaining cases of hypertension that do have a defined cause are known as **'secondary'** hypertension. These are always important to consider because even though they are rare, they are frequently amenable to treatment.

Secondary causes of hypertension

- **Renal causes**: these account for **>80% of cases of secondary hypertension**. They cause inappropriate retention of salt and water and inappropriate elevation of plasma renin levels. They may be split into:
  - *Renovascular*
    Renal artery stenosis
  - *Renoparenchymal*
    Chronic glomerulonephritis
    Chronic pyelonephritis
    Diabetic nephropathy
    Adult polycystic kidney disease
    Chronic tubulointerstitial nephritis

- **Endocrine causes**: there are eight . . .
  - Conn's syndrome (excess mineralocorticoid) → **(b)**
  - Cushing's syndrome (excess glucocorticoid)
  - Acromegaly (excess growth hormone)
  - Adrenal hyperplasia (congenital)
  - Phaeochromocytoma
  - Hyperthyroidism
  - Hypothyroidism → **(c)**
  - Hyperparathyroidism
- **Cardiovascular causes**: the most important is coarctation of the aorta (also polycythaemia rubra vera)
- **Pharmacological causes**: including the oral contraceptive pill, corticosteroids, monoamine oxidase inhibitors (paroxysms when eating tyramine-containing foods), cocaine, amphetamines, vasopressin, etc.
- **Pregnancy**
- **Raised intracranial pressure (ICP)**: an acute rise in ICP causes the 'Cushing phenomenon' or 'reflex', which is essentially a rise in systemic blood pressure in response to the increased intracranial pressure. Commonly occurs in head injury or intracranial haemorrhage → **(d)**

To impress examiners with your knowledge of secondary causes of hypertension, also mention **GRA (glucocorticoid remediable aldosteronism)**. In this condition there is a crossover mutation and fusion of the adrenocorticotrophic hormone (ACTH)-regulatory element of the 11-β–hydroxylase gene and the aldosterone synthase gene, meaning that every time the body attempts to manufacture steroid, it instead produces aldosterone, causing profound hypertension via salt and water retention. Once discovered, the treatment is simple: give exogenous dexamethasone to switch off the need for endogenous steroid production, thereby switching off inappropriate aldosterone production.

(e) Malignant hypertension is said to occur when the BP rises suddenly and precipitously to levels above 140 mmHg diastolic. There is characteristic fibrinoid necrosis of vessel walls and rapid progression to renal failure. There are marked changes in retinal vessels, and grades 3 and 4 on the Keith–Wagener classification of hypertensive retinopathy are diagnostic of malignant hypertension, but *only in the presence of a diastolic BP > 140 mmHg*.

[3] (a) F (b) T (c) F (d) F (e) F

(a) Although nitrates do not have the marked effect of

lessening chest pain in acute MI that they do in stable angina, they are still able to noticeably lessen the pain of acute MI when given sublingually, buccally or intravenously.

(b) So-called '**silent**' infarcts occur in the elderly, diabetics and patients with a long history of hypertension. Instead of presenting with pain, these infarcts **present with dyspnoea** from development of acute pulmonary oedema, **syncope or coma** from dysrhythmias, **acute confusional states, diabetic hypoglycaemic crisis, hypotension** or **shock**.

(c) Although administration of morphine (or more correctly diamorphine) is an important early manoeuvre in treating acute MI (since it produces analgesia and lessens subjective distress from dyspnoea), it should be given **intravenously** (or orally if access is difficult) and not intramuscularly. This is because should the patient later be thrombolysed, significant internal or external bleeding can occur if intramuscular injections have been recently given.

(d) Myocardial infarction should be *suspected* on the history, but is should only be diagnosed in the presence of either positive ECG findings, or a raised level of cardiac enzymes on testing the blood an appropriate interval after onset of symptoms.

(e) The first change of acute MI visible on the ECG is a point of contention, although it most certainly is **not** the appearance of Q-waves.

ST-segment elevation is said to occur within minutes of the onset of acute MI and can persist for up to 2 weeks. If elevation persists over 4 weeks, this suggests formation of a ventricular aneurysm.

Occasionally **T-wave inversion** is said to be the first visible ECG change of acute MI. This tends to persist longer than ST-elevation, yet it is still usually only a transient change. T-wave inversion that occurs without subsequent formation of Q-waves is typical of sub-endocardial infarction (non-Q-wave infarction).

The final ECG change associated with acute MI is the appearance of **pathological Q-waves**. These are broad (>1 mm), deep (>2 mm) negative deflections that start the QRS complex. They occur physiologically in aVR, I and III. Pathological Q-waves develop over hours or days, and are the hallmark of transmural infarct. They reflect electrical silence of infarcted cardiac tissue, causing a window through which the normal endo- to epicardial activation of the opposite, non-infarcted ventricular wall is 'seen'. They are **almost always permanent**.

[4] (a) F (b) F (c) T (d) T (e) T

The complications of myocardial infarction can be thought of under five main headings . . .

1. *Further chest pain*
   - A bruised sensation and musculoskeletal pain are common within the first 48 h, especially if the patient has undergone **CPR** or repeated attempts at **DC cardioversion**
   - **Pericarditis** may develop in the first 1–3 days post-MI; it is commoner with full thickness infarcts and may cause an audible rub ('like walking in fresh-laid snow'); treat with high dose aspirin
   - **Infarct extension** may occur; look for further ST-elevation; treat with repeated thrombolysis or urgent coronary angioplasty
   - It may simply be **post-infarction angina**; this usually develops within 10 days of the acute episode and can be treated with standard medical therapy, i.e. nitrates, β-blockers and Ca^{2+}-channel antagonists

2. *Fever*
   - Fever commonly peaks 3–4 days post-MI and is due to **myocardial necrosis**
   - Other causes of fever must be considered, e.g. infection, thrombophlebitis, venous thrombosis, drug reaction, pericarditis, etc.
   - **Dressler's syndrome** occurs weeks or even months after MI and consists of the triad of pericarditis, fever and pericardial effusion; it is actually an **autoimmune response** to the damaged myocardium; it may necessitate administration of anti-inflammatories. → **(c)**

3. *New systolic murmur* (four to consider)
   - **Pericardial friction rub** secondary to inflammation of the infarcted myocardium
   - **Long-standing murmur** that was missed at presentation
   - **Ventricular septal defect**: this classically occurs 5–10 days post-MI and presents as sudden collapse, pulmonary oedema and hypotension; usually diagnosed on echo, where colour flow shows left to right flow across the septum; requires emergent surgical repair
   - **Acute mitral regurgitation** occurs 2–10 days post-MI due to infarction and rupture of papillary muscle; can cause torrential regurgitation and sudden death, but if the patient survives, emergent surgical repair is vital

4. *Post-MI arrhythmias* (four to consider)
   - **Sinus bradycardia** is common, especially in inferi-

or or posterior MI; treated first with atropine, then with electrical pacing
   - **Atrioventricular blockade** is also common; if the infarction is an inferior one, the blockade is often temporary and does not require treatment; however, if the infarction is an anterior one and 2nd or 3rd degree block/bifascicular block arises, then prophylactic pacing is indicated
   - **Ventricular ectopics** post-MI have a poor prognosis as they frequently herald the development of ventricular tachycardia or fibrillation; there is no evidence that treatment of these alters prognosis, but it may be prudent to correct PaO_2, K^+ and Mg^{2+}; if ectopics continue, a magnesium sulphate infusion may be set up
   - **Ventricular tachycardia** may arise, and it should be treated in the usual way (Mg^{2+}, lidocaine, amiodarone, synchronized DC shock). VT in the first 24 h post-MI has a less sinister prognosis than VT arising later in the post-MI course. Should ventricular fibrillation develop from VT, prompt DC cardioversion should be instigated

5. *Hypotension and shock post-MI*
   - Common in large MIs; treatment is with *cautious* plasma volume expansion (i.e. 100–200 mL colloid over 10 min), and then inotropes if the BP should remain low despite adequate filling pressures

Other complications of MI worth considering are **thromboembolism** secondary to prolonged inactivity or cardiac mural thrombus, **left ventricular aneurysm formation** (think persistent ST-elevation), heart failure and, of course, death.

- Sheehan's syndrome is pituitary necrosis due to circulatory collapse following severe post-partum bleeds, and is nothing to do with MI → **(a)**
- Acute aortic regurgitation is not a complication of acute MI. It happens more often in dissecting aortic aneurysms or with valve destruction associated with the vegetations of bacterial endocarditis → **(b)**
- Electromechanical dissociation (EMD) occurs when the ECG is relatively normal and yet there is no mechanical activity of the heart (*normal ECG but no output*) → **(d)**

The causes of EMD can be grouped into the **4 Hs** and the **4 Ts** . . .

H	Hypothermia	T	Tension pneumothorax
H	Hypoxia	T	Thromboembolism (pulmonary)

H	Hypovolaemia	T	Tamponade (cardiac)
H	Hypo- and hyperkalaemia	T	Toxins (i.e. drugs)

[5] (a) F (b) F (c) F (d) F (e) T

(a) Inferior infarcts cause ST-segment **elevation** in leads **II, III and aVF**. Remember: infarction causes elevation, ischaemia causes depression. Inferior infarcts usually reflect occlusion in the RIGHT coronary artery or one of its branches.

(b) Pericarditis causes **'saddle-shaped' ST-segment elevation** in all leads of the ECG. Downward-sloping ST-segment depression indicates myocardial ischaemia, whereas upward sloping ST-segment depression is non-specific.

(c) Atrial fibrillation causes the ECG to show fine oscillations of the baseline (**F-waves**) and **no clear P waves at all**. The QRS segments occur in an irregularly irregular fashion, and at a rapid rate. The causes of AF can be recalled by remembering that **PIRATES** were often dehydrated after long spells at sea . . .

Dehydration

> P   Pulmonary disease
>
>> I   Ischaemia, infarction
>>
>>> R   Rheumatic heart disease
>>>
>>>> A   Anaemia, atrial myxoma
>>>>
>>>>> T   Thyrotoxicosis
>>>>>
>>>>>> E   Ethanol
>>>>>>
>>>>>>> S   Sepsis

(d) First-degree heart block is manifest on the ECG as **simple prolongation of the PR-interval**. In health, the PR-interval should be between three and five small squares on the ECG, i.e. 0.12–0.2 s. If it is longer than this, then first-degree heart block is present. NB In first-degree heart block, the **PR interval is *constant*** even though it is prolonged, and **a QRS complex follows *every* P-wave**. Broad QRS complexes suggest a rhythm of ventricular origin OR a supraventricular rhythm with concomitant bundle branch block.

(e) Ventricular aneurysm characteristically produces persistent ST-segment elevation in all leads for greater than 1 month's duration.

[6] (a) F (b) F (c) F (d) T (e) F

(a) Flow rate within a vessel is, in fact, governed by **Poiseuille's law**, which states that the flow within a vessel is proportional to the **fourth power** of the radius. The Fick principle is a means of indirectly calculating cardiac output by dividing total body oxygen

consumption by the ... of arterial and mixed ... used in operating the ... parameters.

(b) Claudication me... the Latin *claudicatio*, t...

(c) Leriche syndrom... which causes absent ... claudication, wasting of buttock muscles and impotence. It can be caused acutely by a 'saddle embolism' at the bifurcation of the aorta, but is more commonly seen in the chronic setting of slowly progressive atherosclerosis.

(d) Rest pain indicates advanced peripheral vascular disease. It occurs most commonly in the **toes and metatarsal heads** on lying down at night. Temporary relief can be obtained by dangling the legs over the side of the bed, or by standing up and walking, because this makes the feet dependent, increasing gravitational hydrostatic pressure, increasing venous pressure and so temporarily enhancing oxygen delivery. Unlike claudication, which is caused by muscle ischaemia, rest pain is caused by **nerve ischaemia**, and it often corresponds to an **ankle:brachial pressure index (ABPI) of <0.4**. It should be differentiated from benign nocturnal cramps, which usually occur in the calf and are not associated with impaired blood flow.

(e) *Arterial ulcers* arise due to arterial insufficiency. They tend to occur **on the toes, heel or dorsum of the foot** in response to minor trauma and are **exquisitely painful**. They have a **punched-out** appearance and a **pale necrotic base**.

Venous ulcers usually occur at the **medial or lateral malleolus** in response to venous pooling. They often cause a brownish discoloration of the skin (haemosiderin deposition), have a **granulating base** and whilst **painful**, do not cause anywhere near as much pain as arterial ulcers. They are associated with significant oedema. Treatment is usually conservative.

Neuropathic ulcers are **painless**, and usually located on the **plantar or lateral aspects of the foot**. They are the direct result of diabetic neuropathy and are often associated with destruction of the ankle joint (Charcot's foot). Because of the nature of diabetes, these ulcers often co-exist with arterial ulceration.

[7] (a) F (b) T (c) F (d) T (e) F

(a) Aortic stenosis is heard best in the **aortic area** (2nd right intercostal space) with the patient **leaning forward** and the **breath held in end-expiration** ('breathe in, old it'). Aortic regurgitation is best heard ... ternal border with the patient sitting forward ... xpiration.

Aortic stenosis causes isolated hypertrophy of the ...t ventricle. The left atrium does not become enlarged or hypertrophied because the mitral valve is intact (unless there is mixed valvular disease).

(c) A water-hammer pulse describes a pulse with a **forcible impulse but immediate collapse**, and is characteristic of aortic regurgitation. It is also known as a **collapsing** pulse. The pulse character associated with aortic stenosis is **slow-rising** because of the resistance encountered by the left ventricle when pushing blood past the stenosed valve.

The character of pulsation may also be described in the following ways . . .

- *Pulsus paradoxus*: an **exaggeration of the normal tendency of the systolic pressure to fall on inspiration** (should be <10 mmHg in health, but is greater than this in pulsus paradoxus); characteristically seen in **severe airway obstruction** (e.g. acute severe asthma), cardiac tamponade and constrictive pericarditis.
- *Pulsus alternans*: alternating **weak then strong** (but regular) beats; characteristic of **severe myocardial failure**, indicating very poor prognosis.
- *Pulsus bigeminus*: **ectopic beats follow each sinus beat**, causing beats to occur in pairs; rhythm is not regular.
- *Pulsus bisferiens*: an arterial **pulse with palpable, separated peaks**; characteristic of **hypertrophic, obstructive cardiomyopathy (HOCM)** and when aortic stenosis co-exists with aortic regurgitation.

(d) The murmur caused by aortic stenosis is a **diamond-shaped ejection systolic murmur**, best heard in the aortic area. It is said to be **rough** in quality, and is longer the more severe the stenosis. It **radiates to the carotids**. A systolic **ejection click** may be heard when the valve opens if it is calcified and has become immobile (severe disease). There may be a **prominent fourth heart sound (S4)** if the left ventricle is hypertrophied and has become stiff.

(e) Aortic stenosis alone is not associated with the development of AF as long as the mitral valve remains intact.

[8] (a)T (b)F (c)T (d)F (e)F

(a) Dehydration and hypovolaemia, whether acute or chronic, are common causes of atrial fibrillation, especially in hospital patients.

(b) Thyroid eye signs (i.e. retro-orbital swelling, proptosis, exophthalmos, limitation of eye movements, visual impairment due to optic nerve pressure) are **only seen in Graves' disease**. All causes of hyperthyroidism, however, may cause atrial fibrillation, because it is the high level of circulating thyroid hormone and *not* the high levels of IgG (thyroid stimulating antibody) seen in Graves' that is responsible for precipitating atrial fibrillation.

(c) Because there is no ordered contraction of the atria in AF (i.e. electrical activity does not start at and is not propagated from the sino-atrial node), there are no P-waves visible on the ECG.

(d) Anti-dysrhythmic agents are traditionally classified into four groups according to the **Vaughan-Williams classification** . . .

- Class 1: Membrane depressants
  - Class 1a: disopyramide, quinidine
  - Class 1b: lidocaine
  - Class 1c: flecainide, propafenone
- Class 2: Antisympathetics
  e.g. β-blockers, the cardioselective (i.e. β-1 specific) ones being metoprolol and atenolol
- Class 3: Prolongers of the action potential
  e.g. amiodarone, sotalol
- Class 4: Slowers of conduction in nodal tissue
  e.g. the non-dihydropyridine calcium channel antagonists—verapamil, diltiazem

Class 1c agents (like flecainide) and all other class 1 anti-dysrhythmics should only really be used in the treatment of **intractable or life-threatening arrhythmias**; they should *never* be used where the patient has significant left ventricular dysfunction (e.g. heart failure), prior history of MI or acute coronary ischaemia.

(e) Treatment of AF can be approached in two ways:

1. *Control the ventricular rate and ignore what the atria are doing*: this is usually achieved using an **AV-nodal blocking drug** (e.g. digoxin, β-blockers or verapamil).

2. *Cardiovert in an attempt to stop the atria fibrillating*: this can be performed **electrically** (80% of patients convert to sinus rhythm with synchronized DC cardioversion) or **medically** (with an IV infusion of class 1a, 1c or 3 drug, usually amiodarone). Recurrent paroxysms can be prevented with prophylactic oral treatment with a class 1a, 1c or 3 drug, again usually amiodarone.

Amiodarone is one of a select number of drugs whose

side effect profile should be known for undergraduate final examinations . . .

- Sensitivity to sunlight (i.e. phototoxicity)
- Corneal microdeposits
- Slate-grey skin discolouration
- Peripheral neuropathy
- Hypo- or hyperthyroidism
- Pulmonary fibrosis (irreversible)

[9] (a)T (b) F (c)T (d) F (e)T

(a) The right main bronchus is **wider, shorter and more vertical** than the left; this is why a swallowed foreign object or aspirated material is more likely to impact in the lower lobe of the right lung rather than the left. Material aspirated when a patient is lying flat is most likely to impact in the middle lobe of the right lung.

(b) The lung has a **dual blood supply**. The bronchi, connective tissue of the lung and the visceral pleura receive their blood supply from the **bronchial arteries**, which are branches of the descending aorta. The alveoli on the other hand receive deoxygenated blood from the terminal branches of the **pulmonary arteries**.

(c) The epithelial lining of the alveoli is mainly made up of type 1 pneumocytes. These form a **thin barrier for gas exchange**. They are, however, derived from **surfactant-producing** type 2 pneumocytes, which are slightly more in number but cover less surface area.

(d) Both lungs have oblique fissures, but **only the right has a horizontal fissure**, hence there are three lobes in the right lung (upper, middle and lower) but only two in the left (upper, lower and the lingula—a redundant segment of pulmonary tissue anterior to the surface of the heart).

(e) In health **the strongest stimulation to ventilation is an increase in the arterial partial pressure of CO_2 ($PaCO_2$)**, which causes an increase in the concentration of hydrogen ions in cerebrospinal fluid (CSF), stimulating the brainstem respiratory centre. Sensitivity to increasing $PaCO_2$ can be lost in chronic obstructive pulmonary disease (COPD) due to chronic over-exposure of the brainstem to high levels of CO_2, and in these patients the chief stimulus to breathe becomes the partial pressure of oxygen (PaO_2), as detected by the carotid and aortic arch bodies. Patients with chronic type II respiratory failure should therefore not be administered high concentrations of oxygen because it abolishes their respiratory stimulus, and they would quickly have a respiratory arrest. Pyrexia, large doses of aspirin and the drug doxapram may directly stimulate the brainstem respiratory centre, whereas severe hypoxaemia and sedatives, especially opioids, may depress it.

[10] (a) F (b) F (c)T (d)T (e) F

On examination of the chest in a patient with a unilateral tension pneumothorax . . .

- Chest wall movements will be decreased on the affected side only → **(a)**
- The mediastinum will be displaced away from the affected side → **(b)**
- The percussion note will be hyperresonant on the affected side → **(c)**
- Breath sounds will be decreased or absent on the affected side → **(d)**
- Tactile vocal resonance will be decreased on the affected side → **(e)**
- There are no added sounds

It is very useful for exams to be exactly sure of the chest signs of the most common respiratory complaints. Recent exams have contained MCQs and EMQs that tested precisely the candidate's knowledge of such signs. A useful table to memorize is shown below, but there is no substitute for having seen/discovered such signs for yourself: find patients with signs and examine them!

Pathological process	Chest wall movement	Mediastinal displacement	Percussion note	Breath sounds	Vocal resonance	Added sounds
Consolidation	Decreased ipsilaterally	None	Dull	Bronchial	Increased	Fine creps
Collapse	Decreased ipsilaterally	Towards	Dull	Decreased or absent	Decreased or absent	None

Continued on p. 56

Pathological process	Chest wall movement	Mediastinal displacement	Percussion note	Breath sounds	Vocal resonance	Added sounds
Fibrosis (general)	Decreased bilaterally	None	Normal	Vesicular	Increased	Fine creps
Pleural effusion (>500 mL)	Decreased ipsilaterally	Away	Stony dull	Vesicular (decreased or absent)	Decreased or absent	None
Large pneumothorax	Decreased ipsilaterally	Away	Hyper-resonant	Decreased or absent	Decreased or absent	None
Asthma	Decreased bilaterally	None	Normal	Vesicular, with prolonged expiration	Normal	Expiratory polyphonic wheeze
COPD	Decreased bilaterally	None	Normal	Vesicular, with prolonged expiration	Normal	Coarse creps plus expiratory polyphonic wheeze

11] (a) F (b) T (c) T (d) F (e) T

(a) COPD describes airways obstruction that occurs **mainly in smokers or ex-smokers**. The clinical distinction between COPD and asthma is blurred, because virtually all patients with COPD have a reversible element to their disease, and is the reason these patients are treated with **bronchodilators** [(β-adrenoceptor agonists such as salbutamol (Ventolin®) and antimuscarinics such as ipratropium bromide (Atrovent®)] and **corticosteroids** (initially prednisolone orally, and if this is successful, wean to inhaled beclamethasone).

(b) Chronic bronchitis is defined on the basis of the *history* as 'cough productive of sputum on most days for at least 3 months of the year, for more than 1 year'. This reflects the nature of the underlying condition: hypertrophy of the mucous-secreting glands of the bronchial tree (mainly large bronchi). Emphysema, however, is defined *pathologically* as 'dilatation and destruction of the lung tissue distal to the terminal bronchioles'. Thus, it affects only the small airways, leading to loss of elastic re-

coil of the lungs, decreased gas transfer, expiratory airflow limitation and air-trapping. Whilst bronchitis and emphysema are described as two separate clinical entities, they usually co-exist in all patients with COPD.

(c) Patients with COPD commonly demonstrate asterixis, which is a coarse, flapping tremor due to chronic retention of CO_2. It is also seen in patients with hepatic encephalopathy ('liver flap'), although it can occur in a wide variety of metabolic and toxic encephalopathies. CO_2 retention also causes the hands to be warm (vasodilatation) and the pulse to be bounding (hyperdynamic circulation).

(d) *Cor pulmonale* is the term used to describe **the process of adaptation and failure the right side of the heart undergoes as a result of lung disease**. Normally the pulmonary vasculature responds to local hypoxia by arteriolar constriction. So, for example, in lobar pneumonia, blood flow to the affected lobe is decreased, minimizing the amount of poorly oxygenated blood reaching the systemic circulation. When the pneumonia resolves, the vasoconstriction ceases and the flow returns to normal. However, if hypoxia is widespread and irreversible, as is the case in COPD, the resultant arteriolar constriction is equally widespread and irreversible, thus causing pulmonary hypertension. Over time the right atrium and ventricle hypertrophy, eventually the limit of the heart's ability to adapt is reached, and the right heart fails, leading to the typical signs and symptoms of right-sided cardiac failure.

(e) Respiratory failure occurs when pulmonary gas exchange is sufficiently impaired to cause **hypoxaemia (PaO_2 < 8 kPa) with or without hypercapnia ($PaCO_2$ > 7 kPa)**. There are two types of respiratory failure.

- **Type I respiratory failure — 'acute hypoxaemic'**
  - mainly due to ventilation–perfusion mismatch
  - PaO_2 low (<8 kPa)
  - $PaCO_2$ normal or low (<5 kPa)
  - Common causes include pulmonary oedema, pneumonia, ARDS, pulmonary embolism (PE)
- **Type II respiratory failure — 'ventilatory failure'**
  - PaO_2 low (<8 kPa)
  - $PaCO_2$ high (>7 kPa)
  - Occurs when alveolar ventilation is insufficient to excrete the volume of CO_2 being produced by tissue metabolism
  - Due to reduced ventilatory effort, inability to overcome increased resistance, failure to compensate for increased dead space or CO_2 production, or a combination of these
  - Most common cause is COPD
  - Other causes include chest wall deformity, respiratory muscle weakness [e.g. Guillain–Barré syndrome, motor neurone disease (MND)] and depression of the respiratory centre (e.g. opioid excess)

[12] (a) F (b) F (c) T (d) F (e) F

(a) $PaCO_2$ is not elevated in type I respiratory failure.

(b) The commonest cause of type II respiratory failure is COPD. Pneumonia tends to cause type I respiratory failure.

(c) Pulsus paradoxus is explained in the answers to MCQ [7], above.

(d) Respiratory failure **does not always present with dyspnoea**, e.g. opioid overdosage, Guillain–Barré syndrome. Chronic retainers of CO_2 may also present drowsy and not obviously dyspnoeic.

(e) The CXR described in the question is one of classical heart failure. The CXR in respiratory failure is one of so-called **non-cardiogenic pulmonary oedema**, where the typical features are no upper lobe venous distension, no septal lines or pleural effusion, a normal heart size and the most reliable sign, which is **peripheral alveolar shadowing and/or an air bronchogram**. The CXR in someone with suspected respiratory failure should also be checked carefully for pneumothorax, consolidation, bronchogenic cancer and oligaemia or wedge-shaped infarcts (i.e. signs of PE). Localized oligaemia on CXR is also known as 'Westermark's sign', and is usually indicative of PE.

The main causes of respiratory failure can be remembered if you remember that **A DIMPLE can cause respiratory failure** . . .

- **A** Asthma, ARDS, aspirin
- **D** Drugs (opiates)
- **I** Infection (pneumonia)
- **M** Metabolic acidosis (e.g. diabetic ketoacidosis)
- **P** PE, pneumothorax
- **L** Left ventricular failure
- **E** Effusions

[13] (a) F (b) F (c) F (d) T (e) F

(a) Asthma is characterized by chronic inflammation of the airways which normally presents with a classical triad of symptoms . . .

1. **Wheeze**
2. **Nocturnal cough**
3. **Dyspnoea**

Within the airways themselves, it has three main characteristics: **bronchial inflammation** (mainly involving eosinophils and mast cells with associated plasma exudation, oedema, smooth muscle hypertrophy and mucus plugging), **airways hyper-responsiveness** and **reversible airflow limitation**. It is important to realize, however, that **with chronic asthma, the airflow limitation does become irreversible to a certain degree**. It is also the case that aspects of the acute severe asthma that continues to kill young people are also irreversible (otherwise no-one would die from asthma as long as they were treated with the correct medications).

(b) Typical asthma attacks occur **after the conclusion of, and not during, exercise**. Cold, dry air cools and dries the epithelial lining of the bronchi, precipitating attacks.

(c) ACE-inhibitors are safe to give to asthmatic patients. ACE-inhibitors *should never*, however, be given to patients with **renal artery stenosis** as they block production of angiotensin II and aldosterone, leading to a decrease in the already threatened renal perfusion, and subsequently to acute renal failure. The drugs that should be avoided in asthmatic patients are . . .

- **β-blockers**: cause bronchoconstriction and activate mast cell mediator release and promote release of histamine, so worsening the symptoms of asthma
- **NSAIDs**: these inhibit the enzyme cyclooxygenase, shifting the precursors from metabolism of arachidonic acid down the lipooxygenase pathway, leading to formation of leukotrienes, some of which are potent bronchoconstrictors

(d) The symptoms of asthma are characteristically **worse at night** due to an exacerbation in the normal circadian preponderance of airways tone to be higher at night.

(e) **β-2 agonists** are used in the treatment of asthma (β-2 adrenoceptors are found predominantly in the **respiratory tract**, whereas β-1 adrenoceptors are found in the **myocardium**). They are delivered direct to the tissues that need them by inhalers. In doing this, they avoid hepatic first pass metabolism, and allow lower doses to be used, with concomitant fewer adverse effects. Examples are salbutamol, terbutaline and salmeterol (longer acting; lasts for up to 12 h). There are five main groups of other drugs used in the treatment of asthma:

1. anticholinergic bronchodilators: non-specific muscarinic antagonists (e.g. ipratropium bromide) are useful bronchodilators because they are parasympatholytic (i.e. the parasympathetic nervous system is responsible for bronchoconstriction). They also cause drying up of secretions and may be added to β-2 agonists for a compound effect on bronchodilation

2. anti-inflammatory drugs: prevent activation of proinflammatory cells, especially in mild asthma. Examples include sodium cromoglycate and nedocromil sodium

3. inhaled corticosteroids: patients who continue to have symptoms despite treatment with all three of the above groups of drugs require inhaled corticosteroids. Examples include beclomethasone, budesonide and fluticasone. Unwanted effects include oral candidiasis, hoarse voice, cataract formation and growth retardation. It is important to realize that asthma itself retards growth

4. oral corticosteroids: necessary if symptoms remain uncontrolled on inhaled corticosteroids. The dose of prednisolone should be as low as possible to limit the side effects (iatrogenic Cushing's)

5. leukotriene receptor antagonists: improve control of symptoms in mild-to-moderate asthma when given with inhaled corticosteroid. An example is montelukast.

[14] (a) F **(b)** T **(c)** F **(d)** F **(e)** T

(a) Tuberculosis (TB) is caused by *Mycobacterium tuberculosis*, but this is a **Gram-*positive*** aerobic bacillus that is extremely slow growing (6 weeks in traditional culture medium). It is revealed as an acid- and alcohol-fast bacillus when stained with **Ziehl–Nielsen** stain. *Mycobacterium bovis* and *M. africanum* can also rarely cause TB.

(b) TB is the **most common cause of apical lung fibrosis**. A chest radiograph demonstrating apical fibrosis is quite a common thing to get in an OSCE, and you should have a list of differentials at the ready—hence the mnemonic **BREASTS** . . .

  B HLA:B27 positive conditions (i.e. the seronegative spondylartritides)
  R Rheumatoid arthritis
  E Extrinsic allergic alveolitis (i.e. farmer's lung, etc.)
  A Aspergillosis, asbestosis
  S Sarcoidosis
  T TB
  S Systemic sclerosis

The causes of generalized pulmonary fibrosis can be remembered using the mnemonic **DADS CRUET** . . .

D Drugs	**C** Cryptogenic fibrosing alveolitis	
A ARDS	**R** Radiation, rheumatoid arthritis	
D Dusts	**U** Uraemia	
S Sarcoidosis	**E** Extrinsic allergic alveolitis	
	T TB	

(c) The granulomas in TB are classically **caseating**, i.e. 'cheesy'. The initial reaction within the lungs to infection with TB is exudation and infiltration of the affected area with **neutrophils**. These are rapidly replaced by **macrophages** that ingest the bacilli. Macrophage interaction with **T-lymphocytes** leads to the development of cellular immunity (seen at 3–8 weeks post-infection). At this stage, the classical pathology of TB can be seen: granulomatous lesions with a central area of cheesy necrosis or caseation, surrounded by epithelioid cells and Langerhan's giant cells, both of which are derived from macrophages. Subsequently, caseated areas heal completely and many become calcified. 20% still contain tubercle bacilli, and are capable of reactivation after a variable period of lying dormant.

Non-caseating granulomas occur in a variety of conditions, including . . .

- Sarcoidosis
- Extrinsic allergic alveolitis
- Primary biliary cirrhosis
- Crohn's disease
- Wegener's granulomatosis

- Polymyalgia rheumatica
- Giant cell arteritis
- Takayasu's arteritis
- Churg–Strauss syndrome
- Hodgkin's lymphoma
- Leprosy
- Brucellosis
- Berylliosis
- Mycoses
- Toxoplasmosis
- Leishmaniasis
- Certain drug ingestion (e.g. allopurinol, procarbazine, aspirin, sulphonylureas)

(d) The Heaf and Mantoux tests are both tests of TB status. They are, however, **different tests**. In the Heaf test, a small amount of PPD (purified protein derivative — inactivated but antigenic TB) is placed on the flexor surface of the left forearm. A 6-point disposable apparatus is then penetrated through the solution, and the reaction is graded between 0–4 depending on the **degree of induration at 7 days**. The Mantoux test involves an intradermal injection of PPD and the **induration is measured at 72 h**. Induration of greater than 10 mm indicates a positive test.

(e) TB is a recognized cause of erythema nodosum (= painful nodes on the extensor surfaces of the lower extremities). Apart from TB, the other causes of erythema nodosum may be remembered if you remember that only the **SLIMeST** patients suffer with this paniculitis of the skin (usually of the shins).

   S   <u>S</u>arcoidosis
   L   <u>L</u>eprosy
   I   <u>I</u>nflammatory bowel disease
  Me <u>Me</u>dications (oral contraceptive, sulphonamides)
   S   <u>S</u>treptococcal infections
   T   <u>T</u>uberculosis

The treatment for TB rests mainly in the hands of four drugs, easily remembered using the mnemonic **RIPE** . . .

R	Rifampicin	side effects: hepatic enzyme induction, red secretions
I	Isoniazid	side effects: polyneuropathy
P	Pyrizinamide	side effects: severe hepatic toxicity
E	Ethambutol	side effects: retrobulbar neuritis and blindness (must see an ophthalmologist prior to commencement of this drug!)

The usual regime is **2 months** of treatment with rifampicin, isoniazid and one of the other two drugs (the intensive phase) and then a **further 4 months** of treatment with just rifampicin and isoniazid (the maintenance phase). Multi-drug resistant (MDR) TB needs treatment with all four agents, or with second line agents like spectromycin, ciprofloxacin and ethionamide for a period of around 2 years. Still 30–50% of patients with MDR TB die of their infection. Strict compliance is the cornerstone to TB chemotherapy, and DOTS (directly observed treatment schedule) is frequently employed to ensure compliance.

[15] (a)T (b)F (c)F (d)F (e)T
(a) The liver can also normally be palpated in the epigastrium in thin individuals.
(b) The superior border of the liver should extend no higher than the 5th–6th intercostal space in health.
(c) Hepatomegaly extends vertically downwards toward the right iliac fossa.
(d) The spleen is NEVER normally palpable in healthy individuals.
(e) Splenic enlargement proceeds diagonally downwards toward the ileocaecal valve.

[16] (a)F (b)T (c)F (d)T (e)T
The recognized gastrointestinal causes of finger clubbing are five in number, and are best remembered as **the 5 Cs** . . .

   C Cirrhosis
   C Coeliac
   C Crohn's (and ulcerative colitis)
   C Cancer (specifically gastrointestinal lymphoma)
   C Cystic fibrosis (CF)

[17] (a)T (b)T (c)T (d)T (e)T
The pain of acute MI often masquerades as epigastric pain, and in an obese patient with a history of gastro-oesophageal reflux disease, it is important never to forget that it may be an MI that is causing the dyspepsia-sounding pain. → **(b)**
Addison's is classically a vague, creeping condition and it is always worth bearing in mind when symptoms do not quite add up to a straightforward diagnosis. → **(c)**
  Other medical causes of abdominal pain include . . .
- Gastroenteritis
- Urinary tract infection
- Diabetes mellitus → **(a)**
- Pneumonia (basal)
- Sickle-cell crises
- Tabes dorsalis
- Phaeochromocytoma

- Herpes zoster
- Malaria
- Tuberculosis
- Typhoid fever
- Porphyria
- Cholera
- Thyroid storm
- Opioid withdrawal
- Lead poisoning → **(e)**
- Bornholm's disease
- Hypercalcaemia → **(d)**

[18] (a) F (b) F (c) T (d) F (e) F

(a) The oesophagus originates at the cricoid cartilage and pharynx in the neck and traverses the posterior mediastinum *behind* **the aortic arch and left main bronchus**.

(b) It has a very short (~3 cm) section that lies in the abdominal cavity before it joins the fundus of the stomach; this section is important in preventing reflux of gastric acid by a 'flap-valve' action, and hence in preventing the symptoms of gastro-oesophageal reflux disease.

(c) Unlike the remainder of the GIT, the oesophagus has **no serosal layer**, a fact that is important in the ease of spread of oesophageal neoplasms, the ease of perforation and the difficulty of reconstruction after operation.

(d) The upper third of the oesophagus is made up of **skeletal muscle fibres**, whilst the remaining two thirds comprises **smooth muscle**; it is therefore remarkable that the oesophagus functions in such a co-ordinated manner to bring about swallowing.

(e) Achalasia is caused by a **failure to relax** of the lower oesophageal sphincter on swallowing, due to postulated **non-firing of the vagus nerve**, leading to a classical *beak-shaped* deformity at the lower end of the oesophagus on barium swallow; this failure to relax can also occur in Chagas' disease, which is American trypanosomiasis, a condition where there is damage to the myenteric plexus of the gut.

[19] (a) F (b) F (c) F (d) T (e) F

(a) Melaena is the passage of altered blood per rectum, classically described as black and tarry, from an upper gastrointestinal bleed. The bleed has to be >50 mL, and the lesion is proximal to the caecum. Other causes of a black stool are iron sulphate tablets, liquorice and Guinness.

(b) Massive upper GI bleeds (e.g. from oesophageal varices) can cause fresh blood to arrive at the rectum even though the lesion is significantly proximal to the caecum.

(c) Although varices are a relatively common cause of upper GI bleed, they are over 5× less common as a cause of upper GI bleeding than are peptic ulcers (i.e. gastric ulcers and duodenal ulcers); the frequency of all causes is demonstrated in the table below.

Cause	% of all cases of upper GI bleed
Peptic ulceration (gastric ulcers and duodenal ulcers)	50
Acute gastric ulcers/erosions (e.g. caused by aspirin, which has a double whammy for causing gastric bleeds in that it has both a direct irritant effect on gastric mucosa as well as an antiplatelet effect that encourages bleeding)	20
Oesophageal varices	5–10
Mallory–Weiss syndrome (= linear laceration at the oesophagogastric junction, associated with bleeding or penetration into the mediastinum and subsequent mediastinitis; caused by severe retching ± vomiting)	5–10
Reflux oesophagitis	5

Continued

Cause	% of all cases of upper GI bleed
Gastric varices	Rare
Gastric cancer	Rare
Hereditary haemorrhagic telengiectasia (a.k.a. Osler–Weber–Rendu syndrome; a disease with onset usually after puberty; multiple small telangiectases and dilated venules develop slowly on skin and mucous membranes that are very friable and bleed easily)	Rare
Blood dyscrasias (= a diseased state of the blood, usually referring to abnormal cellular elements of a permanent character)	Rare
Angiodysplaisia	Rare

(d) Octreotide **decreases both splanchnic blood flow and gastric acid secretion** so is especially useful in immediate management of upper gastrointestinal bleed. Prior to this, volume resuscitation of the patient is vital to avoid progression to hypovolaemic shock. Also, identification of the cause of the bleed by endoscopy should be performed early, and if identified, treatment initiated in the form of local tamponade/banding/injection/coagulation of bleeding areas. A useful mnemonic to remember the signs and symptoms of shock is '**ASP SHOCK!**' . . .

  A Anxiety
  S Shivery cold
  P Pallor
  S Sinus tachycardia
  H Hypotension
  O Oliguria
  C Clammy
  K 'K'apillary refill > 2 s

(e) Haematemesis is commonly described as 'coffee-ground', usually when the blood has been altered by the acidic environment of the stomach.

[20] (a) F (b) F (c) F (d) F (e) F

(a) Unlike duodenal ulcers (DUs), **gastric ulcers (GUs) are not caused by acid hypersecretion**; 80% of GU patients have a **normal or even a low gastric acid secretion level**. The exact aetiology of GUs is far from perfectly elucidated. It is believed to be at least in part

due to the presence of a defective gastric mucosal barrier, potentially caused by *Helicobacter pylori*-mediated antecedent gastritis. Other postulated mechanisms include delayed gastric emptying, alkaline reflux of bile, a defective pyloric sphincter and increased H^+ back-diffusion.

(b) Unlike the pain of DUs, GU pain is usually **easier when fasting** but is exacerbated by the ingestion of food. Like DU pain, however, GU pain is located in the epigastrium and may radiate through to the back. The pain of GU may be sufficient to cause the patient to become anorexic and malnourished, contrary to the DU patient who may eat more and gain weight in an attempt to alleviate his/her symptoms.

(c) Gastric ulcers **relatively frequently transform into gastric carcinomas**, whereas DUs rarely undergo malignant change. This is why, at endoscopy, it is vitally important to take multiple biopsies of both the centre and periphery of GUs for histology, whereas it is rarely indicated that a DU should be biopsied.

(d) Medical treatment alone actually **cures fewer than 50% of gastric ulcers**, whereas it heals greater than 90% of duodenal ulcers.

(e) These are actually **ulcers of the duodenum that follow severe burns and head injury**, respectively, due to increased gastric acid output (usually in ICU patients). Any severe and life-threatening condition can, however, cause a 'stress gastritis', which may predispose to gastric ulceration.

[21] (a) F (b) F (c) F (d) T (e) T

(a) The commonest (75%) of all gallstones are the **mixed type**, i.e. contain both cholesterol and bile pigments. Of the rest, 20% are of the **cholesterol type** (often solitary and referred to as cholesterol solitaires) and 5% are of the **pigment type**. Pigment stones are occasionally split into the further subdivisions of **black pigment** stones (associated with sterile bile in circumstances of haemolysis and cirrhosis; mainly found in the gallbladder itself; hard) and **brown pigment** stones (associated with infected bile; mainly found in bile ducts; soft)

(b) Cholesterol and mixed gallstones very rarely contain sufficient quantities of calcium to be visible on AXR (only **10%** of gallstones are traditionally said to be radio-opaque). Conversely, pigment stones commonly contain enough calcification to render them radio-opaque.

(c) Choledocholithiasis means **stones within the bile duct**. The most common cause of this is ejection of stones from the gallbladder. Primary bile duct stones, whilst rare, occur more commonly in patients with bile stasis or infection within the biliary tree.

(d) Gallstones occur more frequently in women in a **3:1** ratio.

(e) **Rapid weight loss** is thought to cause gallbladder stasis and hyperconcentration of bile, hence increasing likelihood of gallstone formation. Other known risk factors for cholelithiasis include:

- **Obesity** (excessive cholesterol formation)
- **Multiparity** (altered steroid metabolism, lithogenic bile, hypomotile gallbladder)
- **High doses of exogenous oestrogens** (altered cholesterol and bile acid production)
- **Conditions that decrease bile acid pool and increase rate of bile acid formation**, e.g. Crohn's disease, resection of the terminal ileum
- **Haemolysis and cirrhosis** (both increase likelihood of pigment stone formation)

The adage 'female, fat, (over) 40 and fertile' used to be used to aid recall of the type of patient in whom gallstones were common.

[22] (a) F (b) T (c) F (d) F (e) F

(a) Cherry-red colour to the skin suggests carbon monoxide (CO) poisoning, and reflects the irreversible formation within the bloodstream of **carboxyhaemoglobin**. CO is a tasteless, odourless gas (from car exhausts, fires and faulty gas central heating) that **decreases the oxygen-carrying capacity of blood** and **inhibits cytochrome oxidase** (impairing utilization of oxygen), both of which combine to produce **severe tissue hypoxia**, eventually sufficient to cause coma and death. Treatment involves giving the patient **high concentrations of O$_2$** to breathe. The half-life of CO in the bloodstream is . . .

- ~4 h breathing room air
- ~1 h breathing 100% O$_2$
- ~23 min breathing 100% O$_2$ at 3 atmospheres pressure (so-called hyperbaric oxygen)

Although theoretically beneficial, hyperbaric O$_2$ is rarely given to victims of CO poisoning.

(b) 'Miosis' is more commonly known as 'pin-point' pupils and is a sign of opiate use at almost any concentration. It is the opposite of **'mydriasis'**, which implies pupillary dilatation. A number of mydriatics are available to facilitate fundoscopy, e.g. atropine, tropicamide, cyclopentolate. It is important to remember that **sympathetic drive causes mydriasis**, not miosis (wide-eyed with excitement!)

(c) Tricyclic antidepressant (e.g. imipramine, amitryptilline, dothiepin) poisoning classically causes ventricular tachycardia. Treatment is ABC, gastric lavage and activated charcoal. Correcting the acidosis with 8.4% sodium bicarbonate avoids further arrhythmias.

(d) Flumazenil is an antidote to benzodiazepine poisoning that should only be used in situations where the benzodiazepine has been iatrogenically administered, e.g. during reduction of a dislocated shoulder. Patients who attend casualty with a suspected benzodiazepine overdose should NEVER be given flumazenil because it is very dangerous in **mixed overdoses** involving tricyclic antidepressants (→ seizures) or in **benzodiazepine-dependent patients** (→ acute withdrawal). Flumazenil has a **very short half life**, and may need to be given as an infusion in patients who have received a significant amount of certain benzodiazepine medications (the half lives of benzodiazepines varies widely, e.g. oxazepam's half life is 4 h, whilst diazepam's is as long as 100 h).

(e) Naloxone is a specific opioid antagonist that will reverse coma and respiratory depression caused by acute opioid overdose, if given in sufficient dosage. However, it has a short half life, and coma and respiratory depression will often recur if it is not given repeatedly or by a continuous infusion.

A good mnemonic for remembering the various **causes of unconsciousness** to consider in the acute situation is **AEIOU-TIPS** . . .

A Alcohol

E Endocrine (Addison's), encephalitis, epilepsy

I Insulin

O Opiates, overdose

U Uraemia

T Trauma

I Infection (meningitis)

P Psychogenic

S Sepsis

[23] (a) F (b) F (c) T (d) T (e) T

(a) The most common cause of acute pancreatitis is **alcohol ingestion** (40% of cases), although the mechanism for this is incompletely understood (it is thought that alcohol causes increased protein concentration of pancreatic secretions, precipitating blockage of smaller pancreatic ductules). The second most common cause is **gallstones** (60% of non-alcohol related cases). Again, the mechanism for this is incompletely understood (it appears that smaller stones are more likely to cause pancreatitis than larger ones). The causes of acute pancraetitis can be remembered using the mnemonic **GET SMASHED** . . .

  G Gallstones

  E Ethanol

  T Trauma

  S Steroids

  M Mumps

  A Autoimmune disease (e.g. polyarteritis nodosa)

  S Scorpion venom

  H Hyperlipidaemia (especially triglycerides), -calcaemia, -parathyroidism, hypothermia

  E ERCP (1% of procedures), emboli (and ischaemia)

  D Drugs (azathioprine, contraceptive pill, thiazides)

   If you like mnemonics and are having trouble remembering the drug causes of acute pancreatitis, remember that **CATS** get smashed—contraceptive pill, azathioprine, thiazides, steroids

(b) The pain of acute pancreatitis is **non-crampy**, located in the **epigastrium** and frequently **radiates to the left or right upper quadrant and through to the back**. It is almost always associated with a significant amount of **nausea and vomiting**. The differential diagnosis includes peptic ulcer disease, gastro-oesophageal reflux disease, cholecystitis, dissecting aortic aneurysm/ruptured abdominal aortic aneurysm and myocardial infarction.

(c) Levels of amylase are usually **higher in patients with biliary pancreatitis** (i.e. that caused by gallstones), because it is usually an **isolated attack,** and pancreatic function and mass are usually normal. Patients developing alcoholic pancreatitis, however, have often had repeated previous bouts of pancreatic inflammation; hence, they have damaged a large proportion of their pancreas and there is little functioning pancreas remaining to produce amylase when it once again becomes inflamed.

(d) One of the first systems for grading severity of an attack of acute pancreatitis was developed by Ranson. The system, known as **Ranson's criteria** (also **'the modified Glasgow criteria'**) uses readily measured lab and clinical variables, and **a score of 3 or more indicates a poor prognosis and should institute transfer to HDU**. The criteria are as follows (score 1 for each) . . .

PANCREAS.

Criterion	Normal reference range
WCC > 15 x 10^9/L	$(4–11 \times 10^9)$
Glucose > 10 mmol/L	(3.5–5.5)
LDH > 600 i.u./L	(70–250)
AST > 200 i.u./L	(5–35)
Urea > 16 mmol/L	(2–7)
Calcium < 2 mmol/L	(2.25–2.65)
Albumin < 32 g/L	(35–50)
PaO_2 < 8 kPa	(>10)

   The other main prognostic index in acute pancreatitis is the **APACHE II** score. It is worth knowing about these to be able to mention them in an OSCE.

(e) Medical treatment of acute pancreatitis can be split into two:

1. General supportive therapy: vast quantities of fluid may be needed to replace that lost due to what is essentially a large retroperitoneal burn. Foley catheter and CVP line assist in monitoring filling. Continue giving fluids to maintain a urine output >30 mL/h. Analgesia (via pain ladder) is vital.

2. Specific treatment of pancreatic inflammation: inhibit pancreatic secretion by inserting a nasogastric tube. Make the patient nil by mouth. Various enzyme inhibitors have been tried to quell the pancreatic inflammation with no success. Similarly, antibiotics, although liberally used, do NOT decrease morbidity or mortality in pancreatitis.

[24] (a) F (b) F (c) F (d) F (e) F

(a) The commonest cause of small bowel obstruction worldwide is **herniae**, whilst the most common cause in industrialized countries is **postoperative adhesions**.

(b) This is the description of an **intussusception**. A volvulus occurs when a length of large bowel becomes twisted on itself, using the mesentery as the axis about which it twists.

(c) In gallstone ileus, a large (>2.5 cm) stone passes from gallbladder or common bile duct into the GIT **through a *fistula***. The stones usually lodge in the terminal ileum.

(d) Bowel sounds are characteristically infrequent, high-pitched and 'tinkling' in small bowel obstruction. They would be absent in paralytic ileus.

(e) In paralytic ileus, there is characteristically **no physical obstruction** to passage of the luminal contents of the bowel, i.e. it is ***functional***. Causes of paralytic ileus include . . .

- Sepsis (either within or adjacent to the peritoneal cavity, e.g. pneumonia)
- Drugs (e.g. opiates)
- Retroperitoneal haematoma
- Electrolyte abnormalities (e.g. hypokalaemia)
- Physical inactivity
- Laparotomy

Paralytic ileus classically demonstrates **absent bowel sounds**, and may be definitively diagnosed from physical obstruction by contrast studies and a history of less abdominal pain.

EMQs

Answer 1

(1) Mitral stenosis with atrial fibrillation

On examination the patient may have a **malar flush** and be in **atrial fibrillation**. There may be evidence of a cerebrovascular accident (hemiplegia, facial weakness). An **opening snap** is followed by a **'rumbling' mid-diastolic murmur**, localizing (often very localized) over the **'tapping' apex beat** (palpable first heart sound). Listen with the patient in the left lateral position with the bell of the stethoscope in several positions over the apex. If difficult to hear, the murmur may be accentuated by asking the patient (if this is possible) to sit up and lie down five times so raising the cardiac output. There is **pre-systolic accentuation only if the heart is in sinus rhythm** and is due to atrial systole.

In addition if **pulmonary hypertension** has developed there may be a . . .

- **Left para-sternal heave** (right ventricular hypertrophy)
- **Loud second heart sound** over the pulmonary area
- Possible murmur of **pulmonary regurgitation** (Graham Steell)
- Murmur of **tricuspid regurgitation** [systolic murmur at lower left sternal edge plus large 'V' waves in the JVP (jugular venous pulse)]
- **Right ventricular failure** (elevated JVP, hepatomegaly, ascites and peripheral oedema)

These findings will also be seen in pulmonary hypertension due to other causes (e.g. congestive cardiac failure, COPD, chronic lung pathology, primary pulmonary hypertension).

Causes of mitral stenosis
- Rheumatic fever (a common cause)
- Congenital
- Calcification

Complications (often the patient is asymptomatic)
- Recurrent chest infections (wet lungs)
- Atrial fibrillation and embolization (stroke)
- Pulmonary hypertension and pulmonary oedema
- Right ventricular failure
- Tricuspid regurgitation
- Bacterial endocarditis

The severity of the mitral stenosis is indicated by:
- Signs of pulmonary hypertension (see above)
- Close proximity of the opening snap after the second heart sound
- The length of the mid-diastolic murmur (directly proportional, however, very tight lesions lead to quiet murmurs)

ECG findings
- Atrial fibrillation
- P mitrale (bifid 'M' shaped P waves best seen in lead II)

CXR appearances
- Prominent left atrium may be the only abnormality
- Calcification of the valve ring
- Possible features of congestive cardiac failure
  - Kerley-B lines
  - Upper lobe venous diversion
  - Bilateral effusions
  - Cardiomegaly
  - 'Bat's wing' oedema spreading from the hilar areas

Management
- Diuretics for symptoms of breathlessness
- Anticoagulation and digoxin if atrial fibrillation develops
- Prophylactic antibiotics for 'dirty' procedures to prevent valve infection (dental procedures or pelvic surgery). Check the British National Formulary for the current recommendations
- Surgical relief of stenosis if secondary pulmonary hypertension develops
- Open surgery can be avoided in those unfit for a general anaesthetic by percutaneous *trans*-septal balloon valvotomy. Here a balloon catheter is passed via a peripheral vein into the right atrium. The atrial septum is then perforated and the balloon is passed across the mitral valve and inflated. Mitral regurgitation is an inevitable consequence. Patients most suitable for this approach include those with:
  - Minimal mitral regurgitation
  - Mobile valves (no calcification)
  - Minimal subvalvular disease

Patients more suitable for formal valve replacement include those with:
- Significant mitral regurgitation
- Extensive valve calcification
- Thrombus in the left atrium

(2) Mitral regurgitation

The patient may be in **atrial fibrillation** (left atrial dilatation). The **JVP** may be elevated if associated with right ventricular failure (secondary to pulmonary hypertension). The **apex is displaced and '*thrusting*'** (a dynamic low-pressure movement indicating volume overload). The **first heart sound is soft**. There is a **pan-systolic murmur heard at the apex radiating to the left axilla**.

There may be a **third heart sound** (volume overload) and a diastolic flow murmur due to the re-entry of the re-gurgitated blood back into the left ventricle.

Clinically the main **differential** will be aortic stenosis causing an ejection systolic murmur, a ventricular septal defect or tricuspid regurgitation which both cause pan-systolic murmurs.

Tricuspid regurgitation, however, will result in prominent V waves in the JVP, a murmur that *increases* during inspiration and possible hepatic pulsations.

Causes of mitral regurgitation
- Myocardial infarction (acute presentation following an acute MI due to rupture of the chordae tendineae)
- Rheumatic fever (acute or old)
- Left ventricular dilatation
  - Severe hypertension
  - Left ventricular failure
  - Cardiomyopathy
- Bacterial endocarditis
- Connective tissue diseases
  - SLE
- Elastic tissue disorders
  - Marfan's syndrome
  - Ehlers–Danlos syndrome
- Prolapsing mitral valve; 'floppy mitral valve'. This occurs in young women. Embolic events and atypical chest pain (localized over the apex) may occur. A mid-systolic click is heard.

The **severity of mitral regurgitation** can be assessed by the presence of a . . .
- Third heart sound
- Mid-diastolic flow murmur
- Left ventricular enlargement
- Thrill

(3) Mitral stenosis

Here the patient is not in atrial fibrillation so there is pre-systolic accentuation of the murmur.

(4) Aortic regurgitation with left ventricular failure

The patient has a **wide pulse pressure** on measuring the blood pressure. The **pulse is collapsing** when the left brachial artery palpated with arm elevated. The **apex beat is displaced** (state the location) and is **thrusting** in character, indicating volume overload.

With the **patient sat forward** and the breath held in end expiration, a short early **decrescendo murmur radi-**

ating down the left sternal edge is heard (listen in several positions down the left sternal edge with the diaphragm). The longer and louder the murmur, the more severe the regurgitation.

In this case, left ventricular failure is suggested by the elevated JVP, displaced apex and bi-basal crepitations. There may be an additional ejection systolic murmur in the aortic area due to increased flow across the aortic valve. The aortic regurgitant jet can cause interference with the anterior mitral valve cusp resulting in a mid-diastolic murmur to be heard at the apex (Austin Flint murmur).

Inspect the patient for Marfan's body habitus, ankylosing spondylitis (kyphosis of the spine) features of rheumatoid arthritis and the small, irregular Argyll Robertson pupils (which react to accommodation but not to light) of syphilis.

Causes of aortic valve regurgitation
- Aortic root dilatation
  - Severe hypertension
  - Connective tissue disorders:
    Marfan's syndrome
    Rheumatoid arthritis
    Ankylosing spondylitis
  - Aortic aneurysm
  - Dissection of the aorta
  - Syphilis
- Valve disruption
  - Congenital (e.g. bicuspid valves)
  - Rupture of the sinus of valsalva
  - Endocarditis
  - Rheumatic fever
  - Ventricular septal defect (loss of support)

Associated eponymous signs
- **Corrigan's sign**: vigorous arterial pulsations in neck
- **De Musset's sign**: head nodding with arterial pulsations
- **Quinke's sign**: visible nail bed capillary pulsations. Partially compress the nail bed and look for pulsations in the subungual capillaries
- **Durozier's sign**: partially compress the femoral artery in the inguinal area with a digit and listen proximally for a regurgitant murmur as blood turbulently flows back under the 'stenosis' during diastole

Patients with aortic regurgitation may have few symptoms until left ventricular failure occurs. It is important to replace the valve before irretrievable ventricular dysfunction occurs as indicated by an enlarging heart on echocardiography. Once the end systolic diameter of the left ventricle has reached 55 mm, then surgery is recommended.

(5) Aortic stenosis
This patient has a **slow rising pulse** and a blood pressure that has a **narrow pulse pressure**. The apex is displaced and **heaving** indicating pressure overload. There may be a **thrill** felt with the ulnar border of the palm over the aortic area (indicating at least a grade 4 murmur and often reflects a pressure gradient across the valve of at least 40 mmHg). An **ejection click** may be heard over the left sternal border indicating the stenosis is occurring from the valves (and not subvalvular or supravalvular in origin) and is due to opening of the valve. A click is especially heard in bicuspid aortic stenosis. Note that clicks may also be heard in pulmonary stenosis or with a prolapsing mitral valve.

An **ejection systolic (rough, sawing, diamond shaped) murmur** is heard all over the precordium, but especially in the aortic area and possibly radiating to the carotids. The **second heart sound is quiet**. The differential diagnosis includes mitral regurgitation, hypertrophic obstructive cardiomyopathy and aortic *sclerosis*.

Aortic sclerosis is simply a noisy valve due to calcification frequently seen in the elderly, and has no abnormal increase of the pressure gradient across the valve. Thus in aortic sclerosis the patient has a normal pulse character, a normal pulse pressure (blood pressure) and a normal apex beat position and character.

Clinical features of aortic stenosis
- Palpitations due to arrhythmias (ventricular)
- Syncope due to arrhythmias
- Chest pain (angina)
- Dyspnoea (left ventricular failure)
- Sudden death (10–20%)

In aortic stenosis the ventricular function is relatively well preserved, unlike in aortic regurgitation. However with significant stenosis exercise fails to improve cardiac output leading to ischaemia and cardiac arrhythmias. For this reason exercise tolerance tests are avoided in these patients. In patients with aortic stenosis **symptoms are a good indication of the disease severity**.

Aortic stenosis is especially prone to bacterial endocarditis as it is a high-pressure valve lesion.

Causes of aortic stenosis
- Valvular
  - Rheumatic fever
  - Calcification
  - Congenital (e.g. bicuspid valve)
- Supravalvular
  - William's syndrome (supravalvular aortic diaphragm, mental retardation and hypercalcaemia)
- Subvalvular
  - Diaphragm below the aortic valve
- Septal
  - Hypertrophic obstructive cardiomyopathy

The severity of aortic stenosis is indicated by:
- A narrow pulse pressure on blood pressure recording
- Reverse splitting of the second heart sound (i.e. pulmonary before aortic)
- A soft second heart sound
- A fourth heart sound (indicating ventricular stiffness due to left ventricular Hypertrophy)
- A thrill
- A heaving apex beat

The **ECG** may show signs of **left ventricular hypertrophy** (R wave in V6 plus S in V2 summate to more than 35 mm) plus signs of **ventricular strain** (ST depression and T wave inversion) in the leads, which look at the left ventricle (leads I, AVL, II, V5 and V6).

The **chest radiograph** may show **post-stenotic dilatation**. There may be **calcification** of the aortic valve. Alternatively there may be feature of **congestive cardiac failure**.

In the **management**, valve replacement is indicated for all patients with symptoms and where the pressure gradient across the valve exceeds 50 mmHg. Balloon valvotomy is reserve for those unfit for surgery or as a temporary measure. Antibiotic prophylaxis is required for surgery.

Answer 2

Know the features for patients with a serious cause for headaches:

History alarm features
- **Morning headache**: improving after getting up
- **Morning vomiting**
- **Pain exacerbated by coughing, straining or bending**: note that this occurs in many headaches to a degree, so avoid using a leading question when asking about exacerbating factors
- **Progressively getting worse**
- **No 'days off'**: relentless daily symptoms suggest a possible serious cause
- **New onset** in middle life (i.e. uncharacteristic, no previous history of headaches)
- **Risk factors for intracranial bleeding:** e.g. anticoagulation, alcoholism, old age
- **Trauma:** recent falls/head injury (frequently the trauma is forgotten)

Examination alarm features
- Any reduction in the **Glasgow Coma Scale**
- **Confusion** (reduction in abbreviated mental test scoring)
- **Focal neurology**: motor/sensory/coordination/visual/meningeal irritation
- **Seizures**
- Purpuric **rash**
- **Signs of meningeal irritation**
- **Fever**
- **Papilloedema**
- **Severe hypertension**

The **diagnosis of headache is made largely on the history**. A good history will pick out those where there should be heightened concern.

(1) Migraine
The features of migraine may be 'classical' in (only) 20%, presenting with a prodrome of visual auras (e.g. flashing lights or zig-zag lines due to cerebral vasospasm) often taking a stereotypical pattern for a given patient. This is followed by a severe unilateral headache with photophobia and phonophobia (intolerance of noise). Nausea and abdominal pain may occur along with focal neurology, e.g. dysphasia, hemiplegia, sensory symptoms.

However, some of these features may be lacking in 'common migraine' and differentiation from tension headaches (the main differential) can be difficult. The approach to first-line treatment is with paracetamol or ibuprofen (or both) used together with an anti-emetic, as gastric stasis during migraine can impair absorption. Codeine is avoided due to its predisposition to cause 'analgesic' headache, in addition to the risk of dependency and side effects such as constipation and drowsiness. Asking about triggers (food, stress, menstruation) and avoidance of these is helpful. Note that there is often a family history in migraine sufferers.

(2) Benign intracranial hypertension

A classical history. The problem is a recirculation disorder of CSF. There is no focal neurology and the CT scan is normal without ventricular dilatation. Prominent papilloedema is found on examination. Enlargement of the blind spot on testing the visual fields occurs; if untreated, blindness can occur. A CT scan is required, however, to exclude mass lesions and other causes of raised intracranial pressure. Treatment involves stopping any causative drugs (e.g. steroids or oral contraceptives), weight loss and thiazide diuretics. Repeated lumbar puncture and shunt operations are second line therapy.

(3) Cluster headache

Typically a pattern of recurrent headaches for a few days or weeks followed by temporary remission occurs. 20% of cases are chronic. The male:female ratio is 5:1. The exact cause is unknown; however, alcohol may precipitate an attack. Sufferers are more commonly smokers. The episodes may be brief (up to an hour) but are recurrent in bouts, often with periods of remission lasting several months. Severe pain occurs behind the eye. A partial Horner's syndrome may occur along with vasomotor dysfunction causing lacrimation and nasal discharge. The treatment is similar to migraine and 5HT (serotonin) antagonists (e.g. sumatriptan) are often helpful. In addition 100% oxygen (which may abort attacks), verapamil, lithium or methysergide are alternatives. Treatment can be very difficult (like some migraine).

(4) Space occupying lesion

This is a worrying history. The progression of focal neurology and seizures suggest an expanding mass lesion. The exact neurological presentation depends on the location; however, common patents of presentation include;
- Features of rising intracranial pressure (headache, vomiting)
- Neurological deficit (see patterns below)
- Epilepsy

  Oedema around the lesion may exaggerate the picture. An urgent CT scan is indicated. Remember the approach to neurology: 'Where is the lesion? Then, what is the lesion?'

Localizing mass lesions
- Frontal lobe
  - Personality change
  - Disinhibition
- Memory/intellect deterioration
- Primitive reflexes return (Plantar response, grasp and suck reflex)
- Expressive dysphasia (Broca's area)
- Anosmia
- Parietal lobe
  - Apraxias (learned movements).
  - Asteriognosis (shape recognition)
  - Homonymous inferior quadrantanopias
  - Extinction (sensory inattention for stimuli on the affected side when both sides stimulated)
- Temporal lobe
  - Receptive dysphasia (Wernicke's area)
  - Memory loss
  - Cortical deafness
  - Homonymous superior quadrantanopias
- Occipital lobe
  - Cortical blindness
  - Homonymous hemianopias

Causes of cerebral mass lesions
- Tumour
  - Secondary > Primary lesions
  - Malignant > Benign
- Abscess
  - Pneumonia
  - Skin sepsis
  - ENT sepsis
- Haemorrhage
  - Extradural haemorrhage
  - Subdural haemorrhage
  - Subarachnoid haemorrhage
- Granulomatous
  - Cerebral sarcoidosis
- Vascular
  - AV malformations
  - Hydrocephalus

(5) Acute bacterial meningitis

From the given history it may seem difficult to separate viral from bacterial meningitis. However, the lack of any viral prodromal illness and the importance of not missing acute bacterial meningitis, make this the best answer. The main other differential diagnoses include encephalitis, subarachnoid haemorrhage, severe migraine, cerebral abscess, subdural and extradural haemorrhage.

Immediate management includes **antibiotics**, which should not be delayed awaiting investigations or even admission to hospital as this is associated with an adverse outcome. Penicillin V 1.2 g should be given immediately. A CT scan should *ideally* be performed before a lumbar puncture ideally to exclude raised intracranial pressure and other differential diagnoses. If meningococcal disease is suspected a lumbar puncture is avoided due to the high risk of coning because of the prevalence of associated cerebral oedema. Blood cultures (several sets) should be taken. The organism can also be looked for on PCR of blood or CSF. General resuscitation measures (IV fluids and oxygen) are required for septic shock, as well as close monitoring and support usually in intensive care. Despite optimum management overall mortality is still around 10%. Early recognition of symptoms is therefore vital.

Presentation of acute bacterial meningitis
- **Headache** (bursting, gradual or abrupt onset)
- **Pyrexia**
- Signs of **meningeal irritation,** e.g. neck stiffness, Kernig's sign
- **Photophobia** (a non-specific feature for meningitis)
- **Rash:** A non-blanching purpuric rash due to disseminated intravascular coagulation (DIC) occurs in meningococcal meningitis only. The lesions may occur anywhere, and the patient should be completely inspected as even a single lesion may be significant
- **Global cerebral dysfunction** (cerebral oedema, toxaemia): confusion/drowsiness/convulsions/vacant staring

- **Focal neurological signs** are possible. Infarction or false localizing signs due to raised ICP (C III, CVI palsy or hemi-paresis)
- **Shock** (septicaemic)
- **Bleeding** (due to DIC) e.g. bleeding from venepuncture sites

Note that many of these features may be absent in certain patients with meningitis and that the disease may present in a non-acute and non-specific manner.

Which blood tests?
FBC/U and Es/CRP/PT/APTT/FDPs (fibrin degradation products), blood cultures.

Which antibiotics?
Penicillin V (2.4 g i.v. or 1 g i.m. stat if no IV access) and **Cefotaxime** (2 g/8 h i.v.). Usually hospitals will have their own policy.

Why CT scan?
- Helps exclude other causes, e.g. IC bleed/subarachnoid haemorrhage/cerebral abscess
- Ideally prior to lumbar puncture to exclude raised ICP

Lumbar puncture patterns
Normal opening pressure: <16 cm manometric height of water.

In general the following apply (for exam purposes):

	Bacterial	Viral	TB	Normal
Appearance	Cloudy	Clear	Clear	Clear
Cells	Neutrophils	Lymphocytes	Lymphocytes	<5/mm^3
Glucose	<1/3 levels in blood	Normal	<1/2 blood levels	1/2–2/3 blood levels
Protein	>1 g/L	<1 g/L	>1 g/L	0.2–0.4 g/L

Answer 3

(1) Pulmonary embolism
The diagnosis of pulmonary embolism relies on a combination of the following . . .

An assessment of the clinical symptoms
- Shortness of breath of abrupt onset (occasionally gradual onset occurs with multiple small emboli)
- Cough

- Haemoptysis
- Chest pain (pleuritic type; a late feature)
- Sudden collapse (cardiac arrest)

An assessment of the risk factors for thromboembolism
- **Plaster casts/immobility***

---

*Major risk factors

- **Postoperative/trauma*** (hypercoaguable state, dehydration)
- **Previous deep vein thrombosis (DVT)/PE***
- **Pregnancy***
- **Poorly (major illness)***
- Oral contraception/oestrogens
- Obesity
- Smoking
- Carcinoma
- Travel
- Old age (PE is rare under the age of 40 years without risk factors)
- Hereditary thrombophilic states:
  - Protein S deficiency
  - Protein C deficiency
  - Antithrombin III deficiency
  - Factor V Leiden (fails to bind Protein C)
- Secondary to other medical conditions:
  - Nephrotic syndrome (renal loss of anti-thrombin III)
  - Diabetic ketoacidosis (dehydration)
  - Antiphospholipid syndrome (poorly understood mechanism; antibodies to phospholipids involved in coagulation occur, the APTT is prolonged *in vitro* but *in vivo* thrombosis occurs)
  - Homocystinuria
  - Paroxysmal nocturnal haemoglobinuria
  - Behçet's disease (arterial and venous thromboses)

An assessment of the clinical findings

- Tachycardia (sensitive sign)
- Tachypnoea (sensitive sign)
- Cyanosis
- Chest findings (often normal):
  - Pleural rub
  - Reduced air entry
  - Hypotension
- Clinical evidence of DVT (frequently lacking)

An assessment of basic investigations

- White cell count; to help exclude infection from the differential diagnosis
- Arterial blood gases; type I respiratory failure pattern (hypoxia with normal or reduced CO_2)
- ECG
  - Tachycardia is the most frequent finding
  - Right axis deviation
  - The classic S1Q3T3 is far less common
- D-dimer
  - Sensitive but not specific
  - Good for excluding PE if normal
  - Should not be performed if there is strong clinical suspicion
- Chest radiograph
  - Often normal
  - Wedge-shaped infarction (opacity) which may cavitate after several days

Assessing the probability of PE

This is assessed by scoring the above as follows . . .

- No other likely diagnosis on the basis of the above clinical findings and the basic investigations? → 1 point
- Presence of a major risk factor (as above in bold)? → 1 point

Definitive tests

- V/Q scan
- Helical CT scanning
- Pulmonary angiography (the most accurate test)

Following the diagnosis of PE anticoagulation is commenced with warfarin by giving a loading dose of 5–10 mg for 2 days, followed by a dose adjusted to give an INR between 2× and 3× normal. Warfarin is continued

---

*Major risk factors

Action	2 points (high risk)	1 Point (medium risk)	0 points (low risk)
Heparinize?	Yes	Yes	Wait
Arrange definitive tests?	Urgent	Soon	Possibly
Alternative diagnosis?	Possible	Likely	Very likely

for 3–6 months. If the PE is a recurrent episode, consideration is given to lifelong warfarin treatment. Following massive PE with collapse, intravenous thrombolysis is given using rtPA or streptokinase.

(2) None of these
Tension pneumothorax on the left pushing all the mediastinal structures over to the right. Patients with tension pneumothorax have respiratory compromise, frequently extreme and rapidly progressive as the 'valve' type leak causes further compromise with each breath. The impedance of venous return to the right side of the heart leads to reduced cardiac output (tachycardia and hypotension) and an elevated JVP. The management involves urgent release using a green needle followed by insertion of an intercostal drain. (See also OSCE 12, p. 244)

(3) Left apical lung fibrosis

Causes
- Old TB
- Silicosis
- Sarcoidosis
- Aspergillosis
- Extrinsic allergic alveolitis
- Ankylosing spondylitis

Differential on CXR of apical opacity
- Pancoast tumour
- TB
- Pneumonia
  - *Klebsiella*
  - Pneumocysti
- Fibrosis (as above)

(4) Right-sided pleural effusion
Stony dull percussion. Normal respiratory rate and lack of cyanosis makes pneumonia less likely. Know causes of effusions (exudates and transudates), CXR appearances of and basic management. (See OSCE 26, p. 271.)

(5) Right lower lobe pneumonia
The patient is breathless, cyanosed with evidence of right lower lobe consolidation. Other clinical features might include pyrexia, tachycardia, herpes labialis. The patient might complain of chest pain that is

pleuritic on closer questioning. Diaphragmatic pleural pain may radiate to the epigastrium and cause confusion with an acute abdomen. Pneumonia is an inflammation of the lung. The causes may be divided into . . .
- Infective
  - Bacterial, viral, fungal
- Allergic
  - e.g. allergic bronchopulmonary aspergillosis
- Physical agents
  - Chemical; aspiration of vomit or caustic material
  - Radiotherapy

Remember the right lower lobe as the most likely location of a pneumonia following aspiration.

(6) Asthma
Beware similar but late acute asthma with respiratory failure and silent chest. Know the blood gases patterns in acute asthma;
- **Type I respiratory failure early** with low PaO_2 and normal (or even elevated) $PaCO_2$ progressing to fatigue and eventual;
- **Type II respiratory failure** and rising $PaCO_2$ and low PaO_2. In asthma, acidosis is an indication that urgent respiratory support (ventilation on ITU) is needed immediately, so call for anaesthetic help. (See EMQ Answers Q24 (4), p.158 and OSCE 1, p. 219.)

Answer 4

Notes
- **Extrinsic pathway**: utilizes factor VII. Tissue factor initiates coagulation
- **Intrinsic pathway**: utilizes factors VIII, IX and XI. Tissue factor/factor VII complex activates
- **Common pathway**: Factor X dependent
- The **PT** (prothrombin time) measures factors II, V, **VII,** and X, i.e. the **extrinsic and common pathways**
- **APTT** (activated partial thromboplastin time) measures VIII, X and **XI**, i.e. the **intrinsic and common pathways**

See diagram overleaf.

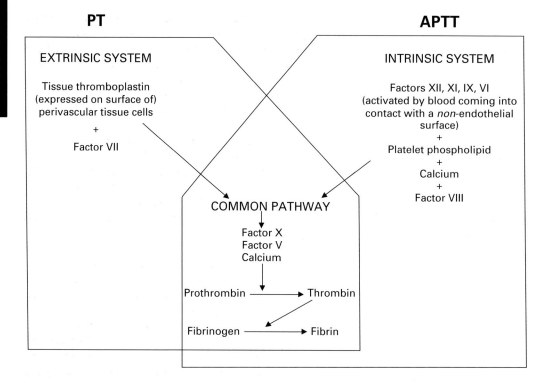

- **Vitamin K** is a co-factor required for the gamma carboxylation of factors II, VII, IX and X, and proteins S and C. This is required so that these factors can bind calcium in the normal process of coagulation. The **intrinsic and extrinsic system** will thus be affected by deficiency of vitamin K. Warfarin inhibits the reduction of Vitamin K epoxide to Vitamin K. As Vitamin K is a fat soluble vitamin (along with vitamins A, D and E) deficiency may arise with cholestatic jaundice. Vitamin K deficiency can also affect the newborn (haemorrhagic disease of the newborn) due to poor placental transfer of the vitamin. For this reason vitamin K is given immediately after birth
- **Coagulation disorders produce:**
  - Bleeding into muscles and joints
  - Large bleeds into the skin
  - Small cuts stop spontaneously but larger deeper cuts do not
  - Healing is delayed
- **Platelet disorders produce:**
  - Multiple small areas of bleeding into the skin (purpura/petechiae)
  - Prolonged bleeding of smaller cuts (which depend on platelet adhesion more than coagulation)

- Bleeding into mucus membranes
- Heavy periods
- Prolongation of the bleeding time

Note that the **platelet count must drop below around 50×10^9 before any bleeding disorder is likely to occur**.

Therefore:

(1) Haemophilia A

Prolongation of the APTT with normal PT and bleeding time. Although the inheritance is X linked recessive, one third of haemophilia A cases are spontaneous mutations without family history. There is a range of severity. Factor VIII:C levels less than 5% are associated with spontaneous haemarthrosis and bleeding into muscles. Restoring factor VIII:C levels to 30% of normal is required in the management.

(2) Haemophilia B, factor IX deficiency (Christmas disease)

As for Haemophilia A, there is prolongation of the APTT, with normal PT and bleeding time. Factor VIII:C levels are normal, however. There is identical inheritance and presentation to Haemophilia A, but the condition is 20% as common as Haemophilia A.

(3) Von Willebrand's disease

Deficiency in factor VIII:WF. Three types occur (Types I and II are dominant; Type II is recessive and produces a severe form of the disease). Chromosome 12. The commonest coagulation disorder. VIII:WF binds platelets, so deficiency behaves like platelet problem. Confusingly factor VIII:C (haemophilia A) may (or may not) also be low, with a resultant prolongation of the APTT. However, haemarthrosis is rare. Ristocetin (an antibiotic) normally clumps platelets, but fails to do so in Von Willebrand's disease and so forms the basis of a the diagnostic test.

(4) Warfarin medication

Although Vitamin K deficiency will produce the same pattern. The raised PT and APTT in this case are suggestive of warfarin therapy given the clinical scenario.

The normal bleeding time counts against liver disease, which causes a coagulopathy via . . .

- Impaired protein synthesis; fibrinogen/coagulation factors
- Malabsorbtion of fat soluble vitamin K due to cholestasis
- Hypersplenism; consumes platelets
- DIC
- Functional platelet abnormalities. Also seen in uraemia/myeloma/scury/antiplatelet drugs/essential thrombocythemia/leukaemia/congenital conditions

(5) Easy bruising syndrome

Common and benign. Reassurance required. Similar to senile purpura in that vessel fragility is to blame. All measurements of coagulation are normal.

Answer 5

(1) Tietze's syndrome

Costochondritis of the sterno-costal junctions. The aetiology is uncertain. Symptomatic treatment and reassurance is all that is required.

(2) Lobar pneumonia

The main differential being pulmonary embolism, given the patient's clear major risk factors for thrombosis. There has been no haemoptysis (although this does not exclude a PE) and septic features dominate the clinical picture. In addition the prodromal symptoms and the 'gradual' onset of breathlessness make pneumonia the more likely diagnosis. She is clearly very unwell given the hypotension (septic shock) and in practice would almost certainly be investigated for both these possibilities. Note that pregnancy does not contraindicate emergency radiography. Other investigations include urgent blood cultures, FBC, U and Es, and arterial blood gases. Intravenous fluids and road spectrum antibiotics (e.g. cefuroxime 1.5 g t.d.s., plus erythromycin 50 mg q.d.s.) are required. Inatropic support may be required on ICU.

(3) Epidemic myalgia (Bornholm's disease)

Coxsackie B virus. A typical history. A seasonal illness often occurring in late summer. The pain may be unilateral and severe ('the devil's grip'). There are no significant clinical findings on examination. Symptomatic treatment is all that is required and resolution occurs spontaneously.

(4) Aortic dissection of the thoracic aorta

The patient has a history of hypertension, which is a major risk factor. Often a history of a valsalva type manoeuvre (e.g. lifting, bending) before the event is obtained. The pain is usually very severe and described as 'ripping' or 'tearing' classically. Two thirds are of the ascending aorta, one third are in the descending aorta. Clinical examination is frequently normal, the diagnosis being made from the history and absence of the acute ECG changes of myocardial infarction (the major differential diagnosis).

Risk factors for aortic dissection

- Hypertension
- Coarctation of the aorta (Turner's Syndrome; XO)
- Marfan's syndrome
- Giant cell arteritis
- Major thoracic trauma

Complications for dissection of the aorta

- Inferior MI (occlusion of the right coronary artery origin)
- Aortic regurgitation (causing cardiac failure)
- Cardiac tamponade (retrograde dissection)
- Dissection of the major arteries coming off the aortic arch leading to strokes and limb ischaemia.
- Rupture of the false lumen back into the aorta or externally (usually resulting in death). In this case pulmonary haemorrhage had occurred

Investigations

- ECG: non-specific changes e.g. tachycardia, left ventricular strain, possible inferior MI

- CXR; wide mediastinum/enlarged aortic knuckle/ pulmonary haemorrhage or normal
- Trans-oesophageal echocardiography (TOE)
- Contrast spiral CT scan
- Angiography

Management

- Analgesia with IV opiates
- Control BP to systolic of around 100 mmHg
- Urgent blood cross match
- Resuscitation with intravenous fluids
- Surgical repair for
  - Ascending dissections
  - Progressive lesions
  - External leaks

(5) Acute pericarditis following myocardial infarction

Characteristically occurs 2–3 days following an acute full thickness (Q waves therefore present on the ECG) myocardial infarction. A pericardial rub (which is continuous) may be heard early, but disappears as an effusion develops. **Cardiac tamponade** may occur in which the myocardium is compressed restricting diastolic filling resulting in systolic hypotension. The speed of accumulation of a pericardial effusion dictates how symptomatic the patient is. Rapid accumulation of 200 mL may cause acute tamponade, whereas 1000 mL may accumulate slowly (e.g. in uraemia) with little compromise to the cardiac output.

Investigations

- ECG; **saddle shaped ST elevation** which is widespread (unlike territorial pattern of myocardial infarction) and without Q waves. In addition QRS alternans may occur in which the cardiac axis swings with each beat due to the heart swinging within a bag of fluid. This gives rise to an alternate complex of different sizes (see below). Low voltage complexes may occur once a significant pericardial effusion develops.

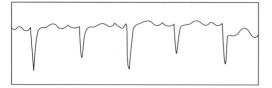

- **Chest radiograph**: classically shows a globular shaped heart

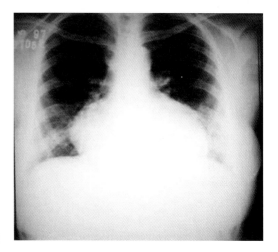

Pericarditis complicating myocardial infarction is managed with rest and analgesia. Warfarin is relatively contraindicated. Treatment with intravenous steroids may be helpful if there are persistent symptoms. Perform pericardocentesis (aspiration) if cardiac compromise occurs.

The following signs are associated with cardiac tamponade . . .

- **Kussmaul's sign** may occur in which there is distension of the neck veins with inspiration (normally the JVP should fall with inspiration due to negative intrathoracic pressure) indicating that the heart chambers are being prevented from expanding (due to a pericardial effusion or a stiff pericardium)
- **Pulsus paradoxus** may occur in which there is a fall in arterial pulse volume (blood pressure) during inspiration, due to compression of the myocardium

In **constrictive pericarditis and restrictive cardiomyopathy** (both lesions cause a fixed ventricular filling volume but are not compressing) Kussmaul's sign can also occur. In addition Friedreich's sign occurs in which there is a rapid diastolic (Y descent) fall in the JVP due to a vacuum effect in diastole. *Pulsus paradoxus, however, does not tend to occur in these conditions as the myocardium is not being compressed.*

Causes of constrictive pericarditis
- Malignant pericarditis
- Uraemic pericarditis
- Tuberculous pericarditis
- Radiotherapy
- Connective tissue diseases

Causes of restrictive cardiomyopathy
- Amyloidosis
- Sarcoidosis
- Eosinophilic myocarditis (Loeffler's syndrome)

Causes of pericarditis
- Infarction
  - Post-MI
  - Dressler's syndrome
- Infection
  - Coxsackie virus
  - Tuberculosis
  - Bacterial (septic emboli)
- Inflammatory
  - Acute rheumatic fever
  - Connective tissue diseases (e.g. SLE, RA)
- Trauma
  - Post-thoracotomy
  - Radiation
  - Seat belt injury
- Metabolic
  - Uraemia
  - Hypothyroidism
  - Gout
- Drugs
  - Hydralazine   (→ drug-induced lupus)
  - Phenylbutazone   (→ drug-induced lupus)
- Neoplastic infiltration

Answer 6

(1) Primary pulmonary hypertension
Pulmonary hypertension is defined as a mean pulmonary artery pressure of greater than 25 mmHg at rest or 30 mmHg on exercise.

Ninety-nine per cent of pulmonary hypertension is **secondary** due to:
- **Increased pulmonary resistance**
  - **Chronic lung disease**, e.g. COPD, pulmonary fibrosis
  - **Chronic hypoxia**
  - **Systemic sclerosis** (20% of cases)
  - **IV drug abuse** ('talc lung')
  - **Chronic pulmonary embolism**
  - **Fenfluramine** (appetite suppressant)
  - **AIDS**
- **Left heart obstruction**
  e.g. mitral stenosis, hypertrophic obstructive cardiomyopathy, atrial myxoma
- **Increased pulmonary blood flow**
  e.g. ASD, VSD, patent ductus arteriosus

One per cent of pulmonary hypertension, however, is primary and occurs without identifiable pre-existing cardiorespiratory pathology. The incidence is 1 per million per year. It is more common in females in the third or fourth decade, and after pregnancy. The condition has a mean survival of approximately 3 years without treatment. Patients present with breathlessness, palpitations and syncope. On examination there are features of right ventricular hypertrophy and right-sided cardiac failure. Pulmonary valve closure is loud and pulmonary as well as tricuspid regurgitation may occur (as here). The JVP is elevated and there is oedema. Hepatomegaly may occur which may be pulsatile if there is tricuspid regurgitation also (as here). Patients are investigated with Doppler echocardiography which allows the pulmonary arterial pressure to be calculated and gives an assessment of ventricular function.

Treatment until recently was only with anticoagulation, diuretics for breathlessness and calcium channel blockers (15% response). Newer treatment involves the use of prostacyclin (or an analogue), which has approximately doubled the five-year survival. This is given by continuous IV infusion. Despite these advances, however, only a heart lung transplant offers a long-term cure.

Causes of breathlessness and a clear chest
(i.e. no crepitations or wheezes)
- Anaemia
- Right ventricular failure
  - Right ventricular infarction
  - Right-sided valve disease, e.g. pulmonary stenosis, tricuspid incompetence
  - Primary pulmonary hypertension
  - Pulmonary embolism (acute or chronic)
- Pneumothorax
- Thyrotoxicosis

- Neuromuscular respiratory failure, e.g. Guillain–Barré syndrome, myasthenia gravis (crisis), botulism
- Anxiety

Causes of sudden onset of breathlessness
(within minutes)
- Pulmonary embolism
- Myocardial infarction
- Pneumothorax
- Arrhythmia, e.g. SVT, VT, fast AF
- Anxiety
- Asthma (note most acute severe asthma develops over several days)
- Anaphylaxis

(2) Hypertrophic obstructive cardiomyopathy

A condition in which asymmetrical septal hypertrophy (ASH) leads to blockage of the aortic outflow tract during systole. The condition can present at any age. There is a 'jerking' pulse due to the sudden throttling of the systolic pressure wave. A double apex beat is felt owing to a palpable atrial systole felt before the main ventricular systole. An 'a' wave is also seen in the JVP and a fourth heart sound may be present due to ventricular stiffness. The clinical picture is variable with many patients being asymptomatic. However, the following may occur:

- Sudden death; complete outflow tract obstruction, ventricular fibrillation, myocardial infarction
- Cardiac failure
- Angina
- Syncopal episodes
- Palpitations: atrial or ventricular arrhythmias
- Bacterial endocarditis

The ECG can take various abnormalities but left ventricular hypertrophy with 'strain' (lateral ST depression and T wave inversion) is typical. There is an association with Wolfe–Parkinson–White syndrome.

The defect is hereditary (autosomal dominant) in around 50% of cases. It is also associated with Friedreich's ataxia and phaeochromocytoma.

Echocardiography shows asymmetrical septal hypertrophy (ASH) and systolic anterior motion of the mitral valve (SAM).

Management
- Anti-arrhythmic agents, e.g. amiodarone
- β-blockers
- Diuretics

- Resynchronization of myocardial contraction using dual chamber pacing
- Surgical resection of the abnormal septal muscle

(3) Atrial septal defect

This is the most common congenital heart defect to remain asymptomatic until into adult life. The classic feature of 'wide fixed splitting' is the give-away piece of information. In normal individuals inspiration causes increased venous return and so delays pulmonary valve closure. In patients with an atrial septal defect, increased inspiratory venous return equalizes across the defect. Thus in atrial septal defects the left to right shunting causes splitting of the second heart sound due to delayed pulmonary valve closure, with no additional delay during inspiration and so the spitting is fixed. A pulmonary ejection systolic flow murmur may be heard. Features of right ventricular failure may also be present.

Note that abnormal splitting due to delayed pulmonary valve closure can occur in:
- Conditions that cause **increase right ventricular flow** (ASD, VSD)
- Conditions that **delay right ventricular systole** (right bundle branch block)
- Conditions that **delay right ventricular emptying** (pulmonary stenosis)
- Conditions which **speed up left ventricular emptying** (mitral regurgitation, VSD)

   However, only ASD has the fixed splitting due to the mechanism discussed above.

Three types of atrial septal defect occur:
1. Ostium secundum defects. These make up 70% of cases and it is these lesions that may present in adult life. Presenting symptoms (which are due to large volume left to right shunting) include . . .
- Fainting
- Fatigue
- Palpitations (atrial fibrillation, SVT)
- Recurrent chest infections (wet lungs)
- Paradoxical embolism
- Later complications
  - Right ventricular failure
  - Eisenmenger syndrome (cyanosis and clubbing) due to shunt reversal consequent upon pulmonary hypertension

The defect is in central fossa ovalis. Right axis deviation and right bundle branch block may occur.

2. Ostium primum defects. These comprise 15% of lesions. Left axis deviation occurs. Mitral and tricuspid valve regurgitation may occur due to the lesion being low down in the septum and associated with valve defects. It is associated with Down's and Noonan's syndromes

3. Sinus venosus defects. These comprise 15%. These are in the septum inferior to the superior vena cava entrance. There is an association with anomalous pulmonary venous drainage

The chest radiograph in ASD shows cardiomegaly with right ventricular hypertrophy, prominent pulmonary arteries and pulmonary plethora.

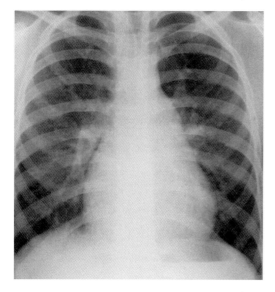

The management of ASD involves valve closure when the pulmonary flow is increased by 50% (pulmonary/systemic ratio of >1.5). Ideally this should be performed in childhood. Previously, small defects were observed, however, recent evidence suggests that some of these lesions may be progressive and therefore some advocate closure for all atrial septal defects.

(4) Chronic pulmonary embolism

This young man had developed features of right ventricular failure as a consequence of pulmonary hypertension. That he abuses IV drugs should be immediately considered given the lesions on his forearms.

Reasons why IV drug abusers might become short of breath include:

- Recurrent pulmonary embolism due to insoluble contaminants in heroin ('talc lung')
- Pulmonary abscesses (*Staphylococcus aureus* septicaemia)
- *Pneumocystis carinii* infection secondary to HIV
- Right-sided bacterial endocarditis
- Anaemia due to malnutrition or chronic ill health
- Tuberculosis

In this case pulmonary hypertension is suggested by the elevated JVP and pulmonary valve incompetence, there are no features to suggest bacterial endocarditis and the chest radiograph is normal making pulmonary embolism the most likely diagnosis. Remember that even in thromboembolic pulmonary embolism 0.5% do not resolve and may lead to pulmonary hypertension.

(5) Pleural effusion

The patient has **systemic lupus erythematosus (SLE)**. An autoimmune disease where the primary problem is autoantibodies directed against DNA. It is more common in females and affects black racial groups more than white races. The brunt of the illness affects the skin in 80%, most commonly with facial erythema and scaling (the butterfly rash). Photosensitivity occurs and sun protection advice must be given. Here it is possible the condition has been drug-induced with minocycline therapy

Clinical features of SLE

- Skin (common)
  - Butterfly rash
  - Vasculitis
  - Photosensitivity
- Joints (Common)
  - Non-erosive arthritis
  - Deformity may occur due to tendon disruption
- Lungs
- Effusions/atelectasis/fibrosis
- Renal
  - Glomerulonephritis/nephritic syndrome
  - Basement membrane IgG deposition (also seen in Goodpasture's syndrome and diabetes). SLE is a cause of membranous glomerular nephritis and nephrotic syndrome. Refractory hypertension is frequently seen
- Heart
  - Myocarditis
  - Libman–Sacks endocarditis

- Pericarditis (tamponade)
- CNS/PNS
  - Psychosis/fits
- Haematological
  - Normochromic anaemia
  - Neutropenia   } pancytopenia
  - Thrombocytopenia
  - Autoimmune haemolytic anaemia (warm — IgG)
- Fever
  - Differential of pyrexia of unknown origin

Investigations

- **ESR**
  Reflects disease activity (unlike CRP)
- **C3 and C4**
  Reduced in active disease
- **Anti-nuclear antibodies (ANA)**
  Occur in 99%, but not specific. They occur also in some cases of rheumatoid arthritis (conferring risk of Felty's syndrome and Sjögren's syndrome), autoimmune hepatitis, Sjögren's syndrome, systemic sclerosis, mixed connective tissue disease, and up to 2% of normal individuals. Note that various recognized stain patterns of the nucleus are seen:

SLE	Homogenous staining pattern
Connective tissue disease	Speckled staining pattern
Scleroderma	Nucleolar staining pattern
CREST syndrome	Centromere staining pattern

- **Anti-double stranded DNA antibodies**
  Specific when in high titres but occur only in 50% of cases
- **Specific anti-nuclear antibodies**
  - Anti-Sm: very specific for SLE but occur only in 20% of cases. Increase the risk of renal disease
  - Anti-Ro: occur in cases of ANA negative SLE. Causes congenital heart block (IgG antibodies are able to cross the placenta)

  Other specific nuclear antigens:
  - Anti-La   Primary Sjögren's syndrome [not due to rheumatoid arthritis (RA)]

- Anti-Jo	Polymyositis
- Anti-centromere	CREST syndrome
- Anti-Scl70	Systemic sclerosis

- **Antiphospholipid antibodies**
  Although up to 40% have anticardiolipin antibodies, only a small proportion develop the arterial and venous thromboses associated with antiphospholipid syndrome.

The criteria given by the **American Rheumatism Association** are widely used to aid diagnosis of SLE. *Four of the following features* are required to make the diagnosis:

1. Malar rash
2. Discoid rash
3. Photosensitivity
4. Oral ulcers
5. Non-erosive arthritis
6. Serositis: pleurisy (pleural effusions) or pericarditis (pericardial effusions)
7. Renal disorders
8. Neurological involvement
9. Haematological disorders
10. Immunological dysfunction
    - False positive syphilis serology
    - Anti-double stranded DNA antibodies
11. Anti- Sm antibodies
12. Antinuclear antibodies

Clinical variants of SLE

- Discoid lupus
  - Benign variant (some mild SLE features)
  - Facial rash but may be more extensive
  - F:M 9:1
  - Photosensitivity
- Drug-induced lupus
  - Dose related
  - Reversible on stopping the offending drug
  - M = F incidence.
  - Causative drugs include . . .
    'HIP DNS': hydralazine, isoniazid, procainamide, dapsone, nitrazepam, sulphonamides

Paper 2 Answers

MCQs

[1] (a) F (b) T (c) F (d) T (e) F
[2] (a) F (b) F (c) F (d) F (e) F
[3] (a) F (b) T (c) T (d) F (e) F
[4] (a) F (b) F (c) F (d) F (e) F
[5] (a) F (b) F (c) T (d) F (e) F
[6] (a) T (b) F (c) T (d) T (e) F
[7] (a) F (b) T (c) T (d) F (e) F
[8] (a) F (b) F (c) F (d) F (e) T
[9] (a) T (b) F (c) F (d) F (e) T
[10] (a) F (b) F (c) F (d) T (e) F
[11] (a) F (b) T (c) F (d) F (e) T
[12] (a) F (b) F (c) F (d) T (e) F
[13] (a) F (b) F (c) F (d) T (e) T
[14] (a) F (b) F (c) F (d) F (e) F
[15] (a) T (b) F (c) F (d) F (e) T
[16] (a) F (b) T (c) T (d) T (e) F
[17] (a) T (b) F (c) T (d) T (e) F
[18] (a) F (b) T (c) T (d) F (e) F
[19] (a) T (b) T (c) F (d) F (e) T
[20] (a) F (b) F (c) F (d) F (e) F
[21] (a) F (b) F (c) T (d) T (e) T
[22] (a) T (b) F (c) F (d) F (e) T
[23] (a) F (b) F (c) T (d) F (e) F
[24] (a) F (b) F (c) F (d) F (e) F

---

[1] (a) F (b) T (c) F (d) T (e) F

(a) The prevalence of heart failure in the UK is **increasing in both sexes**, but this is **more marked in females**. This is because hypertensive heart disease predominantly causes heart failure in females, which modern medicine is relatively ineffective at treating. In contrast, ischaemia is the commonest cause of heart failure in men, which medicine is becoming increasingly adept at treating, through angioplasty and coronary artery bypass grafting (CABG).

(b) **High output cardiac failure** is caused by such conditions as Paget's disease, thyrotoxicosis, fever, Gram-negative septicaemia, pregnancy and anaemia, where the extra demands placed on the heart cannot be met and it fails. This is less common than **low output heart failure,** which refers to the usual situation whereby the ventricles have been damaged/impaired, leading to diminished cardiac output, low blood pressure and inadequate organ perfusion.

(c) The valve lesion that commonly leads to a pulsatile liver is *tricuspid regurgitation*. The tricuspid valve is located between the *right* atrium and *right* ventricle, and should it become incompetent during ventricular systole, blood flows back at high velocity into the right atrium and subsequently into the great veins, with a knock-on effect throughout the venous system. This leads to (amongst other things) a severely elevated JVP and a pulsatile liver. Incompetence of the mitral valve does not cause a pulsatile liver since this is a left sided valve, and any back-flow impinges on the left atrium and pulmonary vasculature.

(d) The **most common cause of right-sided heart failure is left-sided heart failure**. Other causes of right-sided heart failure include . . .

- Chronic lung disease (cor pulmonale)
- Pulmonary embolism (acute cor pulmonale)
- Pulmonary hypertension
- Tricuspid or pulmonary valve disease
- Left-to-right shunts (e.g. atrial or ventricular septal defects)
- Isolated right ventricular cardiomyopathy

In comparison, the commonest cause of left-sided heart failure is ischaemic heart disease, followed by systemic hypertension, mitral/aortic valve disease and cardiomyopathy.

(e) Treatment in heart failure aims to **decrease both pre- and afterload**, both of which have usually become inappropriately high due to the body's vain attempts to maintain a normal circulation. In chronic heart failure, there is increased and inappropriate levels of four hormones . . .

1. Angiotensin II (causes vasoconstriction and direct damage to vascular endothelium)

2. Noradrenaline (causes vasoconstriction)

3. Vasopressin (also known as ADH—causes sodium and water retention at the kidney)

4. Endothelin (promotes vasoconstriction and fluid retention)

Between them, these hormones attempt to correct the hypotension and decreased cardiac output associated with heart failure, but instead they eventually exacerbate the problem leading to preload and afterload too high for the heart to cope with. Hence, a large part of the treatment in heart failure aims to decrease both the pre- and afterload to more physiological levels, to allow the heart to function to its maximal, albeit failing, capacity. Diuretics and venous vasodilators (e.g. nitrates) reduce preload, whilst arterial vasodilators (e.g. hydralazine) reduce afterload. ACE inhibitors and angiotensin II receptor antagonists reduce both pre- and afterload. β-blockers are also thought to have a vasodilating effect, and the initial effect of loop diuretics such as furosemide is thought to be mediated through vasodilatation, not through their diuretic effect, which commences later.

[2] (a) F (b) F (c) F (d) F (e) F

(a) Because the treatment of hypertension is with life-long pharmacological preparations, the label of 'hypertensive' should not be given to a patient without due consideration. The 'white-coat' syndrome affects most patients and each BP recording you do should be viewed in context.

A reasonable way to diagnose hypertension is if the BP is **persistently elevated over levels of 160/100** (i.e. on three or more occasions over 3 months). If this is the case, treatment should be instituted.

Blood pressures persistently below 140/90 do not require treatment.

The difficult patients are those with BPs in the region 140–160 systolic, over 90–100 diastolic, and the decision whether to start them on antihypertensive medications should be guided by the presence of other risk factors, such as age, cholesterol level, smoking status, presence of diabetes, lipid profile and family history of cardiovascular disease. Risk tables are available to give a level of risk of a major cardiovascular event occurring over the next 10 years (based on **Framingham** data). The patients whose BP is in the 'difficult' range who *should* be started on antihypertensives are those with a >15% risk of a major coronary or cardiovascular event occurring over the next 10 years, *or* those that are diabetic, *or* those with obvious target organ damage (eyes and kidneys).

The aim of antihypertensive treatment should be to lower the BP to <140/85 in otherwise healthy subjects, or to <140/80 in diabetic hypertensives.

(b) Afro-Caribbean populations have a higher mean BP than Caucasian populations.

(c) Although commonly ascribed to increased BP, headaches are very rarely caused by hypertension unless the levels of BP are sky-high (usually over 220/120), as is seen in **malignant hypertension**, where striking headache is a classical feature. Most hypertension is entirely asymptomatic and symptoms (if seen) usually reflect long-standing or severe disease. Such symptoms include epistaxis, nocturia, dyspnoea, light-headedness, angina and congestive cardiac failure. If there are associated attacks of palpitations and sweating, then consider **phaeochromocytoma**. The main symptoms of 'phaeo' can handily be remembered if you remember the mnemonic **the 5 Hs** . . .

H Hypertension

H Headache

H Hot

H Heart (palpitations)

H Hyperhidrosis (sweating)

(d) Radio-femoral delay signifies **coarctation of the aorta**, a recognized secondary cause of hypertension.

(e) The ECG of the hypertensive patient demonstrates taller than normal QRS complexes in the anterior chest leads (V1–V6). Cardiologists have different criteria for diagnosing left ventricular hypertrophy on ECG, but a commonly used one is: add the number of squares in the biggest positive QRS deflection above the isoelectric line in leads V5 or V6 to the number of squares in the biggest negative QRS deflection in lead V1. If the total is **more than 35 small squares/more than 7 big squares** then it is very likely that left ventricular hypertrophy is present, and that the possible cause of this is systemic hypertension.

[3] (a) F (b) T (c) T (d) F (e) F

(a) Myocardial ischaemia occurs due to an imbalance in myocardial oxygen supply and demand, due to . . .

1. Mechanical obstruction of blood flow to myocardium [e.g. atheroma, thrombus, spasm, embolus, coronary ostial stenosis, coronary arteritis (resulting from SLE)]

2. Low flow of oxygenated blood to the myo-

cardium (e.g. anaemia, carboxyhaemoglobinaemia, hypotension)

3. Increased myocardial oxygen demand (e.g. thyrotoxicosis, left ventricular hypertrophy, Paget's, pregnancy)

In the UK the commonest cause of myocardial ischaemia is **coronary atherosclerosis**.

(b) High levels of thyroid hormone have both an increased inotropic and chronotropic effect on the heart, increasing the likelihood of angina in the susceptible patient.

(c) Coronary artery disease is the **single most common cause of death in the UK**, contributing 60 deaths per 100 000 population.

(d) Foam cells are actually **macrophages** that accumulate at sites of vascular endothelial dysfunction where oxidized lipoproteins have built up and triggered the early stages of atherosclerosis. Foam cells are so called because the macrophages take up lipids at the site of atherosclerosis, giving them a 'foamy' cytoplasm on microscopy.

(e) HDL particles are considered to be the 'goodie' in the lipoprotein world. They carry 20–30% of the cholesterol found in the blood (being produced by the liver and the intestine) from cell membranes in peripheral tissues to the liver for use or excretion. This is the opposite of the function of LDL particles, which deliver cholesterol to the peripheral cells from the liver, leading to atherosclerosis.

[4] (a) F (b) F (c) F (d) F (e) F

(a) The dose of aspirin given in acute MI is 300 mg. Patients often refer to 75 mg of aspirin as a 'junior' or a 'children's' aspirin, and is sub-optimal for use in acute MI.

(b) The treatment of MI, once diagnosed, should proceed without delay. Portable chest radiograph is indicated at the first convenient opportunity to assess for such things as cardiac size, pulmonary oedema and mediastinal enlargement.

(c) Of patients receiving thrombolytic treatment, 1–1.5% will have a cerebrovascular accident as a result. Therefore, it is important, no matter how acute the situation, that you warn the patient and get verbal consent to proceed. The indications and contraindications for thrombolysis should be remembered, as you frequently have to make the decision whilst under stress.

The indications for thrombolysis are . . .
- Typical cardiac-sounding chest pain for >30 min

- <12 h since onset of pain
- ST elevation in two or more contiguous leads (>1 mm in inferior leads; >2 mm in anterior or lateral leads) *or* new left bundle branch block on ECG

The contraindications to thrombolysis are as follows . . .
- Cardiopulmonary resuscitation for >10 min
- Significant haemorrhage or surgery within the last month
- Stroke or transient ischaemic attack (TIA) within the last 6 months
- Head injury within the last 6 months
- Any intracranial haemorrhage ever
- Bleeding diathesis (INR > 3)
- Hypertension (>200/110)
- Proliferative diabetic retinopathy
- Pregnancy
- Possibility of aortic dissection (rule in/out with CXR)

(d) Clopidogrel (Plavix®) is an antiplatelet drug that is believed to be synergistic with aspirin when given as a one-off in the setting of acute MI. It is contentiously believed to be less irritative to the gastric mucosa than aspirin, and hence may be an alternative in patients with a strong history of upper gastrointestinal bleeding. Glycoprotein IIb/IIIa receptor antagonists (e.g. eptifibatide, tirofiban) may also be given in the setting of acute MI along with aspirin and low molecular weight heparin (e.g. dalteparin, enoxaparin) to limit cardiac myocyte damage.

(e) Thrombolysis is **maximally effective if given within 12 h** of the onset of cardiac chest pain. It may still be given between 12 and 24 h after the onset of chest pain, but only to patients who show continuing chest pain or other signs of clinical deterioration. If patients re-develop symptoms of chest pain and the criteria for thrombolysis are once again fulfilled, there is no problem re-thrombolysing them. Be cautious about the immunogenicity of streptokinase: it should not be given again between 5 days and 1 year after administration of an initial dose, due to the potential presence of antibodies to the drug, limiting it's effectiveness and causing an immune reaction.

The initial medical management of acute MI can be remembered using the mnemonic **MOAN B.A.** (remember the A-team?) . . .

　M Morphine, or better, **diamorphine**, to control pain, limit subjective sensation of dyspnoea and relieve anxiety (always with an anti-emetic)

O Oxygen; give as much as is available, ideally through a fixed-performance mask. Always consider patients with type II respiratory failure (abolishment of hypoxic respiratory drive will make these patients retain CO_2 and eventually stop breathing)

A Aspirin, given for its irreversible anti-platelet effect

N Nitrate; sublingual or intravenous glyceryl trinitrate should be given to relieve cardiac chest pain in all except the hypotensive patient. This does not have any significant effect on mortality (ISIS-4 trial)

B β-blockers given early in intravenous form have been shown to be beneficial for limiting infarct size and reducing mortality (ISIS-1 trial)

A ACE-inhibitors have been demonstrated to reduce mortality and the incidence of severe heart failure in patients with acute MI (ISIS-4 trial)

Once you have worked through this mnemonic, it will be time to consider thrombolysis or emergency percutaneous transluminal coronary angioplasty (PTCA)—make sure you have called for senior help by then!

[5] (a)F (b)F (c)T (d)F (e)F

(a) Q-waves do not follow inversion of T-waves if the infarct is a partial thickness or **non-Q wave infarction (a.k.a. a subendocardial infarction)**. Q-waves result from total coronary occlusion causing **transmural infarction**. However, early reperfusion (either naturally or medically mediated) limits damage to the myocardium and the infarct does not extend transmurally, hence Q-waves do not develop. The diagnosis of non-Q wave MI depends on typical history and a rise in cardiac enzymes. ECG changes may be non-specific, usually being confined to ST-depression. Compared with Q-wave infarcts, non-Q wave infarcts demonstrate a **lower in-hospital mortality** (10% compared with 15% for Q-wave MIs), **lower initial incidence of heart failure**, **more frequent post-infarct angina**, a *higher* incidence of infarct extension or early recurrent infarction (40% cf. 8%), and a *higher* 1-year mortality (65% cf. 35%). Hence, post-infarct management should be much more aggressive for non-Q wave MIs, involving Holter monitoring, stress testing, angiography, PTCA and/or surgical revascularization. Non Q-wave MIs are more commonly referred to as non-ST segment elevation MIs (NSTEMIs)

(b) The small Q waves (<1 mm wide and <2 mm deep) in the left ventricular leads occur physiologically due to the natural left-to-right depolarization of the inter-ventricular septum. Pathological Q waves are >25% of the height of the partner R wave and/or they are greater than 1 small square in width or 2 small squares in depth.

(c) One of things to watch out for in the hours and days following acute MI is a change in the direction of the electrical axis of the heart. It can indicate evolution of infarction or a new infarct occurring.

(d) Creatine kinase is becoming increasingly marginalized in the investigation of acute MI because of its **poor sensitivity and specificity** for the acute event. Serum levels of this enzyme usually rise within 4–8 h of the event, peak at 24 h and are usually back to normal within 48 h, giving a relatively small window in which to assay the enzyme. There is a false positive rate of ~15% associated with alcohol intoxication, myocyte damage, trauma, vigorous exercise, convulsions, intramuscular injections, hypothyroidism and pulmonary embolism. The CK-MB isoform is more specific for myocardial disease, yet this is also found in small quantities in other tissues, including skeletal muscle, tongue, diaphragm, uterus and prostate. The MM isoform is more specific for skeletal muscle.

(e) Troponins T and I are myofibrillar proteins which have a very high specificity for cardiac injury. They are **released early** in the course of MI (within 2–4 h of the initial event) and **remain elevated for up to 2 weeks**, giving a long-lasting, highly sensitive means of diagnosing MI. Troponin T is also raised, however, in some patients with unstable angina, cardiac tachyarrhythmias and those who have chronic renal failure, meaning that it is not pathognomonic for acute myocardial infarction. Raised troponin T over a certain level may be pathognomonic of acute MI, but the level at which this occurs is the topic of much debate.

[6] (a)T (b)F (c)T (d)T (e)F

(a) Lateral infarcts are reflected by ST-segment elevation in chest leads **V5** and **V6**, and in limb leads **aVL** and **I**. There may be reciprocal changes evident in leads that 'look' at the other side of the heart, i.e. aVR, V1 and V2.

(b) Septal infarcts are reflected by ST-segment elevation in leads **V3** and **V4**.

(c) The right coronary artery supplies the right side of the heart which in-situ lies inferiorly, therefore infarction due to right coronary occlusion is reflected by ST-segment elevation in **II**, **III** and **aVF** (the inferior leads).

(d) Old infarcts are revealed by the development of permanent Q-waves in the leads initially affected. If the old infarct was a septal one, then the Q-waves would be expected to appear in V3 and V4.

(e) Saddle-shaped ST-segment elevation is caused by **pericarditis**, not by VT. VT is a **broad complex tachycardia**, defined as three or more consecutive ventricular beats occurring at a rate of over 120/min. Certain ECG features allow VT to be differentiated from it's major imitator, which is supraventricular tachycardia (SVT) with bundle branch block (BBB). These features seen in VT are . . .

- *Very* wide complexes (>3.5 small squares or >0.14 s)
- **Atrioventricular disociation** with *capture beats* (pathognomonic); the definition of a capture beat is where the atria regain temporary control of the ventricles after a period of AV disociation
- QRS *concordance* (all QRS complexes point the same way and are of approximately same size in all chest leads)

[7] (a) F (b)T (c)T (d) F (e) F

(a) Infective endocarditis is an infection of the lining layer of the heart (endocardium). It most commonly occurs in the **subacute** form (SBE, subacute bacterial endocarditis), running an insidious course. It more rarely occurs as an acute, fulminant infection.

(b) Bacterial endocarditis is **more common in developing countries**. Lower levels of sterility employed during invasive medical, dental and social (e.g. tattooing) procedures, and hence higher incidences of bacteraemia, probably play a large role in this differing incidence.

(c) Bacterial endocarditis occurs much more commonly on rheumatic, congenitally abnormal, artificial or previously damaged heart valves.

(d) Many organisms have the potential to cause bacterial endocarditis. However, the most common cause is the α-haemolytic *Streptococcus viridans* that is responsible for 50% of cases. It is a normal part of the flora of the pharynx and upper respiratory tract, and infection often follows dental extraction or cleaning, tonsillectomy or bronchoscopy. Other common causes of bacterial endocarditis are . . .

- *Enterococcus faecalis:* a normal part of the perineal and faecal flora; infection is commoner in older males with prostatic disease, and in females with genitourinary infections or following pelvic surgery.
- *Staphylococcus aureus:* this can cause SBE, but more commonly causes **acute** bacterial endocarditis with a high mortality rate (30% compared with 15% for *E. faecalis* and 5% for *S. viridans*). It is commoner in patients with central venous catheters, Swan-Ganz catheters and in those who inject drugs intravenously,

since it is a normal commensal of the skin. Unlike all other causes of endocarditis, *Staphylococcus* endocarditis usually affects the *right*-sided heart valves.

- *Streptococcus bovis:* strangely, endocarditis caused by this bacterium is very commonly associated with colonic carcinoma, thus if it is discovered, recourse to colonoscopy should be considered.

Streptococcus pyogenes is a Lancefield Group A β-haemolytic streptococcus, commonly responsible for skin rashes such as cellulitis, erysipelas, impetigo and pyoderma, but not SBE.

(e) Bacterial endocarditis is *more common on left-sided heart valves*, with mitral and aortic regurgitation being the commonest valve lesions complicated by endocarditis.

[8] (a) F (b) F (c) F (d) F (e)T

(a) By definition, syncope is **temporary**. The actual definition of syncope is as follows: 'temporary loss of consciousness and postural tone caused by a diminished cerebral blood flow, i.e. **transient global cerebral hypoperfusion**'. There are many different causes of syncope, but they may generally be divided into . . .

1. Arrhythmias: VT, rapid SVT, AV nodal block, sinus arrest and artificial pacemaker failure may all lead to hypoperfusion sufficient to cause a syncopal attack.

2. Obstruction: stenotic valve lesions (especially aortic stenosis), HOCUM, PE, atrial myxoma, defective prosthetic valve, and many other obstructing lesions may obstruct cerebral blood flow sufficiently to cause a syncopal attack.

3. Situational: another name for this mechanism of syncope is 'neurocardiogenic syncope'. It occurs when there is sudden reflex bradycardia and systemic vasodilatation leading to loss of consciousness. Commonly occurs in response to prolonged standing, venesection, pain, fear or after micturition (especially in older men at night).

Whenever dealing with suspected syncope, it is important to remember the possible differential diagnoses, the presentation of which may be very similar to syncope, e.g. epileptic fit, panic attack, hypoglycaemia, TIA, etc.

(b) Onset of syncope classically occurs **over seconds**, not instantaneously.

(c) Jerking movements, although rare, may occur in syncope (due to hypoxia), so do not exclude the diagnosis based on a history of a few jerking movements. Classical violent and rhythmical jerking along with tongue-biting and incontinence make epilepsy much more likely.

(d) Syncopal attacks due to cardiac dysrhythmias (**Stokes–Adams** attacks) may be heralded by palpitation. The classical sort of dysrhythmia that causes syncope is a **paroxysmal bradycardia**, although certain ventricular tachyarrhythmias may also cause syncope (NB it is rare for supraventricular tachycardias to cause syncope due to the presence of the atrioventricular node).

(e) The treatment of syncope is to attempt to restore cerebral blood flow as soon as possible by **lying the patient flat** and **elevating the lower limbs**. The actual cause should then be sought and treated. However, in cases where the cerebral blood flow cannot be restored, e.g. patient fixed in dentist's chair or continuing arrhythmia, a syncopal episode can be followed by cerebral infarction.

[9] (a)T (b) F (c) F (d) F (e)T

(a) Mitral stenosis occurs almost exclusively due to rheumatic heart disease; at least 50% of sufferers have a positive history of rheumatic fever or chorea of unknown cause. The mitral valve is affected in >90% of patients who develop rheumatic valvular disease.

(b) In mitral stenosis, the **left ventricle remains normal in size**. This is in contrast to mitral regurgitation where the left atrium and ventricle become dilated to maintain cardiac output.

(c) In order to maintain sufficient cardiac output in mitral stenosis, the left atrium hypertrophies and becomes dilated, leading to an increase in pulmonary venous, pulmonary arterial and consequently right heart pressure. The increase in pulmonary vascular pressure can lead to development of **cardiogenic pulmonary oedema**. This is resisted by alveolar and capillary thickening and by pulmonary arterial vasoconstriction, leading to 'reactive pulmonary hypertension'. This has the knock-on effect of causing right ventricular hypertrophy, dilatation and eventually failure. Dilatation of the right ventricle can enlarge the tricuspid annulus, leading to tricuspid regurgitation.

Non-cardiogenic pulmonary oedema is caused by hepatic disease, renal disease, severe burns, pneumonia, excessive intravenous fluid administration, chemotherapy, altitude and Hodgkin's lymphoma.

(d) Mitral stenosis frequently causes complications such as atrial fibrillation (AF), systemic embolization of thrombus (stroke), pulmonary hypertension, chest infection, infective endocarditis (not as common as with regurgitant lesions), tricuspid regurgitation and right-sided heart failure.

(e) Mitral stenosis causes a **tapping** apex beat (a sudden, brief impulse).

[10] (a) F (b) F (c) F (d)T (e) F

(a) In health the pleural space is a **potential** space that does not exist due to the close apposition of the parietal and visceral layers of pleura. It only becomes a true space when the layers become separated by fluid, pus or blood in disease processes, e.g. pleural effusions.

(b) The diaphragm is lined by the parietal pleura superiorly and the peritoneum inferiorly. Its muscle fibres originate from the lower ribs and insert into a central tendon. Motor and sensory nerves arrive separately via the *phrenic* nerve.

(c) The **visceral pleura is not innervated by nerve fibres**. The stretching or irritation of the parietal pleura is what causes classical pleuritic chest pain, because it is supplied by branches of the intercostal and phrenic nerves.

(d) In health, expiration is an **entirely passive** process: the intercostal muscles relax and the lung collapses under the influence of its own elastic fibres.

(e) Doxapram is not used to treat hyperventilation. It is a **respiratory stimulant**, or *analeptic* drug, given intravenously usually to expedite spontaneous postoperative ventilation. It rarely can be given as a continuous intravenous infusion in patients with respiratory failure, but only under strict supervision and usually only to patients in whom other methods of ventilatory support are contraindicated.

[11] (a) F (b)T (c) F (d) F (e)T

Examination of the chest in a patient with unilateral consolidation would reveal . . .

- Decreased chest wall movements on the affected side → **(a)**
- Undisplaced mediastinum → **(b)**
- Dull percussion note over the affected area ('stony dull' should be a term reserved for the percussion note in pleural effusion) → **(c)**
- 'Bronchial' breath sounds (get an idea of what these are like by placing your stethoscope over your trachea and breathing in and out) → **(d)**
- Increased vocal resonance over the affected area → **(e)**
- Added sounds in the form of fine crackles

[12] (a) F (b) F (c) F (d)T (e) F

(a) Viruses causing the common cold are usually '**rhinoviruses**'. Rubella is an example of a togavirus.

(b) Sinusitis is usually caused by *Streptococcus pneumoniae* or *Haemophilus influenzae.* Treatment should be with antibiotics, e.g. co-amoxyclav (amoxycillin + clavulanic acid)

(c) *Seasonal* allergic rhinitis is caused by pollens. *Perennial* allergic rhinitis is usually caused by the house dust mite, animals (via aerosolized proteins on their coat from licking), or industrial dusts, vapours or fumes. Treatment of allergic rhinitis is to **avoid the stimulus**. However, as this is often not possible, the alternative is medical treatment with **histamine-H1 receptor antagonists** (e.g. loratidine), **decongestants** (e.g. oxymetazoline), **anti-inflammatories** (e.g. nedocromil sodium, sodium cromoglycate) and, if necessary, **corticosteroids**.

(d) Pharyngitis, or the common sore throat, is usually caused by **adenoviruses**, and therefore is usually self-limiting.

(e) Tonsillitis is caused in **50% of cases by viruses, 50% of cases by bacteria**. As a consequence, the use of antibiotics is debatable. If they are to be used, a 10-day course of penicillin V 250 mg q.d.s. should be employed. It is important to remember that if there is any possibility of the sore throat being caused by the Epstein–Barr virus (as is the case in *all* sore throats) then ampicillin and amoxycillin should be avoided otherwise an unsightly maculopapular rash will result.

[13] (a) F (b) F (c) F (d) T (e) T

(a) COPD is a disease mainly limited to smokers or ex-smokers.

(b) Although used in the past, the distinction between blue bloaters and pink puffers is now very rarely utilized. However, as with all historical things in medicine, it is important that you have some degree of understanding of the details of this older classification of COPD . . .

- **Pink puffers** (type A COPD, 'fighters'): although the pink puffer is very breathless, arterial tensions of O_2 and CO_2 are relatively normal and there is no cor pulmonale; these patients are thought to be suffering predominantly from emphysema
- **Blue bloaters** (type B COPD, 'non-fighters'): these patients do not appear to be breathless, but have marked arterial hypoxaemia, hypercapnia, secondary polycythaemia and cor pulmonale; they are thought to be suffering predominantly from chronic bronchitis

If you are struggling to remember this classification, remember that all the Bs go together: **Blue Bloater, type B, Bronchitis.**

(c) People in type I respiratory failure should *always* be given 100% O_2 to breathe. They are in acute hypoxaemic failure and require as much oxygen as can be delivered. Patients in type II respiratory failure often require hypoxia to stimulate ventilation and should not be given high fractions of inspired oxygen (FiO_2). If you are in doubt, give the patient 100% O_2 until you are in possession of a set of arterial blood gases that will give you a better idea of the patients acid–base situation, and hence if they are in type I or II respiratory failure.

(d) COPD is the most common cause of cor pulmonale.

(e) Patients with COPD often develop a degree of **appropriate polycythemia** (increased haemoglobin concentration) due to hypoxic simulation of erythropoietin production at the kidney. Erythropoeitin causes increased numbers of bone marrow progenitor cells to commit to dividing (erythropoeisis).

[14] (a) F (b) F (c) F (d) F (e) F

(a) Pleural effusions are **only clinically detectable when their size is >500 mL**, although they are detectable on plain chest radiograph when they exceed 300 mL in size. They are defined as *'an excessive accumulation of fluid in the pleural space'* (this fluid can be blood, pus or lymph).

(b) On auscultation of an area of lung where there is a pleural effusion, there will be greatly reduced or absent breath sounds. However, in the area just above an effusion where the lung is compressed, breath sounds will be bronchial.

(c) The neurovascular bundle of the ribs lies on the inferior border of the interior aspect of each rib. In order to minimize risk of damaging this bundle when aspirating a pleural effusion, the draining needle should be inserted **just above the *superior* aspect of the rib** where the effusion is suspected to be.

(d) Typically, **transudative pleural effusions are bilateral**. If a transudative pleural effusion is unilateral, it usually affects the right side (e.g. **Meig's syndrome**, which is an isolated right-sided transudate associated with ovarian cancer). They have a low protein content (<30 g/L) and a low LDH content (<200 i.u./L). Causes of a transudative pleural effusion include . . .

- **Increased venous pressure** (e.g. in heart failure, constrictive pericarditis, fluid overload)
- **Hypoproteinaemia** (e.g. liver disease, nephrotic syndrome)
- **Hypothyroidism**

(e) Typically, **exudative pleural effusions are unila-**

teral (can be bilateral if the pathological process causing it is diffuse, e.g. widespread lung metastases) and have a high protein (>30 g/L) and LDH content (>200 i.u./L). Causes of an exudative pleural effusion include . . .

- **Inflammation** (e.g. infection—pneumonia, TB; rheumatoid arthritis; SLE; pancreatitis; pulmonary infarction; asbestosis)
- **Malignancy** (e.g. bronchial cancer, metastases, mesothelioma, lymphoma)

Fluid samples from a pleural effusion should be drained under aseptic conditions. It should be inspected and then sent for microbiological (microscopy, culture and sensitivity), biochemical, cytological and immunological (if indicated) tests.

[15] (a) T (b) F (c) F (d) F (e) T

(a) Asthma appears to develop in patients who have a greater than normal ability to raise IgE antibodies to common environmental stimulants.

(b) IgE becomes attached to *mast cells*, and when it recognizes specific antigens it triggers the **mast cell to release histamine**, which is a powerful smooth muscle and vasoactive mediator. β-**agonists (like salbutamol) inhibit mast cell mediator release**, as well as producing bronchodilation. Eosinophils do not release histamine. Instead, when they are activated, they release a number of substances that are toxic to epithelial cells. Eosinophils are decreased in both number and activity by inhaled corticosteroids.

(c) Expectoration of yellow sputum is common in asthmatic patients who do not have a chest infection. Their **sputum is yellow in colour because it contains large numbers of eosinophils**.

(d) The wheeze associated with asthma is classically described as **'polyphonic'** because it is generated from the narrowing of a large number of airways of various different sizes. Monophonic wheeze is characteristic of a single fixed obstruction to air flow, such as a foreign body, a lymph node (e.g. sarcoidosis), or a malignant lesion.

(e) Salbutamol causes intracellular movement of potassium ions, and is useful in the acute treatment of hyperkalaemia. This hypokalaemic effect can also be a troublesome side effect, especially in patients with long-standing COPD who require a large number of β-agonist inhalers/nebulizers each day.

It is important that you know in detail the treatment of hyperkalaemia, because it is a very common problem in hospital patients and is potentially fatal. A potassium level greater than 6.5 is a medical emergency and is associated with classical ECG changes . . .

- Flattened P-waves
- Broad, bizarre QRS complexes
- Tall, tented T-waves

Eventually, hyperkalaemia causes **hyperpolarization of all cell membranes**, leading to decreased cardiac excitability, hypotension, bradycardia and eventually asystole. Management should begin with a 12-lead ECG recording . . .

If ECG changes are present, *protect the myocardium* by giving 10 mL of 10% **calcium gluconate** i.v. This can be repeated every 10 min until the ECG normalizes (no more than 5×). The Ca^{2+} ions protect cell membranes from the effects of the potassium, but do not lower the level of potassium (K^+) itself. This has to be achieved by one of four methods . . .

- Drive K^+ into cells by giving nebulized **salbutamol** 5 mg prn (can cause a disturbing muscle tremor at doses required)
- Drive K^+ into cells by giving 50 mL 50% **dextrose** over 30 min. Accompany this with 10 i.u. Actrapid insulin if the patient is diabetic (if they are not, they will produce their own insulin)
- Correct acidosis by giving **sodium bicarbonate**—this stops K^+ coming out of cells in an attempt to correct for the excess H^+ ions
- Deplete body K^+ by giving **calcium resonium** orally or as an enema—this increases gastrointestinal losses of K^+, but can take up to 24 h to work and is exceedingly unpleasant to take

In general, all the above measures are simply buying time to either correct the underlying disorder that caused the increased K^+, or to arrange dialysis, which is the definitive treatment for hyperkalaemia.

[16] (a) F (b) T (c) T (d) T (e) F

The spleen . . .

- Is never normally palpable in health (has to enlarge by 2× or 3× before it becomes palpable in the left hypochondrium)
- Enlarges obliquely toward the right iliac fossa
- Cannot be palpated above (is tightly apposed to the diaphragm)
- Has a notch → **(a)**
- Is dull to percussion
- Moves 'early' on inspiration (soft sign)
- Is not palpable bimanually (not ballotable)

The **causes of splenomegaly** can be recalled by the mnemonic Her Mother Is A Complete Imbecile . . .

H Haemolysis (sickle cell, spherocytosis)

M Myeloproliferative disease

I Infection (TB, Epstein–Barr, malaria, kala-azar)

A Amyloidosis

C Cancer (lymphoma, leukaemia, secondary deposits)

I Inflammation (SLE, rheumatoid arthritis, endo-carditis, sarcoidosis, hepatitis with portal hypertension)

The kidneys . . .

- Can potentially be palpated in thin healthy individuals
- Enlarge inferiorly on the ipsilateral side → **(d)**
- Have a rounded, less sharply defined edge
- Do not have a notch
- Move 'late' on inspiration
- Are palpable bimanually (ballotable) → **(c)**
- Can be palpated from above
- Are resonant to percussion (due to overlying gas-filled bowel) → **(b)**

The liver . . .

- Can potentially be palpated in the right hypochon-drium and epigastrium in thin healthy individuals, especially on deep inspiration
- Enlarges vertically downward towards the right iliac fossa
- Cannot be palpated above
- Is dull to percussion
- Should extend superiorly (causing dullness to percus-sion) no further than the 5th–6th intercostal space

The **causes of hepatomegaly** can be recalled using the mnemonic C_3HATS . . .

C Cancer (usually secondary deposits)

C Cirrhosis (only in the early stages)

C Congestive cardiac failure

H Hepatitis

A Amyloidosis

T Tricuspid regurgitation

S Sarcoidosis

[17] (a)T (b) F (c)T (d)T (e) F

(a) The inflammation caused by appendicitis can cause a real or apparent mass in the right iliac fossa (RIF).

(b) Myelofibrosis causes splenomegaly, which may pro-ceed to such an extent that the spleen reaches a point in the RIF (myelofibrosis is a disease where the bone mar-row becomes generally fibrosed, associated with myeloid metaplasia of the spleen and other organs, anaemia and thrombocytopenia). Remember that anything begin-ning with myel- or myelo- refers to the bone marrow, from the Greek *myelos* for medulla or marrow.

(c) Fifty per cent of patients with Crohn's have ileocolic disease, implying that both small and large intestines are involved in their disease. This commonly includes **termi-nal ileal involvement**, the transmural inflammation of Crohn's causing a palpable inflammatory mass in the RIF.

(d) TB commonly affects the ileocaecal region of the GIT, with the pathognomnic caseating granulomas and inflammation causing a palpable RIF mass.

(e) Sister Mary Joseph's nodule refers to a **malignant intra-abdominal neoplasm that has metastasized to the umbilicus**, causing a palpable mass.

[18] (a) F (b)T (c)T (d) F (e) F

(a) Many factors impinge unfavourably on wound heal-ing, including . . .

- **Local factors:** wound haematoma, necrotic tissue, for-eign body (e.g. suture), obesity (due to poor local blood supply)
- **Systemic factors:** advanced age, shock (because of the associated hypoxia and acidosis), diabetes mellitus (due to impaired neutrophil mobility), malnutrition (e.g. in alcoholics), corticosteroids, antineoplastic chemotherapy, immunosuppressant agents (e.g. post-transplant)

(b) Ferric iron, present as part of the haemoglobin mol-ecule, **enhances bacterial growth** and **diminishes the efficacy of neutrophilic eradication of pathogens**; this is why it is surgically important to rid wounds of blood before closure in theatre.

(c) Operations greater than 2 h in length have a 40% higher infection rate than those less than 1 h in length.

(d) The **most common cause of early postoperative fever is infection in the pulmonary tract**, usually sec-ondary to poor tidal volumes from anaesthesia, analgesia (especially opioids) or the presence of pain from an oper-ative incision. More serious pulmonary problems associ-ated with surgery include pneumonia secondary to atelectasis, ventilator-induced pneumonitis and aspira-tion of gastric contents.

(e) An infected wound must always be opened, pus evacuated, fibrin debrided and subcutaneous suture material removed. Systemic antibiotics are *never* an alternative to drainage and debridement when a wound is genuinely infected.

[19] (a)T (b)T (c)F (d)F (e)T

(a) Sliding, or type I, hiatus herniae allow a portion of the stomach continuous with the oesophagus to slide into the mediastinum through the oesophageal hiatus of the diaphragm. They are associated with **severe reflux symptoms**. Rolling, or type II, hiatus herniae occur when part of the fundus of the stomach herniates independently through the diaphragmatic hiatus causing symptoms of reflux to be rare, but more dangerously, the herniated portion is prone to incarceration and strangulation.

(b) Ninety per cent of hiatus herniae are of the sliding type.

(c) Medical and surgical treatment of sliding hiatus herniae depend on the degree of reflux symptoms that they cause. However, **all rolling hiatus herniae should be repaired** upon discovery because of the danger of incarceration and strangulation

(d) Gastro-oesophageal reflux disease (GORD) symptoms are caused by *normal* **pH gastric acid** being in the wrong place.

(e) The majority of GORD pain is caused by the direct action of gastric acid on the oesophageal mucosa, which GTN would not affect. However, there is a component of the pain of GORD that is caused by **oesophageal spasm**, which is relieved by GTN.

[20] (a)F (b)F (c)F (d)F (e)F

(a) The stomach has two sphincters, but only one of these—the pyloric sphincter—is an actual demarcated anatomical sphincter; the other—the lower oesophageal sphincter—is merely a physiological sphincter without well-demarcated sphincteric musculature.

(b) The stomach is supplied by the gastric, short gastric, gastroepiploic and gastroduodenal arteries, the majority of which arise from the **coeliac trunk**, a direct branch of the abdominal aorta.

(c) The vagus is a **parasympathetic** nerve which innervates the stomach via the anterior and posterior *nerves of Latarjet* from the **lesser curvature**; these stimulate the parietal cell mass to **secrete HCl** and also cause **increased gastric motility**.

(d) Although mucus-secreting goblet cells are found diffusely throughout the stomach, the parietal (HCl-

and intrinsic factor-secreting) and chief (pepsinogen-secreting) cells are mainly concentrated in the gastric fundus.

(e) The duodenum is split into . . .

1. **Duodenal bulb**
2. **Descending duodenum**
3. **Transverse duodenum**
4. **Ascending duodenum**

. . . before it finally ends at the **ligament of Treitz** (a.k.a. 'the suspensory muscle of the duodenum'), which is a broad, flat band of smooth muscle attached to the right crus of the diaphragm at one end and to the duodeno–jejunal junction at the other.

[21] (a)F (b)F (c)T (d)T (e)T

(a) Gastric carcinoma is very prevalent in Japan, China and Chile, and is not so common in Europe and North America. Immigrants appear to gain the endemic risk of the area to which they move, suggesting at least in part an **environmental aetiology**.

(b) The autosomal dominant Peutz–Jehger's syndrome can be associated with gastric polyps, but more commonly the polyps of Peutz–Jehger's are **found in the small intestine**, especially the jejunum. These polyps are **benign hamartomas** that **very rarely become malignant** (occurs in <3% of cases). The main problems that they cause are intestinal obstruction and bleeding. The vital clue to a patient with Peutz–Jehger's is the melanous spots on the lips and buccal mucosa. Conservative treatment of the polyps is indicated.

(c) Gastric cancer is more common in patients who are blood group A.

(d) Patients with pernicious anaemia develop gastric achlorrhydia and extreme atrophic gastritis, and **40% of them subsequently develop gastric cancer**. Ideally, patients with this condition should undergo yearly endoscopy. Other premalignant conditions for gastric cancer include adenomatous polyps, chronic inflammatory gastritis and caustic injury (usually due to lye ingestion).

(e) **Krukenberg's tumour** is the term used for **metastatic gastric carcinoma which has spread to the ovaries (usually bilateral)**. Spread of gastric cancer is also associated with **Virchow's node** (a firm supraclavicular lymph node, especially on the left, sufficiently enlarged that it is palpable from the skin surface) and **Sister Mary Joseph's nodule** (general term referring to spread of any intra-abdominal neoplasm to the umbilicus, but usually

ANSWERS 2

used in reference to the umbilical spread of gastric cancer).

[22] (a)T (b) F (c) F (d) F (e)T

(a) Biliary colic is **constant** and moderately severe, associated with nausea and vomiting, and located in the right upper quadrant/epigastrium. It is a 'visceral' type of pain and usually lasts 1–4 h, often beginning postprandially (especially after large fatty meals) and causing the patient to be **restless**. It is caused by **transient obstruction of the cystic duct** by a gallstone, not by acute inflammation or infection. The pain of biliary colic is seldom relieved by anything other than potent analgesics and time. Classically, the patient is fit and well immediately before and immediately after the episode.

(b) Pruritis, a common symptom of jaundice, is actually caused by the deposition of *conjugated* bile acids within the tissues secondary to extrahepatic obstruction to bile outflow. It is classically associated with darkening of the urine (overflow of excess conjugated water-soluble bilirubin) and pale stools (lack of stercobilin, a by-product of bacterial bile breakdown in the faeces).

(c) Acute cholecystitis is caused by inflammation of the gallbladder.

(d) Murphy's sign is positive in patients with acute cholecystitis. It is defined as 'pain on palpation of the right subcostal area upon inspiration', and it occurs when the visceral peritoneum over the gallbladder becomes inflamed, but the inflammation has not yet spread to the more superficial parietal peritoneum. Once inflammation spreads to the parietal peritoneum, local signs of peritonitis occur, including localized guarding and rebound tenderness.

(e) This is essentially **Courvoisier's law**. The gallbladder in a jaundiced patient with a stone in the common duct is very unlikely to distend because of multiple previous episodes of inflammation and scarring. However, a patient with cancer of the head of the pancreas and a normal gallbladder will have a noticeably enlarged gallbladder as soon as the cancer grows big enough to occlude the common duct.

[23] (a) F (b) F (c)T (d) F (e) F

(a) Hepatitis reflects *inflammation* of the liver parenchyma. **Any agent that causes parenchymal liver damage can lead to hepatitis**, and whilst alcohol and viruses are the most common causes, it can also be caused by bacteria (*Coxiella burnetii*, also known as Q-fever), pharmacology (e.g. paracetamol, halothane), poisons (e.g. aflatoxin, calcium tetrachloride), Wilson's disease and pregnancy.

(b) Hepatitis viruses A, C, D and E are indeed RNA viruses. **Hepatitis B virus is a DNA virus**.

(c) Hepatitis A replicates in the liver, is excreted in bile and then in the faeces of an infected person for 2 weeks before and 1 week after the onset of the clinical illness, being maximally infective just before the onset of jaundice. It is the most common type of viral hepatitis, and is spread by the *faeco-oral* route, infection commonly arising from the ingestion of infected food or water (especially shellfish). Importantly, *there is no carrier state*. It is a notifiable disease in the UK.

(d) Hepatitis B is **spread by the intravenous route and by close personal contact** (e.g. sexual intercourse) — it is found in high concentrations in semen, vaginal secretions, blood and saliva. Vertical transmission is another major route of spread worldwide. Unfortunately, **10% of those acquiring the acute infection go on to become chronic carriers** of the virus . . .

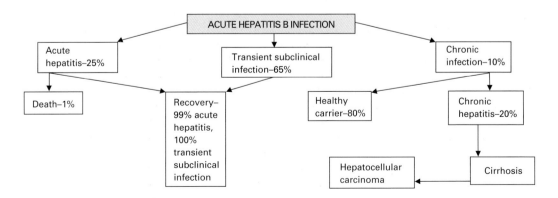

(e) The actual proportion of patients developing acute hepatitis C going on to chronic liver disease is in the region of 60–80%. Cirrhosis develops in 20–30%, and of these 15% develop hepatocellular carcinoma (HCC).

[24] (a) F (b) F (c) F (d) F (e) F

(a) and (b) Primary biliary cirrhosis (PBC) is a disease where there is **chronic progressive destruction of the bile ducts**, eventually leading to cirrhosis. Ninety per cent of patients developing PBC are **females** (as with almost all autoimmune conditions, it is more common in females). The characteristic features are an increase in serum **anti-mitochondrial antibody** (AMAs), and clinically **long-standing pruritis** that precedes the development of jaundice by a number of years. There is also commonly a **raised alkaline phosphatase** (may be the only abnormality in liver function tests), and portal tract infiltrates on liver biopsy ± granulomas. Liver transplant is the only definitive treatment.

(c) Hereditary haemochromatosis is an inherited disease of excessive iron deposition within organs and tissues of the body, causing fibrosis and eventual organ failure. It often **presents in the fifth decade** of life (earlier in males than females) with the classical triad of **bronzed skin, hepatomegaly and diabetes** (due to pancreatic in-volvement). It can be treated by repeated venesection or iron chelation with **desferrioxamine**.

(d) Wilson's disease is caused by a defective copper transporter leading to **failure of biliary copper excretion**, common where there is consanguinity. It typically presents with signs of **chronic liver disease and signs of basal ganglia involvement** (tremor, dysarthria, involuntary movements and eventually dementia). Keyser–Fleischer rings in the eyes are a pathognomonic sign, caused by corneal copper deposition (a greenish-brown ring at the corneo-scleral junction, often requiring a slit lamp to visualize). Wilson's can also affect the kidneys (tubular degeneration) and bones (erosions). It is treated by lifelong copper chelation with **penicillamine** (severe side effect profile).

(e) α_1-antitrypsin deficiency is an **autosomal dominant** deficiency of the serine protease inhibitor ('SERPIN') α_1-antitrypsin, normally synthesized in the liver, diffusing to the lungs via the blood. Its main role in health is to **inhibit neutrophil elastase**. Deficiency causes 10–15% of patients to develop cirrhosis, and 75% to develop lung damage, usually in the form of basal emphysema. The only treatment is liver (and lung) transplantation, depending on the degree of damage. Patients must uniformly stop smoking, otherwise lung damage will be rapid and devastating.

EMQs

Answer 7

(1) Motor neurone disease

A disease in which there are mixed upper motor neurone (UMN) and lower motor neurone (LMN) signs occurring variably together due to **degeneration** of:
- The **motor nuclei** (UMN)
- The **motor neurones of the spinal cord** (UMN)
- The **anterior horn cells** (LMN)

Three disease patterns occur which reflect the mix of the above lesions. These are descriptive rather than clinically distinct entities . . .

1. Amyotrophic lateral sclerosis (ALS): a spastic paraparesis (both legs) or tetraparesis (all the limbs) but with the added LMN features of wasting and fasciculation

2. Progressive bulbar palsy: a mixture of bulbar palsy (LMN), giving weakness and fasciculation of the tongue and pseudobulbar palsy (UMN) giving a brisk jaw jerk

3. Progressive muscular atrophy: here LMN features predominate in the limbs

The disease is more common in the elderly with an incidence of 1 in 10 000 of those over 65 years of age. Ten per cent of cases are familial (various syndromes) and tend to be more severe, and affect a younger age group.

MND does not cause:
- Cerebellar signs
- Palsy of the external ocular muscles
- Sensory system damage
- Incontinence (spared pelvic floor muscles)
- Dementia (except rarely)

Diagnosis

The diagnosis of MND, which is devastating, is based on largely clinical grounds and must be given to the patient with confidence after exclusion of treatable alternatives. Investigations include:

- CT or MRI scan of brain and cord to exclude a structural lesion or cord compression.
- Electromyography (EMG), which shows normal nerve conduction velocity (to exclude peripheral motor neuropathy), chronic partial denervation and fasciculation.
- Muscle enzymes (CPK) to exclude a myopathy, although levels may be slightly raised
- Syphilis serology
- Lumbar puncture and examination of CSF for oligoclonal bands (multiple sclerosis, MS), cell count and protein estimation for inflammatory conditions

Treatment

The treatment of MND is largely supportive and symptomatic.

Riluzole, which is currently licensed in the UK for the treatment of ALS, inhibits the release of glutamate (a neurotransmitter), which has been found to help preserve motor neurones from damage. Liver function tests must be monitored regularly. Randomized controlled trials have found a prolongation of the time to tracheostomy, so justifying its tremendous expense on health economic grounds.

The life expectancy depends upon the progression to ventilatory failure and death often occurs from hypostatic pneumonia.

(2) Myasthenia gravis

Weakness and easy fatigue of proximal limb, bulbar and ocular muscles occur, due to IgG antibodies directed against acetylecholine receptors on the motor end plate. The history may be prolonged prior to diagnosis and mistaken for functional symptoms. Fatigability has to be sought during the examination by asking the patient to repeatedly abduct the arms and then resist adduction by the examiner. There may be a family history of associated autoimmune disease (Grave's disease, rheumatoid arthritis, pernicious anaemia). The disease may seen temporarily following treatment with D penicillamine and these patients are negative for acetylcholine (ACH) antibodies.

Investigations

- Specific ACH receptor antibodies (IgG) occur in 90%
- Tensilon (edrophonium; a short acting anticholinesterase) test. Transient improvement in the weakness occurs over 5 min. The test can occuasionaly provoke anaphylaxis
- Nerve stimulation tests. A gradual trail off in action potentials occurs with repeated nerve stimulation
- CT scan of chest for thymoma or thymus hyperplasia
- Spirometry to assess for respiratory muscle weakness

Crises may occur due to 'stress' (infection, surgery, drugs), with respiratory failure being the most important complication.

Treatment

- Pyridostigmine (long-acting anticholinesterase)
- Steroids for moderate or severe myasthenia or myasthenia not responsive to anticholinesterases
- Azathiopine and cyclosporin as steroid sparing agents
- Thymectomy: younger patients (<40 years) who are antibody positive may benefit from removal of the thymus even if the gland is normal. Seventy per cent have thymus hyperplasia. Older patients may require removal if a thymoma is present (10%) however, improvement of the symptoms may not occur

(3) Multiple sclerosis (see also OSCE 11, p. 242)

The give away is the previous neurological complaint, even though this may be resolved. It is highly suggestive of the typical relapsing and remitting pattern of MS, with an intervening asymptomatic period. In any patient presenting with weak legs, a lesion compressing the spinal cord must be excluded (MRI or CT scanning) as a matter of urgency.

The differential diagnosis of a spinal cord lesion causing paraparesis

- Compression
  - Trauma
  - Tumour (secondary > primary)
  - Abscess (TB or pyogenic)
  - Spondylosis
  - Disc prolapse
- Inflammation (myelitis)

- MS
- Infections, e.g. TB, syphilis, viral, HIV infection
- Vitamin B12 deficiency
- Carcinoma (a paraneoplastic syndrome)
- Infarction
  - Vasculitis (PAN, SLE, syphilis)
  - Dissecting aortic aneurysm

(4) Subarachnoid haemorrhage (SAH)

(see also OSCE 38, p. 293)

SAH is diagnosed given the history of acute onset of occipital headache. SAH accounts for 10% of cerebrovascular accidents.

Causes of SAH

- **Berry aneurysms** (70%): 80% are on the anterior aspect of the circle of Willis. These are found incidentally in up to 5% of people at post-mortem. Fortunately, however, the incidence of SAH is much less common (1 in 10 000 per year). There are many associations of berry aneurysm, e.g. aortic coarctation, polycystic kidney disease, Ehlers–Danlos syndrome, neurofibromatosis I, Marfan's syndrome
- **AV malformations** (5%)
- **Unknown**

The aneurysms are clinically silent until rupture. Thirty per cent of patients have a 'herald bleed' presenting as a resolving severe headache, several days before the main rupture. SAH presents as a severe headache that occurs with an abrupt onset, is often occipital and is described as being like a 'blow to the head'. These patients have features of meningeal irritation (neck stiffness and photophobia) and acute bacterial meningitis is often the main alternative diagnosis in practice. False localizing signs such as 3rd and 6th cranial nerve palsies as well as ipsilateral hemiplegia may occur due to raised intracranial pressure.

Risk factors for bleeds in patients with berry aneurysms

- Smoking
- Hypertension
- Alcoholism
- Family history of SAH

Complications of SAH

- **Coning:** raised ICP causing medullary compression by cerebellar tonsils, leading to Cushing's triad as above (hypertension/bradycardia/respiratory depression)
- **Re-bleed** due to clot contraction at around day 10 in 30% of cases
- **Focal neurological loss** (like any stroke)
- **Vasospasm** presenting as a stroke at day 2–4 in 25%
- **Syndrome of Inappropriate ADH** production causing a low sodium and rarely pulmonary oedema (neurogenic pulmonary oedema)
- **Arrhythmias** due to massive adrenergic response/ long QT syndrome (torsade de pointes)
- **Hydrocephalus** due to a block in CSF circulation through the aqueduct or the fourth ventricle
- **Glycosurea:** in an unconscious patient with glycosuria think of diabetic ketoacidosis, sub-arachnoid haemorrhage or salicylate overdose

The medical management of SAH is supportive (ABC) and observing for complications (as above). Nimodipine (a calcium channel blocker) is used to help prevent vasospasm. Neurosurgical clipping is used selectively in patients with smaller bleeds (no focal neurology) at around day 2 to prevent re-bleeds.

(5) Cervical spondylosis causing cervical myelopathy

This is the most likely diagnosis, although any compressive lesion cannot be excluded from this history. Gradual stenosis of the spinal canal leads to distil upper motor neurone weakness below the lesion. Associated nerve root compression at the site of the lesion (often C5/6 or C6/7) leads to mixed UMN and LMN features in the upper limb. This can produce the so-called 'inversion of reflexes'; testing the supinator reflex, results in an absent reflex of supination (LMN response), but paradoxically produces brisk finger flexion (UMN response). The dorsal columns (position and vibration) are more frequently compromised than the spinothalamic tracts (pain and temperature) resulting in upper limb 'drift' (the patient is asked to maintain position of arms outstretched with palms up-turned with the eyes closed).

Answer 8

The common metabolic bone disease pictures:

	Calcium	Phosphate	Alkaline phosphatase
Osteoporosis	NR	NR	NR
Paget's disease	NR (unless rested)	NR	↑↑
Hyperparathyroidism	↑	↓	↑
Osteomalacia	NR or ↓	NR or ↓	↑
Myeloma	↑	Any	NR

(1) Multiple myeloma

A malignancy (monoclonal) of plasma cells producing an abnormal amount of immunoglobulin (gammopathy) that is usually IgG or A, but occasionally IgD. Light chains are excreted in the urine in 66% and are termed Bence Jones proteins and are toxic to renal tubules. Pancytopenia, raised ESR and hypercalcaemia with *normal* alkaline phosphatase are very suggestive of myeloma.

The clinical features of myeloma
- **Marrow failure**
  - Due to plasma cell infiltration, causing . . .
  - Bleeding, anaemia and infections
- **Bone destruction**
  - Bone pain, fractures and hypercalcaemia
- **Renal impairment** due to:
  - Light chain direct nephrotoxicity
  - Light chain cast formation (5% present as ARF)
  - Hypercalcaemia
  - Hyperuricaemia
  - Amyloidosis
  - Contrast nephropathy if given
- **Hyperviscosity symptoms**
  - Headaches
  - Blurred vision
  - Tiredness

Investigations
- Immunoelectrophoresis of urine for Bence Jones proteins (66%)
- Serum electrophoresis shows a monoclonal band (M band)
- Lytic lesions (small irregular and 'punched out') on skeletal radiographs, e.g. skull

Differential diagnosis of lytic skull lesions
- Myeloma
- Hyperparathyroidism
- Metastatic deposits
- Leukaemia
- Sickle cell disease
- Histiocytosis
- Sarcoidosis
- Paget's disease
- Infections, e.g. TB

(2) Paget's disease

Characteristically gives a very high alkaline phosphatase with normal calcium and phosphate. Hypercalcaemia may occur if patient is on bed rest. The aetiology is unknown; however, it is more common in northern England, and with increasing age (10% of 90-year-olds). Canine distemper virus has been suggested as the cause. Increased bone turnover with abnormal remodelling leads to irregular, bulky, vascular and weak bone. Enlargement of the skull vault, and bowing of the weight-bearing long bones occurs.

Although Paget's is frequently asymptomatic, **clinical features include** . . .
- Bone pain
- Fractures
- Closure of foramina resulting in deafness, optic atrophy and lower motor neurone facial nerve palsy.
- Sarcoma (1%) suspect if more bone pain and swelling occurs together with a rapid rise in alkaline phosphatase

The management of Paget's disease
- Analgesia
- Bisphosphonates to prevent bone turn over

Other causes of skull enlargement
- Rickets
- Achondroplasia
- Congenital hydrocephalus
- Thalassaemia

(3) Osteomalacia

Proximal myopathy is noted in this Asian female, who is at risk of dietary and photosynthetic vitamin D3 deficiency. There may be few symptoms in osteomalacia. Bone softening may produce pain. In children the typical deformity of Rickets may develop. Suspect osteomalacia if:
- *Calcium low*
  consequence of low vitamin D3
- *Phosphate low*
  Raised PTH secondary to low calcium
- *Raised alkaline phosphatase*
  Although not as high as Paget's
  Bone radiographs may show Looser's zones, 'pseudo-fracture' like band demineralization, often in the upper femur or pubic rami.

Vitamin D is a fat-soluble vitamin. As a steroid hormone it has an intracellular receptor in the target cell influencing the synthesis of mRNA. Most vitamin D is derived from manufacture in the skin using sunlight in the conversion of 7-dehydrocholesterol. A small proportion is obtained from the diet. Next, 25 position and then 1 position hydroxylation occurs in the liver and kidney, respectively, to produce the metabolically active 1,25 dihydroxycholecalciferol.

Actions of vitamin D
- **GIT:** increases calcium absorption
- **Bone:** increases bone uptake of calcium
- **Parathythroid gland:** acts to inhibit the release of parathormone in response to any given calcium level. In effect it makes the threshold for parathormone release a lower (predicted) level of serum calcium

Excess vitamin D therapy will cause hypercalcaemia.

Causes of low vitamin D3 (osteomalacia)
- Poor sun exposure
- Malnutrition
- Malabsorption e.g. coeliac disease, gastric surgery
- Hepatic failure (25 hydroxylation)
- Renal failure (1,25 hydroxylation)
- Vitamin D resistance (X-linked dominant); phosphateuria (due to secondary hyperparathyroidism) and low serum phosphate levels occur
- Drugs: barbiturates, phenytoin induce the hepatic metabolism of vitamin D

(4) Primary hyperparathyroidism

In this case, symptoms of hypercalcaemia, a very raised calcium (therefore not secondary hyperparathyroidism), low phosphate and raised PTH indicate primary hyperparathyroidism. Hyperplasia of the parathyroid glands or a single parathyroid adenoma is responsible for the excess parathormone production. Note that it is possible for some tumours (e.g. bronchogenic small cell tumours) to produce ectopic parathormone. Also note that parathyroid hyperplasia may be part of multiple endocrine neoplasia type I (MEN I, along with pituitary adenomas, pancreatic insulinomas, adrenal and thyroid non-functioning adenomas).

An elevated parathormone in the presence of raised calcium indicates hyperparathyroidism. Hand radiographs may show sub-periosteal erosions in the phalanges. The other main differential diagnoses of raised calcium include . . .
- Metastatic bone disease
- Myeloma
- Sarocoidosis
- Thyrotoxicosis

Diagnosing hypercalcaemia

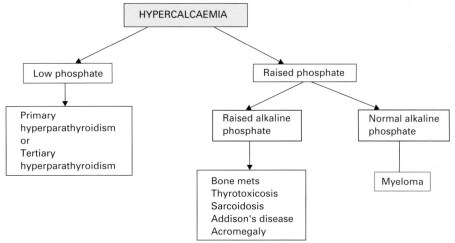

Malignancy is suggested by low albumin, low chloride, alkalosis and a raised alkaline
phosphatase.

Acute management of hypercalcaemia

For any calcium > 3.5 mmol/L or symptomatic with
calcium > 3.0 mmol/L):

- IV fluids
  N saline 3 L 24 h diuresis, monitor fluid balance
- Furosemide
  80 mg day
- Bisphosphonates
  Malignancy (especially valuable)
- Steroids
  Sarcoidosis/vitamin D excess/myeloma
- (calcitonin)
  Rarely used due to flushing/nausea and short-lived
  action
- Investigate and treat the cause

(5) Osteoporosis with pathological fracture

The history suggests osteoporotic vertebral crush
fracture. There may not be a history of trauma. Clinically
the main differential would be metastatic disease.
Osteoporosis produces no imbalance of bone biochemistry. Clinically it is usually silent. Its importance lies in
predisposition to fracture risk both spontaneously and
from minor trauma (neck of femur and forearm
fractures) and the impact this has upon health service
resources.

Risk factors for osteoporosis

- Females
- White
- Post-menopausal/early menopause
- Immobility
- Obesity/underweight
- Malnutrition
- Smoking
- Heparin treatment
- Steroid usage/Cushing's disease
- Metabolic: causes of hypercalcaemia (see diagram
  above)

The diagnosis of osteoporosis relies upon thinking of
the possibility of the condition in a patient, then performing bone densitometry in those with risk factors or
following a low trauma fracture.

Management of osteoporosis

- Health education
- Diet (1.5 g calcium daily and 800 i.u. of vitamin D)
- Exercise
- Stop smoking
- Bisphosphonates
- Hormone replacement therapy

Answer 9

There are several important concepts to understand in acid–base balance:

The anion gap

- Negative charges and positive charges in the body are equal
- An acid is a proton donor and so is negatively charged (anion)
- Anion gap $= (Na + K) - (HCO_3 + Cl) = 10{-}18$ mmol/L
- The anion gap approximates the number of other negatively charged, e.g. proteins, phosphates, sulphates and ACIDS not measured in routine U and Es
- So, if in the presence of an acidosis the **anion gap is raised**, it suggests an **unmeasured acid (anion) is the cause**. This may be either endogenous (e.g. renal failure or ketoacidosis) or exogenous acid (e.g. salicylate overdose)

Causes of an acidosis with a raised anion gap

- Renal failure
- Lactate:
  Hypoxia
  Hepatic failure
  Metformin therapy
- Ketosis:
  Starvation
  Diabetic ketoacidosis
- Exogenous acid:
  Salicylate
- If in an acidosis the **anion gap is normal**, an acid is not the cause. The cause will usually be **bicarbonate loss** (Na^+/HCO_3^-); a *balanced* loss of anions and cations has occurred thus there is no change to the calculated anion gap as above.

Causes of acidosis with a normal anion gap

- Loss of HCO_3^-:
  Diarrhoea/fistulae
- Ureterosigmoidostomy
- Renal tubular acidosis (H^+/CL^- retention $=$ *balanced* loss of cations and anions)
- Acetazolamide therapy (carbonic anhydrase inhibitor $= HCO_3^-$ loss)

Henderson–Hasselbach equation

$$H^+ + HCO_3^- \longleftrightarrow H_2CO_3 \longleftrightarrow CO_2 + H_2O$$

Buffers

- Absorb H^+ in times of excess
- Therefore they are weak acids by definition
- Buffers in the body
  - Intracellular (50%):
    HCO_3^-
    Tissue protein
    Phosphate
  - Kidneys (30%):
    HCO_3^- (via carbonic anhydrase)
    Ammonium
    PO_4^-
  - Extracellular fluid:
    HCO_3^-
    PO_4^-
    Protein
  - RBCs:
    Hb binds H^+
    HCO_3^-

(1) Metabolic acidosis (acidosis plus evidence of hyperventilation)
Low HCO_3^- due to consumption by buffering. The CO_2 is low as it is 'blown off' by hyperventilation giving high O_2 (therefore not type I respiratory failure). Therefore, acid overload is the primary problem. See notes above for causes. We cannot tell where the acid is coming from based on the information given, i.e. there is no information with which to calculate the anion gap.

(2) Respiratory alkalosis (alkalosis plus evidence of hyperventilation)
Hyperventilation can be seen by the depressed CO_2 again. The low O_2 may cause confusion here; it is not pertinent to a description of the problem as asked. The cause of the hyperventilation cannot be determined. Here the patient had pneumonia with painful pleurisy giving hyperventilation plus a type I respiratory failure pattern.

(3) Compensated respiratory acidosis
Type II respiratory failure with a normal pH (only just) but raised HCO_3^-, demonstrates compensation for pre-existing acidosis. Here COPD with chronic respiratory acidosis. Other causes of respiratory acidosis include:
- Severe asthma with (type II) respiratory failure due to fatigue
- Obesity
- Postoperative (abdominal pain)
- Obstructive sleep apnoea

- Opiate overdose
- Neuromuscular respiratory failure, e.g. Guillain–Barré syndrome

(4) Respiratory alkalosis

CO_2 and HCO_3^- are blown off, and O_2 is high due to hyperventilation. Causes include:

- Anxiety
- Pain
- Early asthma due to hyperventilation (before fatigue has occurred)
- Early salicylate overdose
- Thyrotoxic crisis
- Over ventilation

(5) Metabolic alkalosis

Alkalosis is indicated without evidence of hyperventilation; it is therefore not respiratory. A left shift of the O_2 dissociation curve and depressed respiration occurs. Mild CO_2 retention occurs. Causes most commonly include acid loss in prolonged vomiting (pyloric stenosis). Efficient renal shedding of HCO_3^- usually prevents base excess alone from causing alkalosis.

The pattern of the **U and Es and blood gases in vomiting** should be remembered because it is common and produces an apparent paradoxical loss of acid in the urine despite the prevailing metabolic alkalosis. Vomiting causes loss of H^+ and Cl^-, but also K^+ and Na^+. A hypochloraemic metabolic alkalosis develops. Usually acidosis leads to acid urine; however, conserving total body K^+ assumes greater importance. K+ is therefore conserved in preference to H^+, which is lost via the renal Na^+/K^+ atpase mechanism. This results in **paradoxical aciduria**.

Remember that chloride exchanges for HCO_3^- across RBC membranes and so levels vary inversely; the so-called 'chloride shift'. Loss of chloride from extracellular fluid will cause alkalosis as HCO_3^- diffuses out of cells.

(6) None of these

This is uncompensated respiratory acidosis.

(7) None of these

This result is an error. High HCO_3^- with a severe acidosis???? Repeat the gases on a different machine.

Answer 10

(1) Mycoplasma pneumonia

A common cause of pneumonia in younger people. Often occurring in epidemics in the community. Clinical features include malaise and headache initially. Respiratory features may be sparse. There is a poor correlation between the chest film (which can be dramatic) and the clinical appearances.

Complications (with useful mnemonic)

• Myocarditis, pericarditis	**MY**
• Erythema multiforme	**RASH**
• Haemolytic anaemia, thrombocytopenia	**HAS**
• Myalgia	**MY**
• Meningo-encephalitis, Guillain–Barré syndrome, transverse myelitis, cranial nerve palsies, cerebellar ataxia	**MENINGES**
• GI features, e.g. diarrhoea and vomiting	**GOING**

The diagnosis can be made by isolation of organism from the respiratory tract or by a four-fold rise in specific IgM antibody titre. Treatment is with erythromycin or tetracycline.

(2) Aspiration causing pneumonia

The question relies on remembering the causes of a non-resolving respiratory tract infection:

- **Wrong diagnosis**
  - PE/CCF/Sub-phrenic abscess
- **Underlying disease**
  - CA/TB/bronchiectasis/CF/HIV
- **Wrong treatment**
  - Antibiotic choice/atypical pneumonia
- **Complication of pneumonia**
  - Abscess/empyema/pleural effusion
- **Recurrent infection**
  - Aspiration/foreign body/intubation/fistula/HIV

Here the patient is previously well suggesting no underlying disease or recurrent problem. The failure of aggressive treatment with broad spectrum IV antibiotic coverage (including for atypical organisms) implies using the wrong treatment is not to blame. Aspiration therefore is the most likely explanation, either of a foreign body (e.g. peanut) or vomit post-alcohol. The right lower lobe is most commonly the recipient of aspirated material as the right main bronchus is a more vertical branch from the trachea than the left main bronchus.

(3) Lymphoma
In this case a recurrent disease with pulmonary and liver deposits plus B symptoms.

Hodgkin's lymphoma
- Reed–Sternberg Cells
- Painless node enlargement
- B symptoms: sweats or weight loss >10%
- Extra-nodal sites may be involved, e.g. liver, lung, bone, spleen
- Staging (± B symptoms, e.g. Ia, Ib, IIa etc.):
  - I   One nodal area
  - II Two nodal areas on same side of diaphragm or one area plus an extra-nodal site
  - III Nodes on both sides of the diaphragm or spleen plus another area
  - IV Widespread extra-nodal disease

Non-Hodgkin's lymphoma
- No Reed–Sternberg cells.
- T or B cells (mostly B cells)
- Extra-nodal involvement more commonly involved than Hodgkin's disease, e.g. bone, GIT, lung, brain
- Staging is less important because the disease is usually widespread at presentation
- Grading:
  - **Low grade**
    Slow growth
    Difficult to cure
    Mature cells
  - **High grade**
    Rapid growth
    Immature cells
    CHOP chemotherapy
  - **Lymphoblastic**
    Very immature cells
    CNS involvement occurs

Differential diagnosis of lymphadenopathy
- **Infections**
  - Bacterial: local or regional
  - Mycobacterial: **TB**
  - Viral: HIV, **infectious mononucleosis**
  - Protozoal: toxoplasmosis
- **Lymphoma**
  Hodgkin's/non-Hodgkin's

- Leukaemia
  Chronic lymphocytic leukaemia (CLL)
- **Malignancy**
  Metastatic or reactive to local tumour
- Miscellaneous
  - Connective tissue disease: rheumatoid arthritis, SLE
  - Sarcoidosis
  - Histiocytosis

(4) Cystic fibrosis
The clinical pattern is of chronic lung disease and malabsorption. This is a recessive (1 in 25 carriers) condition. The defective gene (delta 508), which is situated on the long arm of chromosome 7, produces cystic fibrosis transmembrane regulator protein (CFTR) resulting in an abnormal chloride concentration in sweat. This results in viscous exocrine gland secretions. (See OSCE 35, p. 289.)

(5) Pulmonary tuberculosis
In this case, post-primary pulmonary TB in a typical at-risk patient.

Primary TB
- No previous exposure or immunity
- A Ghon focus occurs (the primary lesion) usually in the mid, upper zones peripherally and caseating hilar lymphadenopathy. The combination of the Ghon focus and hilar lymphadenopathy is termed the Primary Complex
- The patient is asymptomatic or has mild respiratory features
- Erythema nodosum may occur
- Self limiting frequently at this stage
- The pulmonary lesion heals with calcification (visible on the CXR)
- Sero-conversion occurs

Post-primary TB
(See also answers to EMQ 18, Q4)
- Maybe years later
- Reactivation and spread of the primary infection to (in descending order of frequency):
  Lungs > bone > lymph nodes > CNS > GIT > renal tract > hepatosplenomegaly
- Weight loss, cough, haemoptysis, pleural effusions and pneumonia all may occur

Diagnosing tuberculosis
- **Chest radiograph**: TB is very unlikely with a normal chest film. Chest radiograph appearance includes:
  - *Apical shadowing*
    (The differential diagnosis of apical shadowing includes:
    Sarcoidosis
    Extrinsic allergic alveolitis
    Pneumoconiosis
    Aspergillosis
    Silicosis
    Ankylosing spondylitis)
  - Lobar pneumonia type collapse and consolidation
  - Effusions
  - Hilar lymphadenopathy
  - Miliary TB
- **Isolating 'acid alcohol fast bacilli'** (AAFBs) from: sputum, pleural biopsy, pleural aspirate bronchoscopy), lymph node biopsy, bone marrow, early morning urine, CSF. Note that mycobacterium tuberculosis is never a commensal, so even identification of just one organism gives the diagnosis.
- **PCR amplification** of TB DNA. The culture of TB (on Lowenstein–Jensen medium) takes several weeks, whereas PCR gives a result in a few days.

Treatment of tuberculosis

	Phase 1		Phase 2		
	Drugs	*Duration*	*Drugs*	*Duration*	*Total duration*
Respiratory and non-respiratory TB	Rifampicin Isoniazin Pyrazinamide Ethambutol	2 months	Rifampicin Isoniazid	4 months	6 months
TB meningitis	Rifampicin Isoniazin Pyrazinamide Ethambutol	2 months	Rifampicin Isoniazid	10 months	12 months

Ethambutol may be omitted from phase 1 initially if the patient is at low risk:
- No immunosuppression (HIV)
- No previous chest disease
- Caucasian
- No contact with drug resistant cases

Anti-tuberculous drug therapy side effects include:
- **R**ifampicin
  - Liver enzyme induction/thrombocytopenia
  - Pink staining of urine
- **I**soniazid
  - Perpheral neuropathy/allergy/rash/hepatitis
  - Give isoniazide with Vitamin B6 (pyridoxine)
- **P**yrazinamide
  - Hepatic toxicity
- **E**thambutol
  - Retrobulbar neuritis (dose related)

Answer 11

(1) Iron deficiency
A microcytic anaemia.

Causes of a microcytic anaemia
Use the mnemonic **ITSA** . . .
- **I**ron deficiency
- **T**halassaemia
- **S**ideroblastic anaemia: a failure of iron incorporation into haem; 'ring sideroblasts' occur in the marrow. It may be:
  - Congenital (sex linked and responds to pyridoxine)
    or
  - Aquired:
    Idiopathic
    Secondary to alcohol, malignancy, lead poisoning or drugs toxicity
- **A**lumninium toxicity, e.g. haemodialysis

Only iron deficiency states have low stores (ferritin). Other causes fail to correct with iron.

Causes of iron deficiency
- **Bleeding,** e.g. upper GI, lower GI, menstrual, GU, epistaxis
- **Dietary deficiency**
- **Malabsorption:** any cause, especially post-gastrectomy as an acid environment is required to keep iron in soluble (absorbable) ferrous form (Fe^{3+})
- **Metabolic:** excess use in pregnancy, hyperthyroidism, psoriasis and malignancy

(2) Options D, E, H, J, L and N
These six options may be associated with a pancytopenia. In this case, the most likely cause is vitamin B12 or folate deficiency in light of the much-raised MCV. Bone marrow biopsy would help differentiate the causes.

Causes of pancytopenia
- **Aplasic anaemia**
  - *Primary*
    Congenital (e.g. Fanconi's syndrome)
    Idiopathic (50% of all)
  - *Secondary*
    Toxic drugs/chemicals:
      Gold
      Chloramphenicol
      Cytotoxics, e.g. cyclophosphamide, doxorubicin
      Immunosuppressives, e.g. azathioprine, methotrexate
    Thymoma
    Pregnancy
    Infections:
      Viral hepatitis
      HIV
      Measles
      Tuberculosis
      Parvovirus
      Paroxysmal nocturnal haemaglobinuria
- **Megaloblastosis**
  - *B12 deficiency*
    Pernicious anaemia (autoimmune)
    Malabsorption:
      Gastrectomy
      Terminal ileal disease, e.g. Crohn's
      Bacterial overgrowth metabolizes B12
      Diphyllobothrium latum
    Poor diet (vegans)
  - *Folate deficiency*

Dietary deficiency
Metabolic use increased (pregnancy, malignancy, thyroid disease)
Malabsorption
Drugs:

Methotrexate	Inhibit
Trimethoprim	dihydrofolate
Pyrimethamine	reductase
Phenytoin	

- **Marrow infiltration**
  - Acute leukaemia
  - Lymphoma
  - Myeloma
  - Carcinoma
  - Myelofibrosis
- **Hypersplenism**
  - Infection (many)
  - Haematological, e.g. CML
  - Portal hypertension
  - Storage disease
  - SLE
  - Sarcoid
  - Amyloid
  - Rheumatoid (Felty's syndrome)
- **Autoimmune**
  - Idiopathic
  - SLE
  - Haematological:
    CLL
    Lymphoma
    Hodgkin's
  - Drugs:
    Cyclosporins
    Methyldopa

(3) Causes A, C, G and H
Macrocytosis alone. Note that alcoholism or just regular alcohol consumption is the commonest cause of a macrocytosis and is often the only evidence of excess use ('the HbA1C of alcohol intake'). Macrocytosis does not necessarily mean megaloblasts in marrow (caused by defective DNA synthesis due to B12 or folate deficiency).

Causes of a raised MCV
- B12 deficiency
- Folate deficiency ⎱ megaloblastic marrow
- Drugs impairing DNA synthesis: ⎰
  - Methotrexate
  - Azathioprine
- Reticulocytosis (large young red cells)

- Haemoylsis
- Haemorrhage
- Leukaemia
- Liver disease/*alcohol*
- Hypothyroidism
- Pregnancy

This is an important list to remember as macrocytosis is common and the differential diagnosis is short.

(4) Primary polycythemia

Primary polycythemia (Polycythemia vera) is suggested here. It is one of the myeloproliferative disorders together with:

- Essential thrombocythemia
- Myelofibrosis
- Chronic myeloid leukaemia

Here all the myeloid cell line (RBCs, platelets and non-lymphocyte WBCs) are raised and this is suggestive of primary polycythemia vera (and not chronic hypoxaemia). In many presenting cases, however, only the Hb may be raised; the WCC is raised in 70% and the platelet count in 50% of cases. Confusingly sometimes iron deficiency anaemia can co-exist, so the packed cell volume (PCV) is a more reliable indicator.

An insidious onset in later life occurs with hypertension, itching and bleeding (abnormal platelet function). Symptoms of hyperviscosity can occur such as vertigo, tinnitus and blurred vision. Strokes, intermittent claudication and angina are more common. On examination there is facial plethora (reddening), splenomegaly (in 70% of cases; due to increased turnover of RBCs) and hepatomegaly (in 50% of cases) may occur.

The differential diagnosis of raised haemaglobin includes **secondary polycythemia** due to raised erythropoietin (EPO), which may be:

- Appropriate
  - Hypoxia
  - Altitude
  - COPD
  - Obstructive sleep apnoea
- Inappropriate and due to ectopic EPO production by various tumours, e.g. renal or cerebellar.

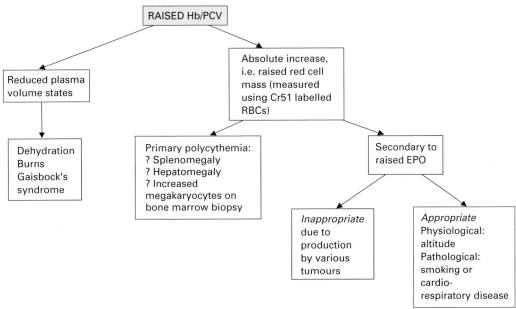

Gaisbock's syndrome is an apparently idiopathic condition often found in middle-aged male smokers. The polycythemia is 'relative' to a reduction in plasma volume.

The investigation of polycythemia includes a **red cell mass** estimation using Cr51-labelled red cells, to decide if the polycythemia is absolute or relative, and **erythropoeitin levels** (which are normal in primary polycythemia).

Management of primary polycythemia

- Repeated venesection
- Hydroxyuria therapy   } Control marrow production
- Radioactive P^{32}

- Allopurinol to prevent gout
- Cimetidine helps controls itch

Prognosis in primary polycythemia
- 30% progress to myelofibrosis
- 5% progress to AML

(5) Options J and K
A normocytic anaemia. Any chronic disease, e.g. renal failure, TB, rheumatoid arthritis, SLE. Also acute bleeding (with fluid replacement) may appear like this before there is time for a marrow response (reticulocytosis/microcytosis).

(6) Options H and N
An isolated neutropenia is the only abnormality.

Causes of neutropenia include:
- Infections: overwhelming or poor reserve (old)
- Drugs
  - Cytotoxics
  - Immunosupressives
  - Carbimazole
- Cyclical: idipoathic/benign
- Racial normal variance, e.g. African races
- Congenital: Kostman's syndrome
- As part of a pancytopenia [see Question 11(2) above]

Question 12

(1) Oesophageal carcinoma
A typical history of progressive dysphagia for solids with weight loss. The jaundice is likely to be due to secondary tumour deposits in the liver. Note that oesophageal varices are not associated with significant dysphagia.

Pathology of oesophageal tumours
- Squamous cell type
  - Upper and middle third
  - High incidence in far east
  - Male sex preponderance, smokers, alcohol, age
  - Predisposing pathologies:
    Achalasia
    Plummer–Vinson syndrome
    Coeliac disease
- Adenocarcinoma
  - Lower third
  - Follows Barrett's oesophagus (intestinal metaplasia)

Clinical presentation
- Often asymptomatic until late
- Progressive solid dysphagia
- Suddern presentation with bolus obstruction may occur
- Pain (late feature)
- Massive weight loss occurs

Investigations
- Endoscopy and biopsy
- Barium swallow shows a long irregular stricture
- Staging CT scanning of the chest and abdomen
- Endoscopic ultrasound is an accurate alternative

Management
- Palliation with stenting at endoscopy
- Radiotherapy and chemotherapy for squamous tumours
- Surgery: radical oesophagectomy; high mortality.

Prognosis
- 2–5% 5-year survival overall
- 10% after surgery

(2) Gastroesophageal reflux disease (GORD)
A very common condition. There is poor correlation between the severity of the symptoms of GORD and the extent of the oesophagitis seen at endoscopy. The lower oesophageal 'sphincter' is a composite of the following mechanisms . . .
- The intra-abdominal section of the last 4 cm of the oesophagus which enters the stomach at an oblique angle creating a flap-valve
- The prominent folds of gastric mucosa around the oeseophageal entry known as the mucosal rosette
- The left and right crus of the diaphragm, which wrap around the lower oesophagus like a sling causing compression

GORD risk factors
- Obesity
- Pregnancy
- Smoking
- Alcohol (relaxes lower oesophageal sphincter)
- Coffee
- Large meals
- Lying flat

Clinical features of GORD

- Burning retrosternal pain, positional (differential of cardiac pain)
- Water brash (an acidic water in the mouth)
- Aspiration (nocturnal cough and wheeze)
- Dysphagia
- Strictures (regurgitation, weight loss, aspiration pneumonia)
- Endoscopic findings vary:
  - Normal
  - Hiatus hernia (NB hiatus hernias are usually asymptomatic)
  - Oesophagitis
  - Plummer–Vinson syndrome

Oesophageal pH probe monitoring with manometry is the definitive investigation and should be performed to confirm the diagnosis if surgery is being considered. A pH value of less than 4, which correlates well with symptoms, supports the diagnosis.

The management of GORD

- Reduce risk factors if possible (especially weight loss, small meals, elevate the head of the bed and alcohol avoidance).
- High dose proton pump inhibitors, e.g. Omeprazole 40 mg o.d. These are now considered safe for long-term maintenance therapy
- Pro-motility drugs that speed gastric emptying, e.g. metoclopramide
- Surgery: Nissen fundoplication [rarely necessary due to the effectiveness of high-dose proton pump inhibitors (PPI) regimens]. Patients must be warned pre-operatively of inability to pass wind and of bloating, which reflect the effectiveness of the procedure

There is no evidence for a role of *H. pylori* in the pathogenesis of GORD, nor eradication therapy producing clinical benefit.

(3) Gastric carcinoma

A typical history is presented here; usually due to an adenocarcinoma in the pyloric region. New dyspepsia in patients over the age of 50 years should be referred for endoscopy as the incidence of gastric carcinoma rises significantly (see OSCE 8, p. 236). Typically the disease presents late with metastases having already occurred. Here Virchow's node (Troisier's sign) is present and is palpated behind the left sternoclavicular joint.

Remember Virchow's node drains the respiratory tract and upper GIT. The rash is acanthosis nigricans (see OSCE 28, p. 279). Gastric lymphoma should be excluded on biopsy which if present carries a better prognosis.

Risk factors for gastric carcinoma

- Smoking
- Alcohol
- *H. pylori* infection
- Lower socio-economic class
- Japanese race
- Blood group A
- Pernicious anaemia
- Previous gastric surgery

(4) Achalasia of the oesophagus

There is an absence of normal oesophageal peristalsis and a failure of the lower oesophageal sphincter to relax. The history is long compared to carcinoma of the oesophagus and dysphagia occurs for both solids and liquids. Retrosternal pain may occurs due to spasm of the oesophagus. Weight loss can occur but is usually slight. Regurgitation and aspiration may occur. A barium swallow examination shows oesophageal dilatation and the classical 'rats tail' narrowing distally (see p. 182). A fluid level may be seen on chest radiograph. Oesophageal manometry shows a failure of lower oesophageal relaxation.

Management of achalasia

- PPIs for reflux symptoms
- Surgery: Heller's myotomy

Differential diagnoses of dysphagia

- CA oesophagus
- Chagas' disease: neural plexus damage due to South American trypanosomiasis. A cardiomyopathy also occurs
- Schatzki ring (benign fibrous ring lower oesophagus)
- Plummer–Vinson web (post-cricoid region; associated with iron deficiency)
- Peptic stricture
- Systemic sclerosis
- Dysmotility problems
  - Myasthenia gravis
  - Stroke
  - Myotonic dystrophy
- Infections

- *Candida* (HIV associated; pain occurs)
- Herpes simplex

(5) Menetrier's disease

Small print but well recognized. The aetiology is un-known. Loss of protein-rich mucus from hypertrophied gastric mucosal folds occurs with resulting hypo-protinaemia and occasional pain may occur. The condition is thought to be pre-malignant.

(6) Globus

The unfortunate term 'globus hystericus' has now been dropped. This is a very common functional illness. A typical history is given in the question. It usually requires no investigation, the diagnosis being made on the history alone. Reassurance is required after a thorough history. There are (should be) no significant findings on examination. Like irritable bowel syndrome and dyspepsia, be careful about diagnosing this for the first time in the elderly when more serious pathology is more likely.

Paper 3 Answers

MCQs

[1]	(a) T	(b) F	(c) F	(d) F	(e) T
[2]	(a) T	(b) F	(c) T	(d) F	(e) F
[3]	(a) T	(b) F	(c) F	(d) T	(e) F
[4]	(a) F	(b) T	(c) F	(d) F	(e) T
[5]	(a) T	(b) F	(c) T	(d) F	(e) T
[6]	(a) T	(b) F	(c) F	(d) T	(e) F
[7]	(a) F	(b) T	(c) T	(d) F	(e) T
[8]	(a) T	(b) T	(c) T	(d) T	(e) F
[9]	(a) F	(b) F	(c) F	(d) T	(e) F
[10]	(a) T	(b) F	(c) F	(d) F	(e) T
[11]	(a) T	(b) T	(c) T	(d) F	(e) F
[12]	(a) F	(b) F	(c) F	(d) F	(e) T
[13]	(a) T	(b) T	(c) T	(d) T	(e) F
[14]	(a) F	(b) F	(c) F	(d) T	(e) F
[15]	(a) T	(b) T	(c) T	(d) T	(e) T
[16]	(a) F	(b) F	(c) F	(d) T	(e) F
[17]	(a) F	(b) T	(c) F	(d) T	(e) F
[18]	(a) F	(b) F	(c) F	(d) T	(e) F
[19]	(a) T	(b) T	(c) F	(d) T	(e) T
[20]	(a) T	(b) F	(c) F	(d) F	(e) F
[21]	(a) F	(b) F	(c) F	(d) T	(e) F
[22]	(a) F	(b) F	(c) T	(d) F	(e) F
[23]	(a) T	(b) F	(c) F	(d) T	(e) T
[24]	(a) F	(b) F	(c) T	(d) T	(e) F

[1] (a) T (b) F (c) F (d) F (e) T

(a) Pulmonary oedema is a frightening, life-threatening emergency characterized by extreme breathlessness. It may first become manifest at night as paroxysmal nocturnal dyspnoea (PND) due to pulmonary congestion following reabsorption of dependant oedema that has accumulated during the day. The relative insensitivity of the respiratory centre at night allows pulmonary congestion to develop to the extent that it only wakes the patient when respiratory impingement is severe. With progression, SOB manifests throughout the day.

(b) Rusty sputum is caused by pneumococcal pneumonia. Pulmonary oedema causes a cough that is characteristically productive of frothy pink (blood-tinged) sputum, which can be copious in amount.

(c) The CXR in cardiogenic pulmonary oedema shows Kerley-B lines, which signify interstitial oedema. Kerley-C lines are the least commonly seen of the Kerley lines, described by the Irish physician of the same name. They are short, fine lines on radiographs seen throughout the lungs, giving a reticular appearance. They may represent thickening of anastomotic lymphatics, or superimposition of many B lines. Kerley-A lines are thin lines that radiate from the hila. They do not branch and do not follow the course of pulmonary or bronchial vessels. It is thought that these lines represent thickening of the central interlobular septa by oedema fluid.

(d) Nebulizers and steroids are the initial pharmacological treatments for airway diseases such as COPD and asthma.

(e) The management of pulmonary oedema is essentially the management of acute heart failure: ABC, and then diuretics. Following this, early transfer to coronary care unit is vital. Diamorphic plus antiemetic help relieve breathlessness. If blood pressure is adequate (>100 mmHg), IV nitrate infusion improves pulmonary oedema. Non-invasive ventilatory support may be indicated if the patient is acidotic or hypoxic.

[2] (a) T (b) F (c) T (d) F (e) F

(a) **True aneurysms** involve all three layers of the arterial wall (intima, media and adventitia). They are associated with atherosclerosis. **False aneurysms** have a wall consisting only of a thickened fibrous capsule. They often arise secondary to trauma or infection and are also known as 'pseudoaneurysms'.

(b) **Saccular aneurysms** are eccentric irregular outpouchings of otherwise normal-appearing arteries. It is **fusiform aneurysms** that are diffuse and symmetrical. Either of these types can occur secondary to atherosclerosis.

(c) An aneurysm is defined as 'a focal dilatation of an artery to >1.5× its normal diameter'. Aneurysms **most commonly occur in the infrarenal aorta**, followed by the iliac arteries and then the popliteal arteries. They can, however, involve any artery of the arterial tree, including the splenic artery, the renal artery, the hepatic artery, the superior mesenteric artery and the coeliac axis.

(d) It is **Laplace's law** which explains how the tangential wall stress within an artery increases with increasing diameter . . .

$$J = (P \times r)/t$$

where J = tangential wall stress, P = intraluminal pressure, r = aneurysmal radius and t = wall thickness.

(e) In patients who are a good surgical risk (i.e. those with little concomitant co-morbidity), it is reasonable to offer repair when the aneurysm exceeds 5 cm in diameter. If the patient has serious risk factors, they are treated more conservatively until the approximate risk of the procedure is less than the risk of aneurysmal rupture. For example, currently the mortality from abdominal aortic aneurysm (AAA) repair in a good candidate is ~2–4%. However, the annual risk of rupture of a 4-cm AAA is approaching 1%, but that of a 5-cm AAA is more than 5%; this is the basis for repairing only those ≥5 cm.

[3] (a)T (b)F (c)F (d)T (e)F

(a) This is an accurate description of Raynaud's disease, which is caused by spasm of the arteries supplying the fingers and toes. This is precipitated by cold and relieved by heat. It is common, affecting 5% of the population.

(b) It predominantly affects young women.

(c) It is usually bilateral.

(d) It affects the digits of the upper limb more severely than those of the lower limb.

(e) Raynaud's can actually be treated by administration of 10 mg nifedipine t.d.s., a dihydropyridine calcium channel antagonist.

[4] (a)F (b)T (c)F (d)F (e)T

(a) The venous system can be divided into a **central system** (including the inferior and superior vena cava, iliac veins and subclavian veins) and a **peripheral system** (including upper and lower extremity veins, and the veins of the head and neck). Extremity veins can then be further divided into **superficial** or **deep**. For example, in the lower extremity, the superficial veins are the greater and lesser saphenous veins, whilst the deep veins are the common femoral, superficial femoral, profunda femoris, popliteal, anterior tibial, posterior tibial and peroneal veins (the last three are paired). The perforating veins in health carry blood **from superficial to deep veins**. Incompetence as a result of scarring or distension allows retrograde flow → varicosities and ulcerations.

(b) Thrombosis of the superficial veins of the lower extremity causes swelling, erythema and tenderness along the course of the involved vein. This situation should be treated with NSAIDs and warm compress. They do not require bed rest.

(c) The major risk factors for DVT are described by **Virchow's triad** . . .

1. **Stasis** (e.g. immobilization)
2. **Hypercoagulable state**
3. **Venous endothelial injury** (e.g. bony and soft tissue trauma to legs, stasis, venous distension, previous DVT)

Other risk factors for DVT may be split into . . .

Patient factors
- Old age
- Obesity
- Varicose veins
- Pregnancy
- Puerperium
- High-dose exogenous oestrogens (e.g. oral contraceptive pill)
- Previous DVT or PE
- Thrombophilia (e.g. antithrombin III deficiency, factor V Leiden, antiphospholipid antibodies, protein C/S deficiency)
- Smoking

Disease or surgical procedure
- Trauma
- Surgery
- Heart failure
- Recent MI
- Infection
- Inflammatory bowel disease
- Nephrotic syndrome
- Myeloproliferative disease

Beck's triad describes the situation in pericardial tamponade, where there is seen to be rising venous pressure, falling arterial pressure and decreased heart sounds. This is also known as the 'acute compression triad'.

(d) **Lasegue's sign** describes the situation where the patient is supine with their hip flexed, and dorsiflexion of the ankle causes pain or muscle spasm in the posterior thigh. It indicates irritation of the lumbar nerve roots or of the sciatic nerve.

(e) Surprisingly, this is true. Warfarin acts by inhibiting the vitamin K-dependant clotting factors, both pro-coagulant (factors II, VII, IX and X) and anti-coagulant (protein C, protein S). The half-life of existing protein C and S within the blood is much shorter than that of the pro-coagulant factors; therefore, for a short time after starting warfarin, the patient's blood will be hypercoagulable. This is why it is important to have heparin cover for 2–3 days when warfarin is first commenced.

[5] (a)T (b)F (c)T (d)F (e)T
(a) Rheumatic fever occurs due to infection with a β-haemolytic, Lancefield Group A *Streptococcus.*
(b) The pharyngeal infection with this bacterium may be followed by the clinical syndrome of rheumatic fever, which is actually due to an autoimmune reaction triggered by the infecting Streptococcus, and not due to direct infection of the heart or the production of a toxin.
(c) The **Aschoff nodule** is the characteristic lesion of rheumatic carditis, i.e. the inflammation of the heart caused by the autoimmune reaction. It is described as a granulomatous lesion with a central necrotic area occurring in the myocardium, especially in the subendocardium of the left ventricle. Also, small warty vegetations may develop on the endocardium, especially the heart valves, leading to varying degrees of regurgitation.
(d) Rheumatic fever is diagnosed using the **Duckett–Jones criteria**. There are five major criteria, and six minor. For diagnosis, you require evidence of antecedent streptococcal infection (e.g. throat cultures), plus either *two major* or *one major and two minor* criteria to be fulfilled.

The *major criteria* are . . .
1. Carditis
2. Polyarthritis
3. Chorea
4. Erythema marginatum
5. Subcutaneous nodules
   The *minor criteria* are . . .
1. Fever
2. Arthralgia
3. Previous history of rheumatic fever
4. Raised ESR/CRP
5. Leukocytosis
6. First-degree heart block on ECG

The Keith–Wagener criteria mentioned in the question are used to evaluate degrees of hypertensive retinopathy.
(e) The skin manifestations of rheumatic fever are twofold . . .

1. **Erythema marginatum**: transient pink rash with slightly raised edges, mostly on trunk or limbs; may coalesce into crescent- or ring-shaped patches
2. **Subcutaneous nodules**: painless, pea-sized, hard nodules, occurring especially under skin over tendons, joints and bony prominences

[6] (a)T (b)F (c)F (d)T (e)F
(a) Mitral regurgitation can indeed be acute (e.g. acute destruction of valve in bacterial endocarditis, rupture of chordae tendinae in MI) or chronic (e.g. due to rheumatic fever, cardiomyopathy, connective tissue disorders, collagen abnormalities).
(b) Regurgitation into the left atrium causes it to dilate, and because a proportion of left ventricular stroke volume is being lost to retrograde flow, it dilates also in order to maintain a normal cardiac output. These factors together lead to the apex beat being laterally displaced, and *'thrusting'*, or *'hyperdynamic'*, in nature. The cause of a 'heaving' apex beat is aortic stenosis.
(c) The murmur caused by mitral regurgitation is described as **pan-systolic**, being loudest at the apex, and radiating widely across the praecordium and into the axilla. This valve lesion also causes there to be a prominent third heart sound (S3) owing to the sudden rush of blood back into the left ventricle in early diastole. An early (or 'ejection') systolic murmur is caused by aortic stenosis.
(d) Long-standing mitral regurgitation does cause the heart size to become enlarged, due to enlargement of both of the chambers of the left side of the heart.
(e) It is mitral stenosis that is said to cause a classic malar flush of the face.

[7] (a)F (b)T (c)T (d)F (e)T
(a) Atrial myxoma is nothing to do with hypothyroidism. It is, in fact, the most common type of primary cardiac tumour (others include rhabdomyomas and sarcomas). Macroscopically it is a polypoid gelatinous structure attached to a pedicle.
(b) It most often develops in the left atrium, but it can arise in any of the chambers of the heart.
(c) It may be associated with constitutional symptoms, including dyspnoea, syncope or mild fever.
(d) It is not malignant in the sense that it does not metastasize. It tends to cause trouble more by obstructing valve orifices, or by being a site of thrombi that then embolize.
(e) Diagnosis is by echocardiography. Treatment is by surgical removal, which should effect a complete cure.

[8] (a)T (b)T (c)T (d)T (e)F

Sinus bradycardia is defined as 'a sinus rate of <60/min during the day, and <50/min at night'. It is usually asymptomatic, and is perfectly normal in athletes and elderly patients. Causes include . . .

- Hypothermia
- Hypothyroidism
- Addison's
- Raised intracranial pressure (the Cushing reflex)
- Drugs (including β-blockers, digoxin and other anti-arrhythmics)
- Sick sinus syndrome (= malfunctioning SA node)
- Acute ischaemia or infarction of the SA node
- Cholestatic jaundice

   Treatment of sinus bradycardia is only necessary if it is acute or symptomatic, and comprises administration of **atropine** (a drug which blocks the effects of vagal parasympathetic efferents on the heart), discontinuation of negatively chronotropic medication (e.g. β-blockers) or even temporary cardiac pacing.

[9] (a)F (b)F (c)F (d)T (e)F

(a) In sick sinus syndrome, the major abnormality is long intervals between P-waves on the ECG (>2s). The length of the PR interval is normal, as is the QRS complex.

(b) In first degree AV block, the major abnormality is simple prolongation of the PR interval to >0.2s (>5 small

squares). Despite this, a QRS complex follows every P-wave (i.e. 1 QRS: 1 P).

(c) The P:QRS ratio in first degree AV block is 1. There are *no* dropped beats, unlike in other forms of atrioventricular nodal block.

(d) In second-degree atrioventricular nodal block, some P-waves conduct through to the ventricle, whereas others do not. In **Wenckebach block phenomenon** (a.k.a. Mobitz type I) there is progressive prolongation of the PR interval, until a P-wave fails to conduct. The PR interval before the blocked P-wave is much longer than the PR interval after the blocked P-wave. In **Mobitz type II** second-degree heart block, there are random dropped QRS complexes that are *not* preceded by progressive PR elongation.

(e) This is false: the PR progressively elongates until eventually one of the P-waves fails to conduct to the ventricle → a 'dropped' QRS.

[10] (a)T (b)F (c)F (d)F (e)T

(a) T-cells comprise approximately 75% of the circulating lymphocyte population, the remainder being made up by B-cells.

(b) All types of immunoglobulin (IgG, IgA, IgM, IgE and IgD) are secreted by B-cells. They are never secreted by T-cells, although they are vitally important in presenting antigens to T-lymphocytes for further recognition and destruction. Characteristics of the five main types of immunoglobulin are detailed in the table below . . .

Ig type	Heavy chain	Mean adult serum levels (mg/mL)	Half life (days)	Complement fixation		Binding to mast cells	Crosses placenta	Mainly found
				Classical	Alternative			
IgG	χ	12	21	++	−	−	+	Serum; the antibody of secondary response; high affinity for antigen
IgA	α	1.7	6	−	+	−	−	Secretions; respiratory, GI and urinary tract
IgM	μ	1.5	10	+++	−	−	−	Intravascular pool; pentameric; major antibody of primary response

Continued

Ig type	Heavy chain	Mean adult serum levels (mg/mL)	Half life (days)	Complement fixation		Binding to mast cells	Crosses placenta	Mainly found
				Classical	Alternative			
IgE	ε	0.0002	2	−	−	+	−	Membrane bound to mast cells and basophils; anti-nematode activity
IgD	δ	0.03	3	−	−	−	−	Surface of B-cells; ? immunoregulatory role

(c) The primary defence against bacterial infection is cells of the polymorphonucleur phagocyte type, also known as neutrophils. T-lymphocytes are much more concerned with defence versus viruses and cancer cells.

(d) Following primary infection with Epstein–Barr virus (EBV) in infectious mononucleosis, EBV remains latent in B-lymphocytes, where it may subsequently become reactivated, especially in the immunocompromized host.

(e) The prognosis in **all** is believed to be poorer if the predominant clone of cells is of B-cell lineage, as opposed to **all** where the predominant clone of cells is of T-cell lineage. Reasons for this are unknown.

[11] (a)T (b)T (c)T (d)F (e)F

(a) The diagnosis of asthma is based on a greater than 15% improvement in either FEV1 or PEFR following the inhalation of a bronchodilator. A relevant clinical history and examination obviously must back this up.

(b) In cases where it is difficult to tell if a patient has COPD (which has a degree of reversibility) or asthma, microscopy of a sputum sample can be helpful. If the sample reveals clumps of eosinophils, then the diagnosis is likely to be asthma.

(c) Inhaled corticosteroids used to treat asthma in children are often blamed for retarding growth. Examples of these drugs include beclomethasone, budesonide and fluticasone. Whilst it is true that these drugs do have a number of side effects, including oral candidiasis, hoarseness and cataract formation, they only retard growth in high doses (>400 µg/day long term). It has been found that asthma itself retards growth in children, regardless of steroid usage.

(d) See answer above.

(e) Status asthmaticus, defined as acute severe asthma uncontrolled by medications, has four classic features that should not be forgotten . . .

1. Inability to complete a spoken sentence in one breath
2. RR > 25 (tachypnoea)
3. HR > 110 (tachycardia)
4. PEFR < 50% predicted or best effort in past

Life-threatening features in this situation include 'silent chest' (total lack of breath sounds on auscultation of the chest), cyanosis, feeble inspiratory effort, exhaustion, confusion or coma (due to CO_2 retention), bradycardia or hypotension, and a PEFR of <33% predicted or previous best effort. The immediate treatment of this situation should be . . .

→ ABC

→ Sit the patient up

→ Give nebulized salbutamol + maximal FiO_2; repeat every 30 min if situation does not improve

→ Add ipratropium nebulizers if no response

Still no response?

→ Salbutamol or terbutaline i.v. over 10 min (aminophylline can be used but it has a narrow therapeutic index)

→ Hydrocortisone i.v. every 4 h

Still no response?

→ Call anaesthetist for intubation and ventilation

→ ITU, consider IV Mg^{2+}

NB Saline nebs have no place in the treatment of acute severe asthma.

[12] (a) F (b) F (c) F (d) F (e) T

(a) Atypical pneumonias account for ~20% of all cases of pneumonia in the UK.

(b) Pneumonia is defined as 'inflammation of the substance of the lungs', and whilst it is usually due to infectious causes, it may also be caused by chemical means (e.g. aspiration of vomit), radiation (e.g. radiotherapy) and allergic mechanisms.

(c) Elderly patients who develop community-acquired pneumonia often have fewer symptoms than do young people, despite having florid clinical and radiological signs.

(d) The CXR in tuberculous pneumonia shows small areas of cavitation without obvious air-fluid levels. It is staphylococcal pneumonia that demonstrates large cavities containing air-fluid levels on CXR (reflects development of abscesses within the substance of the lung). Staphylococcal pneumonia has an exceedingly poor prognosis

(e) Aspiration pneumonia is indeed usually due to infection with anaerobic organisms. If the patient was erect when they aspirated, the most commonly involved portion of lung is the lower lobe on the right. If, however, the patient was lying down at aspiration, as is common in hospital, it is likely to be the middle lobe of the right lung that is involved. Aspiration pneumonia usually presents as insidious, low-grade fever, with a cough productive of foul-smelling sputum. The CXR typically shows consolidation preferentially in the lower lung fields.

[13] (a) T (b) T (c) F (d) T (e) F

(a) Bronchiectasis is defined as 'chronic and permanent dilation and destruction of bronchi or bronchioles as a sequel of inflammatory disease or obstruction'.

(b) It is the commonest cause in the UK of massive haemoptysis (>200 mL of fresh blood expectorated in any 24 h period), due to rupture of the associated high-pressure systemic bronchial arteries. Other causes of massive haemoptysis include pulmonary TB, aspergilloma, lung abscess and primary or secondary malignancies.

(c) Over 50% of cases of bronchiectasis are idiopathic, i.e. of no known cause. Around 30% occur post-severe infection. CF only causes around 3% of cases.

(d) Kartenager's syndrome causes a mucociliary clearance defect as in CF, which eventually leads to bronchiectasis. It is an autosomal recessive condition with variable penetrance that causes complete situs invertus, as well as bronchiectasis and chronic sinusitis due to impaired ciliary mucus transportation in the respiratory epithelium. The mechanism of the reversal of laterality remains an enigma.

(e) Bronchiectasis is *not* associated with Eisenmenger's syndrome, which is cardiac failure with significant right to left shunt producing cyanosis due to higher pressure on the right side of the shunt. Usually due to the Eisenmenger complex: a ventricular septal defect with right ventricular hypertrophy, severe pulmonary hypertension and frequent straddling of the defect by a misplaced aortic root.

[14] (a) F (b) F (c) F (d) T (e) F

(a) The fibrosis in CFA is diffuse, and occurs throughout both lung fields. It may show a preponderance for the lower lung fields.

(b) The onset of CFA is typically in late middle age — patients are usually in their 50s.

(c) CFA causes progressive and inexorable dyspnoea, progressing to cyanosis and eventually **type II respiratory failure** and cor pulmonale.

(d) Bilateral fine end-inspiratory crepitations are the hallmark of lung fibrosis on auscultation of the chest.

(e) CFA is incurable and inexorably leads to death, the median survival from diagnosis being ~5 years. Treatment with prednisolone and immunosuppression (azathioprine and cyclophosphamide) is given, but has demonstrated no benefit in appropriate clinical trials. Supportive therapy includes domicillary oxygen. In certain cases, single lung transplantation can be offered. New classification of diffuse parenchymal lung disease terms CFA 'usual interstitial pneumonia' or UIP.

[15] (a) T (b) T (c) T (d) T (e) T

(a) All types of bronchial carcinoma are indeed more common in males. However, the rising mortality has levelled off in males, whereas it continues to rise in females. The association of cigarette smoking and bronchial carcinoma overshadows all other aetiological factors.

(b) Small cell bronchial carcinoma is the most aggressive form of bronchial cancer, taking on average 3 years from initial diagnosis to death, compared with ~10 years in non-small cell bronchial carcinoma.

(c) Small cell bronchial cancer accounts for ~25% of all lung cancers, with non-small cell bronchial cancer accounting for the majority of the rest.

(d) Small cell bronchial carcinoma is also known as 'oat-cell carcinoma' because of the histological appearance of the cancer cells.

(e) Small cell bronchial carcinoma arises from endocrine cells that are members of the amine precursor uptake decarboxylase (APUD) system. This explains why these tumours secrete many polypeptide hormones, causing small cell bronchial cancer to be considered a systemic disease. Common endocrine disturbances caused by non-small cell bronchial cancers include ectopic ACTH production, syndrome of inappropriate ADH production (SIADH), hypercalcaemia (excessive release of PRP, or parathormone-related peptide), hypoglycaemia, thyrotoxicosis and gynaecomastia.

[16] (a) F **(b)** F **(c)** F **(d)** T **(e)** F
(a) Vice-versa! At least 4× more common in males.
(b) Their incidence varies more than any other carcinoma known — in certain areas of China (e.g. Linxian county) their presence is almost endemic; this is believed to be due to high levels of nitrosamines in fungus-infected food.
(c) It is common due to the absence of a serosal layer in the oesophagus; the serosa acts as a barrier to local spread everywhere else in the GIT.
(d) Followed by odynophagia; constant pain is usually an ominous sign of mediastinal invasion.
(e) The prognosis of oesophageal carcinomas is abysmal — the overall cure rate is just 5%, mainly because of the lack of early symptoms and hence late presentation of these tumours.

[17] (a) F **(b)** T **(c)** F **(d)** T **(e)** F
(a) Most infections of the GIT are self-limiting, and often the only treatment that is required is oral rehydration with a salt-containing solution.
(b) This gram + cocci causes gastroenteritis via a toxin, and accounts for 5% of all UK cases of food poisoning. Infection is characterized by persistent vomiting.
(c) There are actually at least five different sorts of *E. coli* that cause gastroenteritis. Of these the only one responsible for bloody diarrhoea is EHEC, or enterohaemmorhagic *E. coli*, especially verotoxigenic EHEC (O157:H7). The other four (ETEC (entero-toxigenic *E. coli*), EPEC (entero-pathogenic *E. coli*), EAEC (entero-adherent *E. coli*) and EIEC (entero-invasive *E. coli*)) all cause diarrhoea/dysentery not particularly associated with blood PR.
(d) *Salmonella typhi* causes typhoid fever, classically split into three weeks by clinical signs/symptoms . . .
• Week 1: insidious onset of headache, 'stepladder' fever and diarrhoea

• Week 2: classical rose-spot rash
• Week 3: the week of complications: pneumonia, haemolytic anaemia, meningitis, polyneuropathy, osteomyelitis, haemorrhage and intestinal peroration
Typhoid fever is classically diagnosed using the Widal test (a serological test for antibodies). Paratyphoid fever is caused by *S. paratyphi* and is clinically indistinguishable apart from being milder. *Salmonella enteritidis* and *S. typhimurium* cause classical salmonella gastroenteritis from eggs and poultry products.
(e) On the contrary, this bug is one of the most common causes of gastroenteritis in the UK, usually associated with ingestion of infected chicken or milk.

[18] (a) F **(b)** F **(c)** F **(d)** T **(e)** F
(a) A mild increase in levels of serum amylase (normal reference range 0–180 somogyi U/dL) is common in patients with inflammation/infection of the gallbladder. However, if the increase in amylase is marked, pancreatitis should be suspected until proven otherwise.
(b) Because secretion of bile is vitally important for adequate absorption of fats and fat-soluble vitamins, long-standing obstructive jaundice would be expected to have an adverse effect on levels of vitamin K within the body. Vitamin K is a vital co-factor in the clotting cascade, hence clotting would be abnormal if sufficient were not being absorbed
(c) Endoscopic retrograde cholecystopancreatogram (ERCP) is a good investigation for demonstrating many aspects of biliary pathology, but it should not be the investigation of first choice. **Ultrasound scan** is the initial investigation of choice when gallstones are suspected, as it **can visualize around 95% of all gallstones** (usually sees all stones >3 mm in diameter). After these initial investigations, there is a wide variety of techniques for investigating biliary pathology . . .
1. **Percutaneous transhepatic cholecystogram** (PTC)
   • Thin needle passed through skin into liver parenchyma → contrast medium injected directly into intrahepatic bile ducts (easier if the ducts are dilated)
   • Especially good for visualizing the proximal ductal system
   • Can be used to obtain cytological specimens, extract stones and site biliary drainage catheters
2. **ERCP**
   • Endoscopic cannulation of the sphincter of Oddi, with injection of contrast to visualize the biliary and pancreatic ductal anatomy

- Most valuable in patients with normal size bile ducts and in those with suspected ampullary lesions (can be biopsied or brushed to obtain histological/cytological diagnosis)
- Useful for performing electrosurgical sphincterotomy to facilitate stone passage
- Useful for removing stones with a dormier basket
- Useful for placing stents in case of stricture, malignant or otherwise

3. **CT/MRI**
   - Both useful second or third line for identifying level and cause of obstruction, and monitoring response to treatment

4. **Oral cholecystogram**
   - The night before the procedure the patient takes oral contrast (e.g. Telepaque, Bilopaque) → enters liver → excreted in bile → concentrated in gallbladder → take radiograph of right upper quadrant to confirm stones in gallbladder
   - Two consecutive non-visualizations almost certainly mean that the gallbladder is diseased

5. **Radionuclide biliary scanning (HIDA scanning)**
   - Radioactive ^{99}technetium is injected i.v. → excreted in bile → enters gallbladder only if cystic duct is patent
   - No filling of gallbladder after 4 h suggests cystic duct obstruction, and supports the diagnosis of acute cholecystitis
   - Also useful for showing bile leak after surgery
   - *Not* useful for showing stones in gallbladder or CBD

(d) A HIDA scan (see above) is another name for a radionuclide biliary scan. Such scans are especially useful for demonstrating filling defects in the gall bladder or bile ducts, and any abnormal bile pathways.

(e) Alkaline phosphatase is synthesized by hepatocytes and biliary tract epithelium. Serum levels increase due to over-production of the enzyme in circumstances of . . .
- Extra-hepatic biliary obstruction
- Cholestasis from drug reactions
- Cholestasis from primary biliary cirrhosis
- Hepatitis of any cause

In addition to this, serum levels of alkaline phosphatase can also be raised by diseases of the bone, and are especially high in Paget's disease of the bone.

[19] (a)T (b)T (c)F (d)T (e)T

(a) There are three common causes of cirrhosis that must never be forgotten . . .
1. Alcohol

2. Hepatitis B virus infection (±hepatitis D)
3. Hepatitis C virus infection

Alcohol is the commonest cause in the developed world, whilst viruses reign supreme worldwide. However, in addition to these, there are many rarer causes, including primary biliary cirrhosis, autoimmune hepatitis, hereditary haemochromotosis, Wilson's disease, Budd–Chiari syndrome, drugs, α_1-antitrypsin deficiency, CF and many much rarer causes.

(b) Cirrhosis may indeed be caused by the Budd–Chiari syndrome, which is defined as 'thrombosis of the hepatic vein with great enlargement of the liver and development of collateral vessels, intractable ascites and severe portal hypertension'. Don't confuse this with the Arnold–Chiari malformation, which is to do with the brain.

(c) β-human chorionic gonadotrophin is used to monitor patients who have a history of malignant testicular tumour, such as seminoma or teratoma. Patients with known cirrhosis should undergo 6-monthly measurements of α-fetoprotein, as well as 6-monthly **liver ultrasound scans**, because long-standing cirrhosis is known to be linked to development of hepatocellular carcinoma (HCC), for which α-FP is a serum marker.

(d) Child's classification grades level of liver function in cirrhotics from A to C (good–bad) based on a number of variables, including presence of jaundice, ascites, encephalopathy and level of serum albumin.

(e) Cirrhotic patients who develop HCC are *not* candidates for liver transplantation because the recurrence rate of HCC is very high. Liver transplantation is however strongly indicated in patients with fulminant hepatic failure of any cause, primary biliary cirrhosis (when bilirubin levels exceed 100), chronic hepatitis B (recurs post-transplant in 60–70%, although immunoglobulin, interferon and anti-virals reduce this figure), chronic hepatitis C (uniformly re-infects the transplanted liver, but prognosis of this infected graft is good compared with hepatitis B re-infection), autoimmune hepatitis, alcoholic liver disease, Wilson's disease, α_1-antitrypsin deficiency and primary sclerosing cholangitis. Liver transplant overall has an 85% 5-year survival rate, mainly owing to developments with cyclosporine, tacrolimus and mycophenolate motetil.

[20] (a)T (b) F (c) F (d) F (e) F

(a) Paracetamol is metabolized in the body by partial conversion to the toxic metabolite N-acetyl-p-benzoquinonamine, which is normally rendered inactive by reduction with glutathione. After a large overdose, however, reduced glutathione is depleted and the toxic metabolite binds covalently via sulphydryl groups onto liver cell membranes, initiating a series of changes that lead to hepatocyte necrosis. Severe hepatocyte necrosis can occur with as little as 7.5 g (15 tablets), and death with 15 g (30 tablets). Patients who are malnourished, have taken alcohol with the overdose, are alcohol dependant, are taking enzyme inducing drugs or have HIV/AIDS all have lower reserves of reduced glutathione, therefore have to be treated at lower levels of plasma paracetamol.

Common drugs which act as hepatic enzyme inducers can be memorized by thinking of the transexual copper, **PC BRAS** . . .

P Phenytoin (epilepsy)
C Carbamazepine (epilepsy)
B Barbiturates (sedative)
R Rifampicin (TB)
A Alcohol
S Steroids and sulphonylureas (diabetes)

(b) The antidote of choice in paracetamol overdose is **N-acetylcysteine (a.k.a. Parvolex)** given in a three-phase IV infusion. This works by providing sulfhydryl groups that increase the availability and recovery of hepatic glutathione to enable it to mop up the toxic metabolite of paracetamol. The decision to treat is based on the plasma paracetamol level taken 4 h after overdose. Oral methionine is an alternative to Parvolex, but absorption and efficacy are unreliable, and so this should only really be given if patient develops a pseudoallergic reaction to Parvolex.

Pabrinex is a combination of B and C vitamins given parenterally for rapid correction of severe depletion or malabsorption, as is commonly seen in alcoholics. Don't get these two mixed up.

(c) Threshold for treatment of the high-risk patients mentioned above is *lower* than normal patients (they should be treated at approximately half the levels of plasma paracetamol that would prompt treatment in otherwise fit, healthy individuals).

(d) Paracetamol levels in the first 4 h post-ingestion are **unreliable**, and blood should be taken at 4- h or thereafter to gain an accurate reflection of true plasma paracetamol levels. Having said this, you should not wait 4 h before commencing treatment, and in the presence of a strong history or suspicion, or an extremely high pre-4 h paracetamol level, treatment should be given anyway. *If in doubt, treat!*

(e) Signs of a particularly poor prognosis in paraceta-

mol overdose include INR > 3, raised serum creatinine and severe acidosis (pH < 7.3). Where it appears that treatment with N-acetylcysteine is going to be useless, super-urgent liver transplantation should be considered.

[21] (a) F (b) F (c) F (d) T (e) F

(a) Pseudocysts are defined as 'accumulations of fluid in a cyst-like loculus that does not have an epithelial or other membranous lining'. The definition given is that of a cyst.

(b) Pseudocysts are the most common complications of acute pancreatitis. They are caused by ductal disruption and gland autolysis, which results in enzymatic fluid collecting in-and-around the pancreas and being walled-off by the surrounding viscera. They mostly resolve spontaneously.

(c) They commonly present with epigastric pain, nausea and vomiting, and occasionally mechanical obstruction of the stomach or duodenum.

(d) Persisting abdominal pain for greater than 1 week, persistent elevation of serum amylase or lipase, and development of a palpable abdominal mass after an episode of acute pancreatitis should all prompt suspicion of pseudocyst formation.

(e) Thirty per cent of pseudocysts resolve spontaneously with conservative therapy, mainly in the form of pancreatic rest (NBM and subsequently TPN). Symptomatic cysts still present after 4–6 weeks require surgical drainage, preferably CT-guided. Internal drainage is preferred, but if unfeasible, external drainage and pancreatic fistula formation are used. Recurrence after drainage is common. Biopsy of the cyst wall should be taken at drainage, as pancreatic cystadenocarcinoma can commonly mimic a pseudocyst.

Complications of pseudocysts, such as infection and haemorrhage, are catastrophic and if suspected should prompt swift drainage and necessary supportive measures (e.g. volume resuscitation).

[22] (a) F (b) F (c) T (d) F (e) F

(a) Herniae are defined as 'the protrusion of any organ, structure or portion thereof through its normal anatomical confines'. An *indirect* inguinal hernia occurs when bowel, omentum or other intra-abdominal organ protrudes through the deep/internal ring within the continuous peritoneal coverage of a patent processus vaginalis. A *direct* inguinal hernia occurs when bowel, omentum or other intra-abdominal organ proceeds directly through the posterior inguinal wall.

(b) Indirect inguinal herniae are the commonest sort of hernia in both sexes and at all ages.

(c) Indirect inguinal herniae emerge laterally to the inferior epigastric vessels, whilst direct ones emerge medially.

(d) The deep inguinal ring is at the mid-point of the inguinal ligament, which is lateral to the mid-inguinal point (half-way between the pubic symphysis and the anterior superior iliac spine). The external/superficial inguinal ring is just above and medial to the pubic tubercle.

(e) Femoral herniae arise below and lateral to the pubic tubercle. Indirect inguinal herniae emerge above and medial to the pubic tubercle.

The relations of the inguinal canal are as follows . . .
• Floor: inguinal ligament
• Roof: fibres of transversalis and internal oblique
• Anterior: aponeurosis of external oblique
• Posterior: laterally, transversalis fascia; medially, the conjoint tendon

The way to distinguish between a direct and an indirect inguinal hernia is as follows: reduce the hernia → place two fingers over the deep inguinal ring (the midpoint of the inguinal ligament) → ask the patient to cough. If the hernia is restrained, it is an indirect inguinal hernia; if it pops out, however, it is a direct inguinal hernia. In practise it is not always this simple and the only real way to tell which sort of inguinal hernia has presented is at surgical exploration.

Other types of herniae include . . .
1. Spigelian: through the semi-lunar line at the lateral border of the rectus muscles
2. Grynfelt's: through the superior lumbar triangle
3. Petit's: through the inferior lumbar triangle
4. Richter's: only involving a portion of the circumference of the bowel wall
5. Littre's: any groin hernia that contains a Meckel's diverticulum
6. Obturator: through the obturator canal
7. Hesselbach's: like a femoral hernia but coursing lateral to the femoral vessels
8. Pantaloon: simultaneous direct and indirect inguinal herniae
9. Incisional: through the incomplete closure of a previous abdominal incision
10. Epigastric: through the linea alba superior to the umbilicus
11. Umbilical and paraumbilical

[23] (a)T **(b)** F **(c)** F **(d)**T **(e)**T

(a) Obstruction of the appendiceal lumen sufficient to cause appendicitis is caused in 60% of cases by lymphoid hyperplaisia, in 35% of cases by obstruction by faecolith, and in 5% of cases by obstruction due to a foreign body. Lymphoid hyperplasia in the young may be related to a viral or a bacterial illness.

(b) The pain of acute appendicitis begins initially peri-umbilically. This is due to initial irritation of the visceral peritoneum that localizes vaguely to the area where all mid-gut pain localizes, i.e. the peri-umbilical region. With subsequent development of the inflammation, the parietal peritoneum becomes involved and the pain then localizes accurately to the point of appendiceal inflammation, almost always the right iliac fossa.

(c) Murphy's sign is pain on deep inspiration whilst the examiner is palpating in the right hypochondrium, and is a sign associated with acute cholecystitis, not appendicitis.

(d) McBurney's point is classically the site of maximal tenderness in acute appendicitis, and is located two-thirds of the way along a point linking umbilicus to anterior superior iliac spine

(e) Rovsing's sign is also known as the 'distant–local' sign. It is elicited by palpating the left iliac fossa, and is positive if pain is subsequently experienced in the right iliac fossa. It reflects peritonism of the right iliac fossa.

[24] (a) F **(b)** F **(c)**T **(d)**T **(e)** F

(a) Crohn's disease is incurable because it potentially involves the whole gut, and unlike ulcerative colitis (UC) which can be cured by pan-proctocolectomy, removal of the entire gut from mouth to anus is not a feasible treatment option in CD. There is also currently no medical cure. Staged surgery can be carried out, but recurrences usually occur, and are usually located *proximally* to the resected portion

(b) The inflammation associated with CD is *transmural*, hence fissures and fistulae are relatively common. Another consequence of the transmural inflammation is fibrosis during periods when the disease is quiescent, with resultant stricture formation and distortion of normal anatomy, with ureteric obstruction being just one of the many subsequent problems encountered

(c) Perianal complications are common in CD and include ulcers, fissures, perianal fistulae and abscesses. These accompany 30–60% of CD patients with colonic disease, and 8–30% of CD patients with small bowel disease.

(d) Smoking makes development of CD twice as likely, and exacerbates flare-ups of the disease. Paradoxically, smoking of cigarettes seems to decrease the risk of developing UC, and makes flare-ups less severe.

(e) Corticosteroids are mainly indicated in the treatment of flare-ups of CD, rather than in prophylaxis, where there is no good evidence for their usage. Other drugs used to combat CD include sulphasalazine (anti-inflammatory) and immunosuppressants (e.g. azathioprine, methotrexate, cyclosporine). These drugs are often referred to as 'steroid-sparing agents' because their appropriate use can decrease the need for higher doses of corticosteroids.

	Ulcerative colitis	*Crohn's disease*
Symptoms and signs		
Fever and abdominal pain	Less prominent	More prominent
Diarrhoea	Severe, bloody +++, mucus +/–	Less severe, bleeding infrequent, mucus ++
Perianal fistulae	Rare	Common
Strictures/obstruction	Uncommon	Common
Perforation	Uncommon	Common
Pattern of development		
Rectum	Virtually always involved	Often normal and uninvolved
Terminal ileum	Normal, unless backwash ileitis present	Diseased in majority of patients
Distribution	Continuous, extending confluently	Segmented, *skip lesions*
Anus	Anal complications rare	Anal complications common
Toxic megacolon	Common	Rare
Appearance		
Gross	Friable, bleeding, granular exudates; pseudopolyps; isolated ulcers; normal thickness bowel wall; ulcers are shallow and wide	Linear ulcers, transverse fissures; cobblestoning; thickening and stricturing; creeping fat; narrow and deeply penetrating ulcers; *rosethorn* ulcers
Microscopic	Inflamed mucosa and submucosa only; crypt abscesses; fibrosis uncommon; granulomas rare	Transmural inflammation; non-caseating granulomas ++; fibrosis ++
Radiological	Lead-pipe appearance—loss of haustral pattern; foreshortening—featureless shortened colon; continuous; concentric	String sign in small bowel indicating stricturing; segmental; asymmetric; internal fistulae common
Course		
Natural history	Exacerbations → remissions → dramatic flare-ups	Exacerbations → remissions → chronic and indolent course
Medical treatment	Initial response high	Initial response less predictable
Surgical treatment	Curative	Palliative
Recurrence	No	Proximal to resected area

Continued on p. 116

	Ulcerative colitis	*Crohn's disease*
Associations		
Smoking	Decreased incidence	Increased incidence
Clubbing	Present	Present
Systemic manifestation	Present to a lesser degree	Present to a greater degree
Complications		
Fistulae	Do not develop	Enterovesical, enterovaginal and enteroenteral, as well as perianal fistulae develop
Carcinoma	Increased risk; prophylactic colectomy of value	Mildly increased risk
Anaemia	Severe	Moderate
Abscesses	Fewer	More, hence fever is more prominent

EMQs

Answer 13

(1) Ovarian carcinoma

This woman has malignant ascites and paraneoplastic cerebellar degeneration. The vague initial history is typical, hence the frequently late diagnosis. Abdominal swelling may occur due to ascites, the tumour or an omental mass.

Central nervous system **paraneoplastic syndromes** occur with several tumours: bronchus (small cell), ovarian, breast and Hodgkin's lymphoma. The mechanism is presumed to be immunological. Tumour resection may result in improvement. There are various patterns . . .
* Encephalitis
* Cerebellar degeneration
* Cord damage: long tract signs
* Dorsal root ganglia: motor neurone disease
* Neuromuscular junction; Eaton Lambert syndrome

The causes of ascites include:
* **Malignancy**
  * Intra-peritoneal
  * Hepatic (secondary > primary)
* **Cardiac**
  * Right ventricular failure
  * Cor-pulmonale
  * Constrictive pericarditis
* **Hepatic**
  * Chronic liver disease
  * Budd–Chiari syndrome
* **Hypoprotinaemia**
  * Hepatic failure
  * Protein loss; gut/renal/skin
  * Malabsorption
* **Inflammation**
  * Peritonitis
  * Perforation
  * TB
  * Pancreatitis
* **Via SIADH**: hypothyroidism

(2) Irritable bowel syndrome (IBS)

A typical history, although the exact symptoms may vary between patients. Typical symptoms include . . .
* Bloating
* Flatulence
* Pain; cramping
* Altered bowel habit
  * Rabbit dropping like stools
  * Diarrhoea or constipation
(See OSCE 37, p. 292)

Inflammatory bowel disease (ulcerative colitis) would be the main differential diagnosis; however, the normal CRP and FBC count against this. Additionally the recurrent pattern and previous set of negative investigations are typical of IBS. Laxative abuse may be expected to cause hypokalaemia, and is again a less likely diagnosis than IBS. Large bowel malignancy is less likely given the age of the patient, the duration of symptoms and the fact that she has has a normal colonoscopy in the recent past.

(3) Inflammatory bowel disease
Bloody diarrhoea has a short differential diagnosis . . .
- **Infective colitis** due to:
  - *Salmonella*
  - *Shigella*
  - *Campylobacter*
  - *E. coli*
  - *Clostridium difficile* (toxin)
- **Inflammatory bowel disease**

(See OSCE 30, p. 282)

(4) Pseudomembranous colitis
Toxin produced by *Clostridium difficile* (a commensal in 5%). It occurs following broad-spectrum antibiotics. The elderly are especially vulnerable. It may be several weeks after treatment before symptoms occur. It presents as profuse watery diarrhoea, with blood in 10%. Yellow plaques (the pseudomembrane) are visible on sigmoidoscopy. The diagnosis is made by isolation of the toxin from the stool. Management is with isolation (patient-to-patient spread possible), oral metronidazole or IV vancomycin if very sick. Mortality may be up to 20%.

(5) Thyrotoxicosis
Probably an overdose of thyroxine. Sometimes deliberate overdosing by patients (to lose weight) or the result of failing to monitor the dose of thyroxine.

Causes of acute diarrhoea (<14 days)
- **Infections**
  - Viral:
    Rotavirus
    Adenovirus
  - Bacterial:
    Salmonella
    Campylobacter
    Shigella

- Protozoal:
  Giardia
  Cryptosporidium
- **Drug side effects**
  - Most drugs have GIT side effects

Causes of chronic diarrhoea (>14 days)
- **Malabsorption**
  - Pancreatic:
    Cystic fibrosis
    Chronic pancreatitis
  - Small bowel:
    Coeliac disease
    Bacterial over growth
    Tropical sprue
    Giardiasis
    Crohn's disease
    Short bowel syndrome (resection >50% of the small bowel)
    Whipple's disease
- **Neuroendocrine tumours**
  - Gastrinomas
  - VIPoma
  - Somatostatinoma
  - Carcinoid
  - Medullary thyroid (calcitonin)
- **Large bowel**
  - Tumours
  - Inflammatory bowel disease
  - Diverticular disease
- **Others**
  - Anxiety
  - Thyrotoxicosis
  - Irritable bowel syndrome
  - Spurious due to faecal impaction
  - Autonomic neuropathy; diabetes (nocturnal)
  - Drugs: virtually any/laxative abuse
  - Osmotic (sorbitol in chewing gum)

Answer 14

(1) Goodpasture's syndrome
Although Wegener's granulomatosis may cause a very similar picture. Anti-glomerular basement membrane antibodies occur. A shared antigen on glomerular basement membrane and pulmonary tissue is presumably responsible for the co-pathology. It classically follows a recent upper respiratory tract infection. Smoking or

hydrocarbon exposure predispose to the pulmonary component of the condition. The pulmonary pathology often precedes the renal involvement by weeks. Intrapulmonary haemorrhage can be seen as fluffy shadowing on the chest radiograph. The resultant haemoptysis may be massive. Renal failure may be rapidly progressive (crescentic). There may be positive p-ANCA. Treatment is for the renal failure (fluid balance, correct hyperkalaemia, dialysis), immunosuppressive therapy (steroids, azathioprine, etc.) and plasmapheresis to remove autoantibodies.

Other causes of pulmonary plus renal disease

- Vasculitis
  - Wegener's granulomatosis
  - Polyarteritis nodosa
  - Micoscopic polyangitis
- SLE
- Pneumonia with septicaemia (causing acute renal failure, ARF)
- Legionnaire's disease
- ARF leading to pulmonary oedema
- Drugs, e.g. NSAIDS (asthma plus interstitial nephritis)

(2) Acute renal failure (ARF) due to angiotensin converting enzyme (ACE) inhibitors

The bruit suggests renal artery stenosis (a potent cause of secondary hypertension via secondary hyper-aldosteronism). Patients on ACE inhibitors are likely to have atheromatous disease in various locations including the renal arteries. Treatment with ACE inhibitors prevents the renin angiotensin aldosterone (RAA) system from acting as a mechanism for maintaining renal perfusion; ARF thus ensues. This is the most common cause of patients presenting with ARF in the UK. It is essential to be able to describe **how to initiate an ACE inhibitor** ...

- Stop any diuretics (these augment hypotension)
- Start with lowest dose, e.g. enalapril 2.5 mg/day
- Advise patient to take them at night to avoid first dose hypotension
- Check U and Es at 1 and 2 weeks
- Slowly increase the dose

The prognosis of ACE inhibitor induced ARF is good on withdrawal of the drug and supportive treatment.

All of the above also applies to angiotensin II receptor antagonists ('A2RAs').

(3) Nephrotic syndrome

The definition of nephrotic syndrome is . . .
- Proteinuria (>3–5 g/day in adults)
- Hypoalbuminaemia
- Oedema
- Hypercholesterolaemia

Here the two most likely causes are NSAIDs and minimal change nephropathy. Confirm the diagnosis using 24 h urinary protein assay.

Complications of nephrotic syndrome

- **Infection** due to loss of immunoglobulins
- **Thrombosis** due to loss of antithrombin III
  - Renal vein thrombosis occurs in 6–8% (loin pain, haematuria, renal failure worsens)
  - DVT
  - PE
- **Hyperlipidaemia**: a by-product of increased hepatic activity synthesizing albumin. However, LDL production is greater than HDL production leading to raised total cholesterol

Causes of nephrotic syndrome

Use the mnemonic '**Please DIP A MAD Cow**' . . .

P Primary glomerular disease of any pattern, but **minimal change** disease is the most frequent cause in children and young adults and **membranous disease** at other ages

D Diabetes mellitus

I Infections, e.g. leprosy, malaria, hepatitis B

P Pre-eclampsia

A Amyloid (rheumatoid arthritis, osteomyelitis)

M Myeloma

A Accelerated hypertension

D Drugs, e.g. penicillamine, gold, captopril, NSAIDs

C Connective tissue diseases, e.g. SLE (membranous glomerular nephritis)

Summary of the management of ARF

- Investigate to remove and then treat any treatable cause (especially hypovolaemia, drugs and sepsis)
- Supportive measures for fluid balance, biochemistry (especially hyperkalaemia) and nutrition
- Prevent complications (as above plus also pericarditis)
- Specific immunosuppressive therapy, e.g. steroids for vasculitis
- Renal replacement therapy (dialysis)

- Monitor progress (U and Es, fluid balance, urine output, daily weight)

Indications for acute dialysis
- pH < 7.1
- K$^+$ > 6.5 mmol/L
- Pulmonary oedema
- Severe uraemia; vomiting/encephalopathy/pericarditis

Causes of ARF
- **Pre-renal**
  Volume loss from any cause leading to ATN; **the main category**
  - **Hypovolaemic shock**
  - **Sepsis**
  - **Cardiogenic shock**
  - **ACE inhibitors** (especially in patients with renal artery stenosis)
- **Renal**
  - Toxic:
    Drugs
    Contrast media
    Rhabdomyolysis
  - Vasculitis:
    Polyarteritis nodosa
    Microscopic polyangitis
  - Glomerulonephritis (any pattern)
  - Intra-renal vascular:
    Accelerated hypertension
    Disseminated intravascular coagulation (DIC)
    Haemolytic uraemic syndrome (HUS)
    Thrombotic thrombocytopenic purpura (TTP)
    Systemic sclerosis
    Myeloma
  - Interstitial nephritis:
    Pyelonephritis
    Drug hypersensitivity, e.g. NSAIDs, penicillins, sulphonamides
    Infections, e.g. leptospirosis, Hanta virus
- **Post-renal**
  - Any obstruction 'from the papillae to the penis'

Is the renal failure acute or chronic?
When a patient presents with deranged urea and creatinine, it is important to decide if the renal failure is new or long standing because ARF *may* be reversible.

Features suggesting that the renal failure is chronic
- **Anaemia;** chronic renal failure causes anaemia due to:
  - Chronic disease related anaemia
  - Erythropoietin deficiency
  - Malnutrition
  - Bleeding tendency
  - Uraemic marrow toxicity
- **Metabolic bone disease** (renal osteodystrophy secondary hyperparathyroidism)
- **Small kidneys** (small scarred kidneys)
- **Apparent patient tolerance of severe uraemia** (very raised U and Es and patient is not acutely unwell)
- **Left ventricular hypertrophy** (long-standing hypertension)
- **Old urea and electrolyte results for comparison**

Features suggesting the renal failure may be acute (or acute on chronic)
- An acute illness in a previously well patient
- An acutely unwell patient
- Hyperkalaemia
- Known recent renal insult
- Absence of the features of chronic renal failure as given above

(4) Acute pyelonephritis
A typical history. The diagnosis is made on the history and examination together with dipstick test of the urine. Antibiotics are started once the MSU sample has been sent. In this case septic shock is present. Blood cultures and intravenous fluids and antibiotics (cephotaxime, ampicillin or gentamycin) will be required. Reflux nephropathy is more common in pregnancy due to progesterone mediated smooth muscle relaxation of the ureters.

(5) Henoch–Schönlein syndrome
An IgA-mediated glomerulonephritis. Purpura, synovitis and abdominal pain (serositis) are characteristic. It is rare but not unknown in adults. Usually produces a focal and segmental glomerulonephritis.

Summary of the glomerulonephritides (GNs)
Note that each type may present in a variety of ways (e.g. nephrotic syndrome, nephritic syndrome, hypertension, haematuria or proteinuria), but equally certain GNs may follow characteristic patterns (e.g. minimal change GN and nephrotic syndrome).

ANSWERS 3

- **Mimimal change GN**

  Children > adults

  Clinically usually gives nephrotic syndrome

  Usually highly selective protein loss (IgG/transferrin ratio low), which is used to predict minimal change disease in children and so avoid a traumatic renal biopsy

  Carries a good prognosis

  Causes include:
  - NSAID
  - Gold
  - Hodgkin's disease
  - Thymoma

- **Focal segmental**

  Focal IgM/IgA deposits

  Middle-aged/obesity associated

  25% go to end stage renal failure (ESRF)

  Causes include:
  - Henoch–Schönlein purpura
  - HIV
  - SABE
  - Polyarteritis nodosa
  - Wegener's granulomatosis

- **Membranous GN**

  Often with nephrotic syndrome presentation

  30% go to ESRF

  5% get renal vein thrombosis

  Causes include:
  - Idiopathic
  - Drugs, e.g. gold, penicillamine
  - Malignancy, e.g. bronchus
  - Connective tissue disease, e.g. SLE, Rha
  - Chronic infections, e.g. hepatitis B

- **Mesangioproliferative**

  Recurrent macroscopic haematuria occurring with upper respiratory tract infections

  The most common GN in adults

  25% go to ESRF

  No response to immunosuppression

- **Mesangiocapillary**

  Type I — acquired due to:
  - Immune complex deposition
  - Shunt (extra-corporeal) nephritis
  - Sickle cell disease
  - α_1-antitrypsin deficiency
  - Kartagener's syndrome
  - Rheumatoid arthritis

  Type II — congenital

  Associated with absent adipose tissue (partial lipodys-

trophy) and raised C3 nephritic factor present in the circulation

- **Diffuse proliferative**

  Causes include:
  - Post-streptococcal infection
  - SLE (poor prognosis)

- **Crescentic**

  Rapidly progressive GN. Patients are acutely unwell and in a catabolic state (rapid weight loss) with ARF or a nephritic syndrome.

  Causes include:
  - Goodpasture's syndrome
  - Wegener's granulomatosis
  - Polyarteritis nodosa
  - SLE

Answer 15

(1) Antiphospholipid syndrome

An autoimmune condition where autoantibodies occur which are directed against phospholipids (β_2-Glycoprotein recently implicated). *In vitro* these autoantibodies act as anticoagulants by inhibiting certain proteins in the coagulation pathway; however, paradoxically, *in vivo* they result in recurrent arterial and venous thromboses. The reason for this paradox is not understood.

There is a curious relationship with SLE. A small number of patients with antiphospholipid syndrome have SLE. However, a large proportion of patients with SLE produce antiphospholipid antibodies (up to 40%), but only a small proportion of these present with the arterial and venous thromboses that are so characteristic of antiphospholipid syndrome.

Features of antiphospholipid syndrome

Use the mnemonic **T TAC VAC** . . .

T Thromboses; arterial (strokes) and venous. Often presenting atypically, e.g. upper limb, hepatic vein thrombosis (Budd–Chiari syndrome)

T Thrombocytopenia

A Abortions; recurrent episodes

C CNS lesions:

Chorea

Convulsions

Migraine

V Valvular heart disease:

Aortic and mitral valve (Libman–Sacks endocarditis)

A Artheroma:
Premature myocardial infarction
C Cutaneous:
Livido reticularis (as here); fine reticular bruise coloured pattern indicating small vessel vasculitis
Splinter haemorrhages
Ulceration and necrosis, e.g. of digits

Antiphospholipid syndrome is suggested by the clinical presentation along with an elevated APTT (which fails to correct when mixed with donor plasma and so is due to **inhibition** of the clotting mechanism and *not* a deficiency of a coagulation factor) and reduced platelets. Anticardiolipin antibodies (measured using ELISA) are diagnostic, however. Patients need investigating for a possible underlying connective tissue disorder (SLE). Management involves anticoagulation with warfarin, or aspirin and heparin during pregnancy.

Note that strokes do present in younger people (<40 years) and must be investigated for an underlying cause.

Causes of stroke in young people
- Vascular malformations
  - Subarachnoid haemorrhage
  - Dissection of carotid ateries
  - Sturge Weber syndrome
- Thrombophilia
  - Antiphospholipid syndrome
  - Protein S or C deficiency
  - Antithrombin III deficiency
  - Homocysteinuria
  - Paroxysmal nocturnal haemaglobinuria
- Vasculitis
  - SLE
  - Wegener's granulomatosis
  - Polyarteritis nodosa
  - Takayasu's arteritis
  - Behçet's syndrome
  - Syphilis
- Infective
  - Abscesses (secondary to pneumonia, endocarditis, IV drug abuse)
  - Granulomas (sarcoidosis, tuberculoma)
  - HIV is associated with an elevated risk of stroke.
- Others
  - Migraine; especially in women on oral contraception

- Pregnancy and oral contraception
- Fibromuscular dysplasia
- Unknown
- Not a stroke; MS, migraine, seizures

(2) Behçet's syndrome
A rare disorder that is more common in Turkey and the Middle East. There is an association with the HLA B55 allele. The disease consists of an inflammatory condition of unknown cause.

Main features
- Oral ulceration (recurrent)
- Genital ulceration (recurrent)
- Anterior uveitis (recurrent resulting in possible blindness)

Occasional features
- Skin
  - Erythema nodosum
  - Vasculitis (affecting both arteries and veins)
  - Pathergy reaction (very specific; red papules or pustules occur following needle stick injury after 24 h)
- CNS
  - Meningoencephalitis
  - Acute confusional states
  - Ataxia
- Joints
  - Large joint non-erosive oligoarthritis
- GIT
  - Anorexia, nausea, vomiting, diarrhoea (may resemble Crohn's disease, i.e. oral ulceration and diarrhoea)

(3) Takayasu's arteritis (pulseless syndrome)
A large vessel arteritis of unknown aetiology affecting the aortic arch and its branches. More common in Japan and amongst young females. Systemic symptoms can occur such as fever, malaise and weight loss. Claudication symptoms can occur affecting the upper limb occur along with features of cerebral ischaemia. Treatment is with corticosteroids but the prognosis is poor.

The gradual onset is against an embolism as a possible cause. In subclavian steal syndrome a stenosis proximal to the vertebral artery results in retrograde flow down the vertebral artery during upper limb exercise. This produces vertebrobasilar ischaemia symptoms, e.g. vertigo.

ANSWERS 3

(4) Polyarteritis nodosa (PAN)

A vasculitis affecting mainly middle-aged males result-ing in inflammation affecting medium-sized vessels with aneurysm formation. **Systemic symptoms** such as fever, malaise and weight loss may be predominant in the early stages. The vasculitis may result in infarction of the affected organ (e.g. stroke, peripheral neuropathy, ischaemic colitis, myocardial infarction, renal failure). There is an association with positive **hepatitis B serology** (in 30% worldwide) and it is presumed the vasculitis is due to immune complex deposition. The diagnosis can be made on the characteristic biopsy findings of **fibrinoid necrosis** within blood vessel walls and demonstrating microaneurysms on arteriography. There is typically a leucocytosis and raised ESR but antineutrophil cytoplasmic (ANCA) antibody is usually negative (90%).

Vasculitis is a generic term referring to inflammation of the vessel wall secondary to various mechanisms . . .
- **Immunological damage**
  - Immune complexes
    e.g. PAN, subacute bacterial endocarditis
  - Autoantibodies
    e.g. SLE
  - Antineutrophil cytoplasmic antibodies
    e.g. Wegener's granulomatosis
  - T-cell damage
    e.g. giant cell arteritis
- **Direct infection**
  e.g. Syphilis, HIV infection

Within the group of conditions causing vasculitis, some have vasculitis as the main pathological mechanism (frequently termed systemic vasculitis or primary vasculitis), whereas other conditions (e.g. SLE, rheumatoid arthritis, dermatomyositis) can cause vasculitis, but this is a variable feature (secondary vasculitis).

Various classifications exist for *primary vasculitis*; however, vessel size is frequently used . . .
- **Large vessel vasculitis**
  - Takayasu's disease
  - Giant cell arteritis
- **Medium vessel vasculitis**
  - PAN
  - Kawasaki's disease
- **Small vessel vasculitis**
  - Microscopic polyangitis*

- Wegener's granulomatosis*
- Churg–Strauss syndrome*
- Henoch–Schönlein syndrome

Those marked with * are frequently ANCA positive. These antibodies can be divided into two types:
- **cANCA** directed against proteinase 3; found in 90% of active Wegener's granulomatosis
- **pANCA** directed against myeloperoxidase. Found predominantly in cases of Churg–Strauss syndrome and microscopic polyangitis. They are, however, also found (variably) in other conditions in which vasculitis is a variable component of the disease, and these diseases are frequently grouped separately. They include:
- SLE
- RA
- Scleroderma
- Dermatomyositis
- Subacute bacterial endocarditis
- Behçet's disease

The exact pathogenic role of ACNA in vasculitis is debated: however, testing is valuable because . . .
- A positive **ANCA is 95% specific** for supporting a clinical diagnosis of vasculitis
- ACNA is **80–90% sensitive** also for detecting vasculitis
- The titre of ANCA can be used to **monitor disease activity**
- ANCA is the leading cause of rapidly progressive, crescentic glomerulonephritis (**predicts problems**)

The **clinical features of vasculitis** can be divided broadly into non-specific features (e.g. weight loss, fever, malaise, anaemia) and those features related to the exact organ(s) affected, the patterns varying between conditions. These include . . .
- **Renal**: glomerulonephritis, hypertension, haematuria, proteinuria
- **Central nervous system**: strokes, epileptic seizures
- **Peripheral nervous system** (involvement of vasa-nervorum): mononeuritis multiplex, cranial nerve lesions, peripheral sensory neuropathy
- **Gastrointestinal**: ischaemic colitis, abdominal pain, haemorrhage
- **Respiratory**: haemorrhage, alveolitis
- **Cardiovascular**: ischaemic heart disease, peripheral vascular disease

(5) Dermatomyositis

Together with polymyositis, these are rare conditions where there is idiopathic inflammation and wasting of proximal muscle groups. Dermatomyositis in addition has associated characteristic skin lesions . . .

- **Purple heliotrope** discoloration around the eyes and eyelids
- **Gottron's papules**: purple vasculitic raised scaly lesions over the knuckles
- Nail bed **vasculitic lesions**
- **Cutaneous calcification**

Muscle involvement in both conditions tends to affect the **proximal muscles** leading to difficulty getting out of chairs and going up stairs. Muscle involvement may also involve the . . .

- Oesophagus: leading to dysphagia
- Respiratory muscles: leading to respiratory failure

There is an **association** with . . .

- Other connective tissue disorders, e.g. RA, SLE and systemic sclerosis
- Internal malignancy *when dermatomyositis occurs in the elderly*

A distinct **childhood form** is recognized with . . .

- Prominent vasculitis (skin ulceration and episodes of abdominal pain)
- Ectopic calcification

Investigations for polymyositis and dermatomyositis

- Muscle enzymes, e.g. creatine phosphokinase (CPK) are elevated
- Autoantibodies
  - Rheumatoid factor positive in 50%
  - Anti-Jo: if positive predicts an acute onset and pulmonary fibrosis
- Muscle biopsy shows myocyte necrosis and regeneration

The **management** involves immunosuppressant with corticosteroids, and agents such as azathioprine or methotrexate.

Answer 16

(1) Sarcoidosis

The patient has pulmonary sarcoidosis with respiratory impairment due to pulmonary fibrosis. The rash is ery-thema nodosum and although this may occur in pulmonary tuberculosis (along with the cervical lymphanenopathy), it is less likely and is also less likely to give pulmonary fibrosis, as indicated here by the spirometric results and suggested by the clinical finding of 'fine end inspiratory crepitations'. Lymphoma is the other main differential diagnosis in a young patient with respiratory symptoms and a palpable cervical lymph node; however, again, this does not fit the case description as well as sarcoidosis.

Spirometry will shows a **restrictive pattern** indicating pulmonary fibrosis (FEV1/FVC > 80%). The chest radiograph may show hilar lymphadenopathy (occasionally with calcification) and/or a reticular (lace like hard lines) pattern of diffuse fibosis (honeycomb lung). (See differential diagnosis, OSCE 22, p. 264.)

The main **causes of hilar lymphadenopathy** include . . .

- Carcinoma
- Sarcoidosis
- Lymphoma
- Tuberculosis

Pulmonary **sarcoidosis is graded radiographically** as follows . . .

- Grade 1   Hilar lymphadenopathy alone
              (best prognosis)
- Grade 2   Hilar lymphadenopathy with lung field involvement (fibrosis)
- Grade 3   Lung field involvement (fibrosis) alone
              (worst prognosis)

The definitive diagnosis of sarcoidosis is made on **transbronchial biopsy,** which demonstrates the **non-caseating granulomas.**

Serum **angiotensin converting enzyme** (ACE) is raised in 70% sarcoidosis, but is not specific being raised in asbestosis, silicosis, lymphoma and TB. It is useful, however, as a **marker of disease activity** along with serum calcium if elevated. Be aware of sarcoidosis as a cause of hypercalcaemia (in 10% of cases) due to 1α hydroxylation of vitamin D by sarcoid granulomas.

The granulomas in sarcoidosis can occur anywhere, hence it is a multi-systemic disease much loved by examiners.

Non-pulmonary sites of sarcoidosis include:

- **The eye**: any layer can be involved
  - Anterior uveitis: acute or chronic problems

ANSWERS 3

- Vasculitis affecting the retinal vessels: retinal infarction and reduced visual acuity
- Granuloma affecting the optic nerve
- **The skin**
  - Erythema nodosum
  - Skin granuloma; red plaques or papules
  - Scar infiltration
  - Lupus pernio
- **The GIT**
  - Parotid gland enlargement
  - Hepatic granulomata (often asymptomatic)
  - Splenomegaly
- **Bone**
  - Granulomata causing swelling, e.g. of the digits
  - Arthritis
- **The CNS** (uncommon)
  - Seizures
  - Cranial nerve palsies (facial nerve most commonly; occasionally bilaterally)
  - Pituitary failure; diabetes insipidus
  - Mass lesions
  - Meningitis
  - Hydrocephalus due to aqueduct obstruction

The prognosis is worse in black people and those with predominantly pulmonary fibrosis. Treatment with steroids is indicated for progressive lung fibrosis and if there is extra-pulmonary involvement.

(2) Bronchogenic carcinoma

The combination of cough and weight loss in a lifelong smoker makes this the most likely diagnosis. The patient probably has early clubbing. Examination findings suggest a left-sided pleural effusion. There is also a suggestion of proximal myopathy as a non-metastatic manifestation of malignancy which is well recognized.

Non-metastatic manifestations of malignancy (paraneoplastic syndromes)

- General
  - Weight loss
  - Anorexia
  - Lethargy
- Musculoskeletal
  - Proximal myopathy
  - Eaton Lambert syndrome
  - Hypertrophic pulmonary osteoarthropathy
- Endocrine
  - Ectopic ACTH production

- Ectopic parathormone (hypercalcaemia)
- SIADH (hyponatraemia)
- Ectopic TSH production
- Gynaecomastia (squamous cell tumours)
- Haematological
  - Normochromic normocytic anaemia
  - Disseminated intravascular coagulation (DIC)
  - Micoangiopathic haemolytic anaemia (and consequent) haemolytic uraemic syndrome)
  - Autoimmune haemolytic anaemia
- CNS
  - Encephalopathy (confusion)
  - Aseptic meningitis
  - MND
  - Peripheral neuropathy
- Skin (see OSCE 28, p. 278)
  - Acanthosis nigricans
  - Pyoderma gangrenosum
  - Dermatomyositis
  - Thrombophlebitis migrans
  - Pruritus

First-line investigations include a plain chest film. A large effusion would be tapped for symptomatic improvement of dyspnoea and to yield fluid for culture and cytology. Bronchoscopy for histology and CT scan for staging are appropriate.

(3) Churg–Strauss syndrome

This is a vasculitis associated with p-ANCA in about 70% of cases. Rhinitis or progressive asthma plus skin vasculitic signs (purpura) suggest the diagnosis. Peripheral neuropathy may occur. Renal complications (unlike other vasculitides) are uncommon. Often the patient has had asthma for years. Withdrawal of inhaled steroids may precipitate the onset of the disease.

Pulmonary eosinophilias

Chest X-ray shadowing with raised peripheral eosinophil count . . .

- **Loffler's syndrome**, due to an allergic response to worm infestations (e.g. *Ascaris lumbricoides, Ankylostoma braziliense*) or to drugs (e.g. aspirin, penicillin and many more). Patchy shadowing on the chest radiograph occurs. It may resolve spontaneously (simple pulmonary eosinophilia) or be prolonged and require treatment with steroids
- ***Aspergillus fumigatus*** illness

- **Tropical pulmonary eosinophilia** due to *Wuchererria bancrofti* (filariasis)
- **Churg–Strauss syndrome**
- **Polyarteritis nodosa**
- **Hypereosinophilic syndrome**: a systemic illness of unknown cause with eosinophil infiltration of various sites including . . .
  - The lungs giving breathlessness and a cough
  - The heart causing a restrictive cardiomyopathy
  - GIT causing abdominal pain

(4) Cryptogenic fibrosing alveolitis (CFA)

Presents typically with insidious onset of dyspnoea in middle to old age. Clubbing and central cyanosis occur. Fine 'end inspiratory crepitations' occur. A restrictive pattern (FEV1/FVC > 80%) is found on spirometry and is typical of fibrotic lung disease with 'shrinking' lung volumes. A type I respiratory failure pattern is found on blood gas analysis. There is an association with other autoimmune disorders. Treatment is with steroids and other immunosuppressive drugs, e.g. azathioprine. The prognosis is poor. Respiratory physicians recognize various sub-groups, e.g. an acute form known as Hamman–Rich syndrome.

Causes of pulmonary fibrosis

(See also OSCE 22, p. 264)
- CFA
- Pulmonary sarcoidosis
- Extrinsic allergic alveolitis; various organic dusts, e.g. farmers' lung, humidifier fever, etc.
- Inorganic dust (coal, asbestos, silica, cotton)
- Drugs, e.g. bleomycin, methotrexate, amiodarone, sulphasalazine
- Radiation
- Mitral stenosis
- Uraemia
- Connective tissue disorders

(5) Pneumococcal pneumonia

An abrupt illness in a previously fit young person. Pleuritic sounding chest pain occurs; the differential diagnosis of this being infection, infarction, malignancy infiltration or pneumothorax. Herpes labialis and rusty-coloured (haemosiderin) sputum are classically pneumococcal in origin. Central cyanosis (type I respiratory failure) and chest signs are consistent with consolidation.

In contrast to this 'typical' presentation, certain organisms produce 'atypical' presentations occasionally with additional systemic features.

Some atypical pneumonias

- **Mycoplasma**
  - Epidemics/young people
  - Chest radiograph may not correlate with clinical state
  - Cold agglutinins in 50%; rouleux (IgM)
  - Various systemic complications:

My	Myocarditis
Rash	Erythema multiforme
Has	Haemolytic anaemia
My	Myalgia
Meninges	Meningo-encephalitis
Going	Diarrhoea/vomiting

  - Erythromycin or tetracycline is used to treat
- **Staphylococcal pneumonia**
  - Frequently follows influenza
  - Intubation
  - Contaminated IV injections in drug addiction
  - Abscesses and septicaemia occur
- *Chlamydia psittaci*
  - Pigeon exposure
  - Can cause an acute or chronic illness
  - Systemic symptoms are prominent
  - Complications include:
    Meningism
    Hepato-splenomegaly
    'Rose' spots
  - The diagnosis is made by detecting a four-fold rise in IgM
  - Erythromycin or tetracycline is used to treat
- *Haemophilus influenzae*
  - Common in COPD patients
  - Thick, green, purulent sputum
  - Treat with cephalosporins
- *Legionella pneumophila*
  - Aerosol distribution from a water reservoir, e.g. cooling systems, showers. Outbreaks occur in institutions or hotels. Respiratory features start with a dry cough that becomes purulent. Shadowing in more than one lobe occurs on the chest film
  - Systemic symptoms include:
    GIT symptoms; diarrhoea
    CNS; confusion
    Renal failure, haematuria
    SIADH; low sodium

- There is a high mortality
- Clarithromycin is used to treat

Prognosis in pneumonia (British Thoracic Society)
The following features are associated with an adverse outcome . . .
- **Clinically**
  - Age >60 years
  - Respiratory rate > 30 b.p.m.
  - BP < 60 mmHg diastolic
  - Confusion
  - Atrial fibrillation
  - Underlying disease
- **Investigations**
  - Urea > 7 mmol/L
  - Albumin < 35 g/L
  - $PaO_2 < 8$ kPa
  - WCC < 4 or > 14×10^9/L
  - Bacteraemia
  - Multi-lobe involvement

Answer 17

(1) Silent myocardial infarction
More common in the elderly or any other patient with autonomic neuropathy. Cardiac pain is mediated via the autonomic nervous system. (See EMQ 20, p. 145) Not only is the typical chest pain absent, but also typical features such as nausea, anxiety and sweating may be lacking due to the failure of sympathetic drive. It should be considered in any (especially) elderly patient presenting with new cardiac failure. Q-waves should be looked for in the ECG.

(2) Acute non-cardiogenic pulmonary oedema
This patient has most likely been given excess volume. This probably occurred as a consequence of his prostate surgery due to absorption of saline used to wash out the prostate resection chippings, and also over generous post-operative intravenous fluids. Patients undergoing surgery are likely to retain fluids due to the 'stress' of the operation resulting in ADH release. Owing to the speed of onset, typical features such as a displaced apex and peripheral oedema will not have had time to develop. There should be an elevated JVP, a third heart sound and bi-basal pulmonary crepitations. The management (after ABC) would include stopping the IV fluids, sitting the patient up and giving intravenous furosemide.

Clinical signs of cardiac failure
- Raised respiratory rate
- Cyanosis
- Tachycardia
- Hypotension (poor sign)
- **Elevated JVP**
- **Displaced cardiac apex**
- **Third heart sound** (the most reliable sign)
- End inspiratory bi-basal crepitations
- Hepatomegaly (right ventricular failure)
- Ascites
- Peripheral oedema

Causes of pulmonary oedema
- **Cardiogenic,** e.g. ischaemic, valve lesions, arrhythmia, tamponade
- **Volume overload**
- **Neurogenic**: via SIADH, e.g. trauma, raised ICP, post-seizure
- **Lung injury**: adult respiratory distress syndrome via increased capillary permeability
- **Low albumin**

(3) Accelerated hypertension
The patient has hypertensive encephalopathy and grade IV hypertensive retinopathy. Chest pain and cardiac failure may also occur. Accelerated hypertension is more likely to be caused by secondary hypertension.

Causes of secondary hypertension
- **Renal**: renal artery stenosis, renal failure, systemic sclerosis causing reno-vascular disease
- **Adrenal**: Cushing's syndrome, Conn's syndrome, phaeochromacytoma
- **Pregnancy**
- **Coarctation** of the aorta
- **Endocrine**, e.g. hyperparathyroidism, acromegaly, thyrotoxicosis or hypothyroidism
- **Polycythemia**
- **Raised intracranial pressure**
- **Drugs,** e.g. steroids, carbenoxolone

When to suspect a secondary cause for hypertension
- **Young** patient
- **Accelerated** hypertension or very raised blood pressure
- **Refractory** hypertension; this is a matter of experience. Note that many patients require two or

three agents especially given the modern treatment targets
- **Target organ damage** at presentation, e.g. renal impairment (proteinuria, haematuria), grade III or IV retinopathy
- **Hypokalaemia**: note the adrenal conditions listed above all tend to cause sodium retention and potassium loss. Check that this is not simply due to diuretic use
- **Abnormal examination,** e.g. coarctation bruit, renal artery bruit, enlarged kidney, pregnancy

Hypertensive retinopathy grading

Grade I	**Silver wiring**; an increased light reflection from the retinal arteries
Grade II	**AV nipping**; retinal arteries pass over the veins and 'nip' at cross-over points
Grade III	**Flame shaped haemorrhages**, **Cotton wool spots** (fluid leakage from vessels)
Grade IV	**Papilloedema**

Microvascular damage in accelerated hypertension results in neurological features and **microangiopathic haemolytic anaemia (MAHA)**. Here there is fragmentation of red cells in the microcirculation due to endothelial damage and fibrin strands 'cheese wiring' red cells as they pass through. Red cell fragments (schizocytes) and spherocytes (red cells forced into a spherical shape by the loss of membrane surface area) occur. Free haemoglobin that is found in the circulation (and urine) binds to haptoglobins, which become reduced in quantity and hence are used as an indirect measure of haemolysis.

Causes of MAHA
- Disseminated intravascular coagulation (DIC)
- Thrombotic thrombocytopenic purpura (TTP)
- Prosthetic valves
- Haemolytic uraemic syndrome (HUS)
- Pre-eclampsia of pregnancy

Management of hypertensive encephalopathy
- ABC and control seizures
- Exclude hypoglycaemia and an intra-cerebral tumour or haemorrhage with a CT scan
- Aim to reduce the blood pressure slowly over 4 h using a β-blocker plus thiazide diuretic plus nifedipine (or IV furosemide or nitroprusside if severe)

- Monitor the urine output, fluid balance and Glasgow Coma Scale
- Investigate for secondary cause as listed above

Differential diagnosis of papilloedema
- Raised intracranial pressure, e.g. space occupying lesion, benign intracranial hypertension, hydrocephalus
- CO_2 retention
- Accelerated hypertension
- Exophthalmus
- Lead poisoning
- Retinal vein thrombosis
- Hypoparathyroidism

(4) Syndrome X
A rare syndrome consisting of . . .
- Typical clinical symptoms of angina
- Abnormal exercise EGC test (typical for angina)
- Normal coronary arteries
- No evidence of coronary artery spasm (i.e. Prinzmetal's angina)

Patients tend to be female and menopausal. They can present repeatedly with typical angina but are often incorrectly labelled as having a functional illness following the finding of normal coronary arteries. Other causes of chest pain, such as musculoskeletal pain, oesophageal reflux or spasm, etc., must be excluded before considering the diagnosis. Recently MRI scanning techniques have suggested microvascular ischaemia as the cause. It may be that low oestrogen levels predispose to abnormal microvascular circulation in some way. However, there is evidence that pain may develop without evidence of myocardial ischaemia, and thus it has also been proposed that some patients have abnormal pain perception. In this respect Syndrome X may represent a heterogeneous group of conditions awaiting future clarification. Conventional therapy (nitrates, beta-blockers, calcium channel blockers) are used in the management. The prognosis is good.

(5) Unstable angina
A patient who has risk factors for ischaemic heart disease and typical chest pain at rest. The **management** of unstable angina, acute coronary syndrome and non-ST segment elevation myocardial infarction (NSTMI) include . . .
- Rest

ANSWERS 3

- Oxygen therapy
- Establish IV access
- Relieve pain with morphine 10 mg i.v. and metoclopramide 10 mg i.v. as required
- Nitrates sublingual whilst establishing an isosorbide mononitrate infusion
- Beta-blockers: aim for heart rate 50–60/min; do *not* use in asthmatics
- Anti-platelet agents using aspirin and clopidogrel in combination
- Anticoagulate using . . .
  - Low molecular weight heparin, e.g. dalteparin (for up to 6 weeks)
  - Glycoprotein IIb, IIIa receptor antagonists in high-risk patients.
- Angiography and revascularization early for **high risk cases** . . .
  - Age >70 years
  - Raised troponin levels
  - Angina >20 min at rest
  - ST changes >1 mm
  - Haemodynamic changes, e.g. hypotension or pulmonary oedema
  - Diabetes

NB There is no role for thrombolytic therapy in acute coronary syndromes such as these unless the patient proceeds to an acute myocardial infarction. The ECG should be repeated every 15 min whilst the patient is symptomatic to watch for this.

Answer 18

(1) Sciatica with intervertebral disc prolapse at the level of S1

Typical nerve root (radicular) pain in the distribution of the S1 dermatome with reduced ankle jerk (S1) and pain in the distribution of the S1 root down the back of the leg and involving the sole of the foot. Most sciatica involves roots L4, L5 and S1. The strong anterior and posterior spinal ligaments usually divert a disc prolapse (which occurs backwards) either left or right posterior-laterally. A simple protrusion of the nuclus pulposus through the annulus may result in pain, but a full prolapse may compress a nerve root. Remember disc protrusions occur in areas of relative spinal mobility: cervical and lumbar.

Remember also that in the cervical area a prolapse will compress the nerve root corresponding to the vertebra **below** (i.e. a C5,6 prolapse will compress the C6 root), but as there are eight cervical roots and only seven cervical vertebrae the pattern reverses below the 7th cervical vertebra. Thus, a prolapse (or other source of compression) at any level below the C7 vertebrae will compress the root corresponding to the vertebra **above** (i.e. an L4,5 disc protrusion will compress the L4 root).

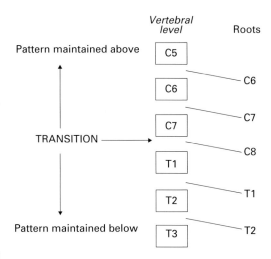

Reflex	Root
Biceps	C5,(6)
Triceps	C6,7
Supinator	C(5),6
Knee	L3,4
Ankle	S1
Extensor hallucis longus	L5

Key dermatomes to remember (the rest can be worked out if these are remembered)

Level	Sensory area
C7	Mid palm, third finger
T1	Medial arm
T5	Nipple
T10	Umbilicus
L2	Below inguinal ligament
S1	Sole of foot and back of leg
S4,5	Perianal area

(2) Cauda equina syndrome due to central disc prolapse

Occasionally the strong posterior spinal ligament does

not divert the prolapsing disc laterally (so compressing the nerve root) and the prolapse occurs directly backwards with resultant compression of the relevant cord structures.

The spinal cord is not as long as the spine and finishes with the conus medullaris, which is located between T9 and L1. Below this, nerve roots T12 to L5, which com-prise the cauda equina (horse's tail), fan out to exit at their respective spinal level.

Disc lesions that compress the **conus medullaris** (**T9–T12**) will produce mixed upper and lower motor features in the lower limbs, e.g. absent knee reflexes and up-going plantars, as they may compress both the cona (UMN) and adjacent nerve roots.

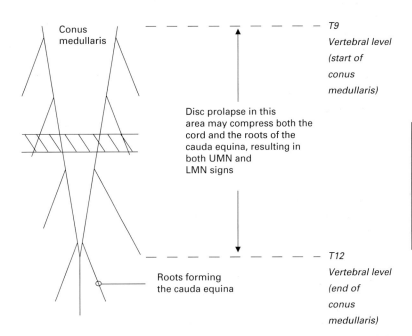

ANSWERS 3

Other causes of up-going plantars and absent knee reflexes (i.e. mixed UMN and LMN signs) include . . .
- Subacute combined degeneration of the cord (vitamin B12 deficiency)
- Friedreich's ataxia
- Motor neurone disease
- Tabes dorsalis
- Diabetes

As the cord finishes at the lower border of the L1 vertebral level and the most common disc protrusions are in the L 4, 5 and S1 area, a central disc prolapse will result in compression of the (**LMN**) **corda equina**. The result is **lower limb sensory loss (in the saddle distribution)**, **wasting paralysis**, **areflexia** and **down-going plantars**. In addition, lower motor neurone denervation of the bladder may occur, leading to loss of the sensation of filling and a large flaccid bladder with overflow incontinence. Emergency decompression is required to avert permanent neurological damage.

Note that the **detrusor muscle reflex arc** consists of stretch receptors with afferent neurones which synapse in the cord at the **S2, S3 and S4** level with the efferent neurones to the detrusor muscle of the bladder wall. The normal urge to void occurs when the bladder contains around 300 mL of urine. Descending higher inhibitory control signals prevent automatic reflex voiding until it is appropriate to do so.

Patterns of neurological dysfunction affecting the bladder
- **The automatic bladder** due to an *UMN* lesion above the level of the reflex arc (i.e. cord lesion above S2, S3 and S4). There is loss of descending higher control of the reflex arc resulting in a small (spastic) bladder that fills and automatically voids.
- **The autonomous bladder** due to *LMN* interruption of the reflex arc (e.g. by lesion at S2, S3 and S4) due to, for

example, a cauda equina lesion or sensory neuropathy. This results in a large flaccid bladder without reflex contraction but with overflow incontinence.

(3) Multiple myeloma

A multi-system condition much loved by examiners. The combination of marrow failure, renal failure and bone pain are highly suggestive of myeloma as the correct answer.

An abnormal proliferation of plasma cells produces large amounts of paraprotein IgG (in 66% of cases), IgA (in 30%) or rarely IgD. Light chains (Bence Jones proteins) appear in the urine in only two-thirds of cases. The plasma cells invade the marrow producing bone destruction (pain, deformity and hypercalcaemia) and marrow failure (bleeding, infections and anaemia). Renal failure is due to deposition of light chains and other causes (see EMQ 8, p. 93). The paraprotein itself may cause symptoms of hyperviscosity, such as headaches, tiredness and blurred vision.

The diagnosis can be made by demonstration of the paraprotein using **plasma electrophoresis**. Bone radiographs show the characteristic lytic lesions. The so-called 'pepper pot' skull has numerous well-defined 5–10 mm lytic areas.

Other paraproteinamias
- **Waldenstrom's macroglobulinaemia**
  - IgM produced: a large protein, so hyperviscosity symptoms are prominent and RBC rouleaux formation occurs
  - Otherwise behaves like myeloma but with the addition of lymph node enlargement like lymphoma
- **Monoclonal gammopathy of uncertain significance (MGUS)**
  - What it sounds like; often in older people with evidence of a low-level paraproteinaemia (raised gammaglobulin with a band on electrophoresis)
  - However, there are no features of an aggressive malignant disease such as bone marrow failure, bone destruction, hypercalcaemia or renal failure. Follow up is required to watch for any progression of the disease and features of myeloma

(4) Tuberculosis

In essence this is a case of spinal cord compression in which the pathological process involves the lymph nodes and respiratory system. The main differential here is lymphoma, although the social history and hilar node calcification and cavitation make TB the more likely diagnosis. The investigation of this case would centre on the positive identification of mycobacterium tubercles or lymphoma, from a biopsy of the superficial cervical node. The histology of the tubercle consists of caseation surrounded by Langerhan's cells (giant multi-nucleate), epithelioid cells and fibrosis.

Following primary tuberculosis, usually in the form of pulmonary infection, healing of the (usually peripheral) focus occurs. There is hilar lymph node enlargement, often with calcification. Cellular immunity develops which is dependent upon T-lymphocytes.

Post-primary TB involves reactivation due to reduced immunity in old age or general disease. There is spread of the mycobacteria within the lung and often to other areas. After the lungs, the bones are the second most common location involved, followed by lymph nodes, the renal tracts and GIT.

Patterns of post-primary TB
- Lung
  - Apical shadowing/fibrosis/cavitation
  - Miliary TB
  - Pleural effusion
  - Pneumonia
- Bone/joints
  - Destruction/osteomyelitis
  - Spinal disease (Pott's disease) may result in vertebral collapse and an acute angulation (the gibbus deformity); 'cold' abscess formation may occur
- Lymph node
  - Hilar/cervical nodes often
  - Sometimes large with skin sinuses (scrofula)
- Renal tract
  - Spread from lesions in the renal cortex causing renal tract fibrosis and strictures. Upper tract obstruction (hydronephrosis) haematuria, dysuria and urinary frequency occur. Early morning urine samples are requested to culture the organism
- GIT
  - Illeocaecal mass
  - Peritonitis
- Skin deposits
  - Lupus vulagris
- CNS
  - Meningitis
  - Tuberculoma

- Adrenal gland
  - Addison's disease

Causes of calcification on a chest radiograph
- Hilar nodes
  - TB
  - Silicosis
  - Sarcoidosis
  - Histoplasmosis
- Pleural
  - Asbestosis
  - Old TB
  - Old haemothorax
- Diffuse
  - Old TB
  - Old Chicken pox pneumonia
  - Healed histoplasmosis
  - Cysticercosis (tapeworm cysts)
  - Chronic venous hypertension (mitral stenosis)
  - Calcified metastases:
    Osteosarcoma
    Chrondrosarcoma
    Mucinous adenocarcinoma of breast or colon
    Papillary thyroid carcinoma
    Carcinoid tumour

Causes of a cavitating lesion on a chest radiograph
Use mnemonic **CAVIT** . . .
  C Carcinoma, e.g. squamous cell tumours
  A Autoimmune, e.g. polyarteritis nodosa, Wegener's granulomatosis
  V Vascular infarct
  I Infections, e.g. Staphylococcal, *Klebsiella*, tuberculosis
  T Trauma

History taking in back pain
The vast majority of back pain is musculoskeletal, usually termed **mechanical**, and indicates an injury to paraspinal muscles and intervertebral ligaments. It is extremely common and a history of unaccustomed exercise or chronic back misuse is usually obtained from an unfit and/or obese patient. The history seeks to confirm this and exclude serous pathology such as . . .
- Metastatic disease
- Infections
- Neurological complications
- Inflammatory spondarthropathies

Ask about . . .
- New or recurrent problems?
- Location?
- Trauma or unaccustomed exercise?
- Pain eased by rest and worse with movement?
- Nocturnal or rest pain?
- Weight loss?
- Fever/sweats/rigors?
- Peripheral neurological symptoms
  - Unilateral 'shooting' pain?
  - Bowel and bladder function?
  - Lower limb weakness?
  - Sensory disturbance?

(5) Ankylosing spondylitis
One of the seronegative inflammatory spondarthritides. The seronegative arthritides are a group of inflammatory arthritides that share several characteristic features . . .
- They are **negative for rheumatoid factor** (NB the group does not include seronegative RA)
- An **asymmetrical large joint** arthritis (oligoarthritis) occurs
- Predilection for the **axial skeleton** (spondarthritis) and sacroiliac joints
- **Inflammation of tendinous insertions** (enthesopathy)
- Association with **HLA B27** (90% of ankylosing spondylitis but also a normal finding in 8% of the normal population so little use diagnostically)

The seronegative arthritides comprise . . .
- **Ankylosing spondylitis**: the brunt of the disease on the axial skeleton (enthesopathy) and sacroiliac joints. Back pain in the morning and stiffness occur. There is progressive stiffness and a decreased range of movement in the spine leading to progressive kyphosis (forward flexion deformity). Radiographs of the spine show calcification of the tendons with loss of the normal lumbar lordosis. Eventual fusion of the spine to form the so-called Bamboo spine can occur. Physiotherapy to prevent this is central in the management. There are several extra-articular manifestations of the disease, which can easily be remembered as **the 7 As** . . .

  A <u>A</u>nterior uveitis
  A <u>A</u>pical lung fibrosis
  A <u>A</u>ortitis (aortic regurgitation due to dilatation of the aortic ring)

A A̲trio-ventricular conduction defects of the heart (heart block)

A Ig̲A̲ nephropathy

A A̲myloidosis

A A̲chilles tendonitis

- **Reiter's syndrome** (see EMQ 23, p. 154)

- **Psoriatic arthritis**: affects 7% of patients with psoriasis (see EMQ 23, p. 154)

- **Enteropathic arthritis:** affects around 10% of patients with Crohn's disease and ulcerative colitis in a pattern of a spondylitis (like ankylosing spondylitis) or an asymmetrical large joint oligoarthritis

Paper 4 Answers

MCQs

[1] (a) T (b) T (c) T (d) F (e) T
[2] (a) F (b) T (c) F (d) F (e) F
[3] (a) F (b) F (c) F (d) F (e) T
[4] (a) F (b) F (c) T (d) T (e) F
[5] (a) T (b) T (c) F (d) T (e) F
[6] (a) F (b) T (c) T (d) F (e) T
[7] (a) F (b) F (c) F (d) F (e) F
[8] (a) T (b) T (c) T (d) T (e) T
[9] (a) F (b) F (c) F (d) F (e) F
[10] (a) F (b) T (c) F (d) F (e) F
[11] (a) F (b) T (c) T (d) F (e) T
[12] (a) F (b) T (c) F (d) F (e) F
[13] (a) T (b) T (c) T (d) T (e) T
[14] (a) T (b) F (c) F (d) F (e) T
[15] (a) F (b) T (c) F (d) T (e) F
[16] (a) F (b) T (c) T (d) F (e) F
[17] (a) T (b) T (c) F (d) T (e) F
[18] (a) F (b) T (c) T (d) T (e) T
[19] (a) T (b) T (c) T (d) T (e) T
[20] (a) T (b) F (c) T (d) F (e) T
[21] (a) F (b) F (c) F (d) T (e) T
[22] (a) F (b) F (c) T (d) T (e) F
[23] (a) F (b) F (c) F (d) T (e) T
[24] (a) F (b) T (c) T (d) F (e) F

---

[1] (a) T (b) T (c) T (d) F (e) T

(a) Heart failure (HF) is one of the causes of simultaneous central and peripheral cyanosis. Peripheral cyanosis occurs due to sluggish peripheral circulation, whereas central cyanosis occurs due to defective oxygenation of blood caused by pulmonary oedema, leading to a relative right to left shunt. Central cyanosis is always accompanied by peripheral cyanosis. The reverse is not true.

(b) Patients with end stage HF often become jaundiced ('icteric') due to hepatic congestion interfering with liver metabolism, especially in cases of predominantly right-sided cardiac failure.

(c) Although now commonplace in the management of chronic HF, where they have been unequivocally proven to improve survival, β-blockers should be avoided in acute HF since their negative ino- and chronotropic effects can be extremely detrimental. They should only be considered once the patient has been stabilized.

(d) Chronic lung disease typically causes *right* HF — cor pulmonale.

(e) 'Cachexia' is a Greek term, literally meaning 'bad condition of the body'. It is defined as 'a general weight loss and wasting occurring in the course of a chronic disease or emotional disturbance'. It is not, as is commonly misconstrued, strictly related to malignancy, and it is commonly seen in patients with long-standing cardiovascular disease.

[2] (a) F (b) T (c) F (d) F (e) F

(a) Rib-notching seen on chest radiograph is most often a sign of coarctation of the aorta. It is defined as 'a smooth defect in the lower border of one or more **upper** ribs caused by enlarged **intercostal collateral vessels**' that develop to carry blood to the lower portion of the body otherwise cut-off by the coarctation.

(b) Thiazide diuretics have a number of well-recognized side effects, including hypercholesterolaemia, hypokalaemia, hyperuricaemia and gout, postural hypotension, and impotence (reversible on discontinuation of treatment).

(c) ACE-inhibitors (tend to end in –*pril*) are well-recognized to cause a persistent dry cough due to **build up** of bradykinin. This occurs because ACE is not only important for converting angiotensin-I to angiotensin-II, but also for breaking down bradykinin into kininogen.

(d) Doxazocin is an α-**blocker** that causes potent post-synaptic α-1 blockade, hence **arterial vasodilatation** and lowering of blood pressure.

Calcium channel antagonists can be split into two groups: the dihydropyridines (class 2, e.g. nifedipine, amlodipine) and the non-dihydropyridines (class 1, e.g. verapamil, diltiazem). All of the calcium channel antagonists block calcium flux into myocardial cells and it's usage within cells. They also all relax coronary arteries, cause peripheral vasodilatation and decrease force of left ventricular contraction (*negatively inotropic*). However (and this is the important bit), **only the non-dihydropyridine calcium channel antagonists are also negatively chronotropic**, i.e. decrease the heart rate as well, and therefore are very useful anti-anginals. However, because of this added effect, *non-dihydropyridine calcium channel antagonists should never be used in combination with β-blockers*. The newer dihydropyridine agents, like amlodipine, have a very smooth pharmacological profile and barely even cause negative inotropism at the correct dosage, leaving a very 'clean' vasodilating agent.

(e) Benign intracranial hypertension is characterized by **marked papilloedema in the absence of a mass lesion or an increase in ventricular size**. It occurs mainly in **obese young *females***, presenting usually with severe headache, visual blurring and palsy of the 6th cranial nerve (the abducens). It is benign only in that it is not fatal; it can cause infarction of the optic nerve leading to **blindness**, especially if it is severe and long-standing. Palliation is with thiazide diuretics, acetazolamide and repeated lumbar puncture. Weight reduction is important and surgical decompression or shunting is sometimes necessary.

[3] (a) F (b) F (c) F (d) F (e) T

(a) In the setting of acute MI, serum readings of cholesterol and HDL (high-density lipoprotein) remain close to baseline for ~48 h before falling thereafter. They take up to **8 weeks** to return to baseline levels, hence cholesterol levels between 2 and 56 days post-MI are not representative of baseline levels.

(b) Cholestyramine is an example of a **bile-acid binding resin** used in the treatment of hyperlipidaemia. It acts as an anion-exchange resin to bind bile acids in the gut, preventing entero-hepatic circulation and increase formation of bile acids from cholesterol in the liver of the treated patient. It has been shown to decrease LDL cholesterol in the blood by 8–15%.

(c) Statins actually block **HMG-CoA reductase**, the enzyme controlling the rate-limiting step in cholesterol synthesis within the body. They have been shown to decrease LDL cholesterol within the blood by 30–40%.

(d) Chylomicrons are synthesized post-prandially in the small intestine and are hence present in large quantities within the blood after every fatty meal. They are the main mechanism for transporting dietary fat to the liver. An isolated raised plasma level is therefore not reflective of a significantly elevated cardiovascular risk. Isolated levels of any blood parameter rarely mean much at all — they should be put in context with other blood parameters and serial measurement of that same parameter.

(e) Statins are recognized to be **hepatotoxic**. Other important side effects include reversible myositis and IBS-like symptoms (abdominal pain, diarrhoea and bloating).

[4] (a) F (b) F (c) T (d) T (e) F

(a) Classical angina is provoked by **physical exertion** and typically comes on **after** heavy meals, especially in cold, windy weather.

(b) Variant/Prinzmetal's angina is angina that comes on without provocation, usually at rest. It is due to **coronary artery *spasm***. Surprisingly, it is more common in females than males.

(c) Myoscans (also known as cardiac scintography) are used for demonstrating the perfusion of the heart. They involve contrast agents (such as technetium[99]) and are performed before and after exercise. The redistribution of the contrast agent is a sensitive indicator of ischaemia. They are particularly useful for deciding if stenoses seen at angiography are indeed causing significant physiological ischaemia.

(d) The side effects of GTN include a throbbing headache, flushing, dizziness, postural hypotension and tachycardia; all are due to the drug's venodilating effects.

(e) β-blockers cause **broncho*constriction*** and should definitely be avoided in asthmatics if at all possible.

[5] (a) T (b) T (c) F (d) T (e) F

(a) PTCA involves multiple inflations of a balloon located inside obstructing coronary atheroma, sited by X-ray fluoroscopy. Surprisingly, although it markedly improves the symptoms of angina, *it provides **no currently demonstrable prognostic benefit***.

(b) Side effects of PTCA include endothelial denudation, local dissection, distal embolization (of attached thrombus or plaque fragments) and acute coronary occlusion (observed in 2–4% of procedures).

(c) The mortality of PTCA is much higher than this: 1/100, or **1%**. There is also a 2% risk of acute MI and a 2% risk of need to move to urgent coronary artery bypass graft (CABG).

(d) This is indeed true: where possible, the left internal mammary artery (LIMA) is used to bypass stenoses. The right internal mammary (RIMA) is used almost as frequently. Reversed saphenous vein grafts are also still commonly used, but the long-term patency of these compared to arterial grafts is less good. Occasionally, the radial or gastroepiploic arteries may also be used where the alternative native vessels are absent.

(e) Long-term patency of arterial grafts is superior to that of venous grafts.

[6] (a) F (b) T (c) T (d) F (e) T

Acute pericarditis has numerous recognized aetiologies, but the most common causes in the UK are **MI and Cox-sackie virus infection**. A comprehensive list of causes is shown below . . .

- **Viruses**
  - Usually the enterovirus Coxsackie virus → **(e)**
  - Sudden onset
  - Usually young adults
  - Lasts only a few weeks
  - Good prognosis, but recurrences and death do occur
- **Post-MI**
  - Occurs in 20%, especially post-anterior MI → **(c)**
  - Clinically hear friction rub, and patient develops recurrence of chest pain and fever
- **Uraemia**
  - Usually only the terminal stages of uraemic disease will cause pericarditis → **(b)**
- **Bacteria**
  - Usually *Staphylococcus* or *Haemophilus*
  - Especially in pneumonia or septicaemia
  - Treat with antibiotics and surgical drainage
  - Usually fatal
- **TB**
  - Typical sign is low-grade chronic fever with signs of pericarditis
  - Aspiration is usually required to make the diagnosis
- **Malignancy**
  - Carcinoma of the bronchus, breast and Hodgkin's disease are the commonest malignant causes
  - Leukaemia and multiple myeloma also associated

[7] (a) F (b) F (c) F (d) F (e) F

(a) SAH describes *spontaneous* (rather than traumatic) *arterial* bleeding into the subarachnoid space.

(b) CT imaging is the investigation of choice in SAH, where subarachnoid or intraventricular blood can easily be seen. Lumbar puncture is not necessary if the diagno-

sis is confirmed by CT, but should be considered where there is doubt. The CSF becomes yellow — '**xanthochro-mia**' — several hours after the initial bleed. This discoloration of the CSF would be expected to last for a matter of days, but certainly not for 3 weeks.

(c) The abducens, or 6th cranial nerve, supplies the lateral rectus muscle, normally causing the eye to abduct. Lesions of the 6th cranial nerve cause a convergent squint, the affected eye being unable to abduct past the midline. There are many causes of a lesion to the abducens nerve because it has a *long intracranial course*. In cases where the intracranial pressure is increased, e.g. SAH, the abducens becomes pressed against the petrous part of the temporal bone causing a palsy. This is not a valuable localizing sign as it simply reflects the generally increased ICP.

(d) The oculomotor, or 3rd cranial nerve, sends motor fibres to . . .

- Four external ocular muscles: superior rectus, inferior rectus, medial rectus and inferior oblique
- Levator palpebrae superioris
- Sphincter pupillae (parasympapthetic)

All of these motor fibres enter the orbit through the superior orbital fissure. There are many causes of a lesion to the oculomotor nerve, but in situations where there is raised intracranial pressure, partial or full coning of the temporal lobe impinges on this nerve, bringing about palsy. This, again, is not a valuable localizing sign because it merely reflects the generally raised intracranial pressure, and not necessarily that the site of the pathology is in the region/course of the oculomotor nerve. A palsy to the 3rd nerve can be recognized by an eyeball facing inferolaterally, unilateral complete ptosis and a dilated pupil.

(e) The causes of SAH are shown in the list below . . .

- **Berry aneurysm (70%)**
- **No lesion identified (20%)**
- **Arteriovenous malformation (10%)**
- Bleeding disorders
- Mycotic aneurysms (endocarditis)
- Acute bacterial meningitis
- Brain tumour (e.g. metastatic melanoma)
- Arteritis (e.g. SLE)
- Coarctation of the aorta
- Connective tissue disorders (e.g. Marfan's, Ehlers–Danlos)
- Polycystic kidney disease (very important)

Berry aneurysms are also known as *saccular* aneurysms. They often form on the circle of Willis and its branches, the commonest sites being on the **posterior and anterior communicating arteries**, and where the middle cerebral artery bifurcates. One in a hundred people are found to have one incidentally at autopsy. Apart from causing symptoms by spontaneous rupture, berry aneurysms cause problems by direct pressure effects on the structures around them, e.g. posterior communicating artery aneurysms may cause a painful 3rd nerve palsy.

Arteriovenous malformations (AVM) are developmental lesions usually existing within the cerebral hemispheres. Patients who survive an SAH secondary to AVM commonly rebleed (recurrence rate being ~15% per annum).

[8] (a)T (b)T (c)T (d)T (e)T

Pancytopenia is described as 'pronounced reduction in the number of erythrocytes, all types of white blood cell, and platelets in the circulating blood'.

The **causes of pancytopenia** are listed below . . .
- Aplastic anaemia
- Drugs
- Megaloblastic anaemia → **(a)**
- Bone marrow infiltration or replacement:
  Hodgkin's and non-Hodgkin's lymphoma
  Acute leukaemia → **(d)**
  Myeloma
  Secondary carcinoma
  Myelofibrosis → **(e)**
- Hypersplenism
- SLE
- Disseminated TB → **(c)**
- Paroxysmal nocturnal haemoglobinuria → **(b)**
- Overwhelming sepsis

Aplastic anaemia is rare but very serious. It is defined as '**pancytopaenia with hypocellularity or aplasia of the bone marrow**'. It can be inherited or (much more commonly) acquired. It occurs due to a **reduction in the number of** *pluripotential stem cells*, together with a fault in those remaining or an immune reaction against them so they are unable to repopulate the bone marrow. The sum effect is a disorder characterized by *anaemia, bleeding* and *infection*.

The individual **causes of aplastic anaemia** are given in the list below . . .
- *Primary*
  Congenital, e.g. Fanconi's anaemia
  Idiopathic acquired (50% of cases)
- *Secondary*
  Chemicals, e.g. benzene
  Drugs, e.g. chemotherapeutic, idiosyncratic reactions
  Insecticides
  Ionizing radiation
  Viral infections, e.g. hepatitis, measles, HIV
  Other infections, e.g. TB
  Pregnancy
  Paroxysmal nocturnal haemoglobinuria

Paroxysmal nocturnal haemoglobinuria is a form of non-immune haemolytic anaemia, where a clone of red cells in the sufferer's circulation is particularly sensitive to destruction by activated complement. These cells are continually haemolysed intravascularly. It is so-called because typically only the urine voided in the morning on waking is dark in colour. The reason for this phenomenon is unclear. These patients are at high risk of having venous thrombotic events. Treatment is conservative, repeated blood transfusions and anticoagulation being the mainstays.

[9] (a)F (b)F (c)F (d)F (e)F

(a) Aortic sclerosis refers to a situation where the murmur of aortic stenosis is present ('diamond-shaped, ejection systolic murmur') **without any of the other stigmata** of aortic stenosis (e.g. no slow-rising pulse, no ejection click, no left ventricular failure).

(b) The symptoms of aortic stenosis only occur at a relatively late stage in the disease (when the valve orifice is more than two-thirds stenosed). It causes **symptoms mainly attributable to increased workload placed on the left ventricle** (including angina and subsequently left ventricular failure), and also **symptoms due to reduced outflow from the left ventricle** (including exercise-induced syncope).

(c) The apex beat in aortic stenosis is **not usually displaced**, because it causes hypertrophy of the left ventricle, not dilatation.

(d) An opening snap is heard in mitral stenosis, occurring just after the second heart sound. Aortic stenosis causes an *ejection click*, just after the first heart sound.

(e) The murmur of aortic stenosis may be audible over the entire praecordium, but is best heard in the aortic area (second right intercostal space, parasternally).

[10] (a)F (b)T (c)F (d)F (e)F

(a) In isolated AV nodal blockade, the QRS complexes usually have a **normal morphology**, as do the P-waves. It is the relationship of the P-waves to the QRS complexes that is abnormal. The only time the QRS complexes may be abnormal in AV nodal blockade is in third-degree heart block with a broad complex escape rhythm.

(b) Mobitz type II is a form of second-degree heart block where **occasionally a P-wave is not followed by a QRS complex**. There is **no pattern** to these so-called dropped beats, and the dropped beats are **not** preceded **by progressive PR elongation**.

(c) Wenkebach block phenomenon (also known as Mobitz type I) is another form of second-degree heart block. There is progressive PR elongation before eventually a P-wave fails to conduct to the ventricles and a QRS complex is 'dropped'. The PR interval before the blocked P-wave is considerably longer than the PR after the blocked P-wave. The mechanism is unknown, but it is believed to be the **most benign** form of second-degree block, as it is associated with a reliable subsidiary pacemaker and a lower chance of progressing to third degree heart block than Mobitz type II or 2:1/3:1 advanced block.

(d) First-degree heart block is simple yet constant prolongation of the PR interval to >0.2 s. However, a QRS complex follows every P-wave. It never requires treatment in isolation.

(e) The conduction of P-waves to the ventricles in third-degree heart block is *not* variable—it never happens! P-waves do fire regularly, but there is no conduction through the 'broken' AV node. The ventricle in this situation is described as 'lonely'. Life is maintained by a spontaneous ventricular escape rhythm that has either a broad or a narrow complex, depending on where it originates in the conduction system.

[11] (a) F (b) T (c) T (d) F (e) T

(a) Each epithelial cell of the upper respiratory tract has around **200 cilia**.

(b) Type I pneumocytes form the thin barrier for gas exchange and make up the majority of the epithelial lining of the lung. Despite this, they are formed from type II pneumocytes, which produce the surface-tension lowering surfactant.

(c) Airflow within the lungs is maximal within the trachea, slowing towards the periphery of the lung and in the terminal airways of the lung, gas flow occurs entirely by diffusion.

(d) Airway tone is under the control of the autonomic nervous system. Bronchomotor tone is maintained by vagal efferent nerves. Sympathetic nerves do *not* directly

innervate the airways. Instead there are many adrenoceptors on the surface of bronchial muscle which respond to circulating catecholamines. **Airway tone shows a circadian rhythm**, even in non-asthmatic, healthy individuals: greatest at 04.00 hours, lowest at 16.00 hours. This rhythm remains the same but is exacerbated in asthmatics; hence asthma symptoms are typically worse early in the morning and late at night (these times are closest to the 04.00 hours nadir).

(e) 'Dead space' describes a situation where there is **ventilation of an area of lung, but no perfusion** of that region with blood. It occurs commonly in situations such as pulmonary embolism, pulmonary arteritis and pulmonary fibrosis. This is in contrast with 'shunt', which is a situation where an area of lung is being perfused with blood, but is not being ventilated. Such is the case in asthma, COPD, lung collapse or consolidation and diseases of the chest wall.

[12] (a) F (b) T (c) F (d) F (e) F

(a) Sinusitis, or infection of the paranasal sinuses, often complicates upper respiratory tract infections. Bacteria such as *Streptococcus pneumoniae* and *Haemophilus influenzae* are the usual cause. It develops mainly in children **over the age of 8 years**. It should be treated with antibiotics.

(b) **Parainfluenza virus** mainly causes croup, although rarely measles virus can be the cause.

(c) Epiglottitis is caused by *Haemophilus influenzae type B*.

(d) Direct inspection should be avoided in acute epiglottitis, especially the use of tongue depressors to visualize the red, swollen epiglottis, because this can distress the child and precipitate acute airways spasm.

(e) Unlike epiglottitis, which can be prevented by immunization with the Hib vaccine, croup cannot be immunized against. Treatment of croup is with inhalation of steam, oxygen and IV fluids. Intubation may be necessary but concomitant treatment with steroids can shorten its duration.

[13] (a) T (b) T (c) T (d) T (e) T

The porphyrias are a heterogeneous group of rare inborn errors of metabolism caused by enzymatic abnormalities in the biosynthetic pathway leading to haem production. Enzymatic errors lead to accumulation of intermediate compounds known as 'porphyrins'. In porphyria, the excess production of porphyrins occurs in either the liver (hepatic porphyrias) or in the bone marrow (erythropoeietic porphyrias). These disorders can also be classified as either acute (associated with neuropsychiatric disorders) or non-acute.

Acute intermittent porphyria is . . .

- an **autosomal dominant** condition that normally presents in early adult life (around the age of 30 years) affecting **more women** than men → **(b), (d)**
- **precipitated by alcohol and a vast range of lipid-soluble drugs**, including the OCP, barbiturates, tetracycline, chlordiazepoxide and furosemide → **(a), (c), (e)**

It usually presents with severe colicky abdominal pain, vomiting and constipation. There is also commonly a mainly motor polyneuropathy. Less commonly, it presents with hypertension, tachycardia and, bizarrely, psychiatric disorders, including depression, anxiety and frank psychosis. Classically, *the urine turns red-brown on standing*. Management acutely is largely supportive, with opioid analgesia and high carbohydrate intake (thought to reduce porphyrin overproduction). During periods of remission, it is important to stress avoidance of precipitating factors, especially drugs and alcohol.

[14] (a)T (b)F (c)F (d)F (e)T

(a) Because the defect in the opening of the critical chloride channel CFTR (which is the pathological basis of CF) is not limited to the lungs, CF affects many of the other organ systems of the body too, including the GIT. **85% of patients with CF have symptomatic steatorrhoea** due to pancreatic dysfunction caused by the tenacity of secretions in CF. Cholesterol gallstones are more frequently observed in patients with CF, as are cirrhosis, peptic ulceration and gastrointestinal malignancy.

(b) Males with CF are almost always infertile because there is **failure of development of the vas deferens and epididymis**. Females *are* able to conceive, but often develop secondary amenorrhoea with disease progression.

(c) *Inhaled* recombinant human DNAse degrades DNA, which is a major contributor to the tenacity and viscosity of the secretions in CF, and can improve the FEV1 by ≈20%.

(d) On the contrary, lung transplant should be **considered early in all patients with CF**.

(e) Because of the gastrointestinal effects of CF, patients should receive pancreatic supplements (including trypsin and lipase to allow fat content of diet to be kept normal), and their nutrition should be optimized, with

regular and thorough dietician input. Calorific input should be 150% of normal, and vitamin supplements should be included in the nutritional package.

[15] (a)F (b)T (c)F (d)T (e)F

Eosinophilia is said to occur when the number of eosinophils is >0.4 × 10^9/L in the peripheral blood.

(a) Eosinophils comprise **up to 5%** of WBC numbers in healthy individuals. Eosinophils are used selectively within the body for fighting **parasitic (particularly nematode) infections**. They are also involved in **immediate hypersensitivity** (allergic) reactions. They have low affinity surface receptors for antibodies of the IgE class.

(d) Eosinophils contain **many large granules** which are cytotoxic when released onto the surface of organisms. These granular structures include major basic protein (directly damages helminths), eosinophil cationic protein (highly toxic to parasites; a potent neurotoxin), eosinophil-derived neurotoxin and eosinophil peroxidase.

(e) Ulcerative colitis does *not* cause an eosinophilia.

A comprehensive list of the **causes of eosinophilia** is given below . . .

- **Parasitic infestations**
  Ascaris
  Hookworm
  Strongyloides
- **Allergic disorders**
  Hayfever (allergic rhinitis)
  Other hypersensitivity reactions, including drug reactions → **(b)**
- **Skin disorders**
  Urticaria
  Pemphigus
  Eczema
- **Pulmonary disorders**
  Bronchial asthma
  Tropical pulmonary eosinophilia
  Sarcoidosis
  Allergic bronchopulmonary aspergillosis
  Churg–Strauss syndrome
- **Malignant disorders**
  Hodgkin's disease
  Carcinoma
  Eosinophilic leukaemia

Eosinophils are slightly larger than neutrophils, and are characterized by a nucleus with usually two lobes and large cytoplasmic granules that stain deeply red (hence the name).

[16] (a) F (b) T (c) T (d) F (e) F

(a) Other bacteria such as *Mycobacterium bovis* and *M. africanum* can cause TB as well as *M. tuberculosis*.

(b) The initial reaction to inhalation of *M. tuberculosis* is exudation and infiltration of the area with neutrophils. These are rapidly replaced by macrophages that ingest the bacilli. Macrophage interaction with T-lymphocytes leads to the development of cellular immunity, which is typically seen at 3–8 weeks. At this stage, the classical pathology of TB can be seen: granulomatous lesions with a central area of cheesy necrosis ('caseation') surrounded by epithelioid cells and Langerhan's giant cells (both of which are derived from macrophages). The alternative name for these lesions is '*cold abscesses*'. Subsequently caseated areas heal completely and many become calcified, but 20% still contain tubercle bacilli. These initially lie dormant, but are capable of reactivation → 'post-primary TB'.

(c) Pott's disease is also known as '**tuberculous spondylitis**', and is defined as 'tuberculous infection of the spine associated with a sharp angulation of the spine at the point of the disease'. Named after Sir Percival Pott, an English surgeon who lived from 1714 to 1788.

(d) Immunization with the live, attenuated TB vaccine derived from *M. bovis* is **only 70% effective** at the current time.

(e) Lupus pernio is, in fact, a skin disorder associated with **intrathoracic sarcoidosis**. It is described as 'chronic indurated purple granulomatous skin clinically resembling frostbite, involving ears, cheeks, nose, lips and forehead'. TB is a classic cause of **erythema nodosum**.

[17] (a) T (b) T (c) F (d) T (e) F

(a) Non-small cell lung cancer (NSCLC) is indeed approximately **3× more common** than the small cell variety. The commonest type of NSCLC is **squamous cell carcinoma**, which accounts for ~**40%** of all bronchial carcinomas.

(b) The **squamous** variety of NSCLC is indeed the most likely to cause cavitation within the lungs.

(c) It is the **adenocarcinoma** variety that is most likely to arise from occupational exposure to asbestos.

(d) **Alveolar cell carcinoma** does have the propensity to cause expectoration of large volumes of mucoid sputum.

(e) NSCLC tends in general to be **much slower at killing victims** than small cell lung cancer: time taken from initial diagnosis to death for NSCLC is ~10 years, compared with ~3 years in small cell lung cancer.

[18] (a) F (b) T (c) T (d) T (e) T

The following is a comprehensive list of causes of a mass in the right iliac fossa (RIF) . . .

- Crohn's disease (commonest)
- Caecal carcinoma → **(b)**
- Caecal diverticular disease
- Carcinoma of the ascending colon
- Appendix mass
- Ileocaecal TB
- Volvulus → **(c)**
- Meckel's diverticulum → **(e)**
- Mesenteric adenitis
- Ovarian mass (+ other obstetric/gynaecological causes) → **(d)**
- Abdominal wall herniae
- (Renal)
- (Amoebiasis)

Meckel's diverticulum is a remnant of the embryonic vitelline duct, which connects the ileum with the umbilicus. It is present in 1–3% of the general population, but only 2% of patients with it are symptomatic. It is 2× more common in men than in women. It is located ~2 feet (90 cm) from the ileocaecal valve. The cells lining it have the capacity to develop into multiple types of mucosa, thus it is common to find heterotopic tissue in the diverticulum. The most common type of lining mucosa is gastric and this has the potential to cause large GI bleeds. The Meckel's may also precipitate intussusception. The most common age for symptoms is <2 years, and it can be very difficult to distinguish it from acute appendicitis.

Sigmoid diverticulitis presents as a mass in the left iliac fossa (LIF). → **(a)**

[19] (a) T (b) T (c) T (d) T (e) T

(a) Alcohol is widely known to be associated with the development of oesophageal carcinoma, especially consumption of the equivalent of >9 g ethanol per day, with spirits being more dangerous than beer/lager.

(b) Smoking (especially at levels >20 cigarettes per day) is well correlated with an increased risk of development of oesophageal neoplasia.

(c) Achalasia is associated with oesophageal malignancy, presumably due to the increased length of time any carcinogens in food are in contact with the mucosa.

(d) Barratt's oesophagus is defined as at least 3 cm of intestinal metaplaisia present at the lower end of the oesophagus, and it arises due to long-standing GORD. It is pre-malignant for adenocarcinoma of the oesophagus,

not the squamous cell carcinoma that generally afflicts the oesophagus in the absence of intestinal metaplaisia.
(e) Plummer–Vinson syndrome is also known as Patterson–Brown–Kelly syndrome. It describes an upper oesophageal web, either asymptomatic or causing dysphagia, that is associated with iron-deficiency anaemia, angular stomatitis and glossitis. It is rare and mainly affects females. The aetiology is poorly understood, but it is known to confer an increased risk of late development of oesophageal carcinoma.

[20] (a)T (b)F (c)T (d)F (e)T

The middle cerebral artery (MCA) is the **largest branch** of the internal carotid artery, coming off the middle portion of the circle of Willis. It initially runs laterally in the lateral cerebral sulcus. Cortical branches supply the **entire lateral surface of the cerebral hemisphere**, except for a narrow strip supplied by the anterior cerebral artery, the occipital pole and the inferolateral surface of the hemisphere, which are supplied by the posterior cerebral artery. The MCA thus supplies all the motor area, except for the 'leg' area. Central branches of the MCA enter the anterior perforated substance, and supply the deep masses of grey matter within the cerebral hemisphere.

Weakness/flaccidity of the limbs of the right side of the body would be expected to occur with an acute left-sided MCA infarction because this vessel is responsible for supplying the vital corticobulbar and corticospinal fibres in the internal capsule of the left side of the brain. These motor fibres then cross over in the brainstem to supply motor function to the right side of the body, hence the contralateral weakness. → **(a)**

Total occlusion of the MCA leads to a phenomenon known as *middle cerebral artery syndrome* . . .
- **Contralateral hemiplegia** (as described above)
- **Contralateral hemianaesthesia**
- **Visual field defect** (here, left homonymous hemianopia — due to a lesion of the optic tract between the optic chiasm and the lateral geniculate body) → **(e)**
- Deviation of the head and the eyes towards the side of the lesion

Left-sided MCA occlusion is more likely to lead to **global dysphasia** (because speech areas are in left frontotemporal regions), whereas right-sided MCA occlusion is more likely to lead to unilateral neglect of the contralateral side (because visuospatial awareness is located in the right temporal lobe). → **(c)**

Branch occlusions of the MCA are common, and may lead to incomplete syndromes. For example, occlusion of an upper branch of the MCA leads to Broca's expressive dysphasia, whereas occlusion of a lower branch of the MCA leads to Wernicke's receptive dysphasia.

Acute occlusion of the left MCA does *not* generally cause . . .
- Left-sided facial paralysis → **(b)**
- Headache: headache in general is not a feature of ischaemic stroke → **(d)**
- Laryngeal paralysis: the larynx is supplied by the right and left recurrent laryngeal nerves, both of which are branches of the vagus nerve.
- Loss of consciousness: although an occasional feature of acute stroke, loss of consciousness is rarely seen in infarction of the MCA as this blood vessel does not supply the reticular activating system of the brainstem.
- Same-day changes visible on head CT: whilst CT scanning of the head would be expected to reveal a haemorrhage from the minute that it occurred, the changes related to infarction of the brain only occur over the ensuing 2–3 days. Over 90% of infarcts are visible at one week post-event. MRI is more sensitive in detecting infarction than is CT.
- Hyperreflexia in the contralateral limbs: initially, the affected limbs (in this case those of the right side of the body) are areflexic. It is only after a variable period (usually several days) that the reflexes recover and become exaggerated, and an extensor plantar response appears.

[21] (a)F (b)F (c)F (d)T (e)T

(a) The hepatic artery has a blood pressure that is equal to systemic blood pressure, whilst the hepatic portal vein, although not a vein in the truest sense of the word, has a pressure much lower than this, in the region of **5–8 mmHg**, with only a small gradient across the liver to the hepatic vein. If the pressure within the portal vein rises above 10–12 mmHg, the compliant venous system dilates and collaterals develop, mainly at the gastro-oesophageal junction (oesophageal varices), rectum, left renal vein, diaphragm, retroperitoneum and the anterior abdominal wall via the umbilical vein (caput medusa).

(b) Patients with cirrhosis and hence portal hypertension have a **hyperdynamic circulation** (→ palmar erythema). This is due to release of mediators such as nitric oxide (NO) that attempt to help the situation by vasodilating the venous system so that collaterals can develop. The vasodilatation causes sodium retention and plasma volume expansion, exacerbating the portal hypertension and formation of ascites.

(c) Balloon tamponade with a Sengstaken–Blakemore tube should only be used with the greatest care when other methods of stopping variceal haemorrhage have failed (e.g. sclerosant injection, variceal banding, vasoconstrictor therapy). The oesophageal balloon of the tube should *never* be used. These tubes have serious and life-threatening complications, e.g. aspiration pneumonia, oesophageal rupture and mucosal ulceration, though in certain circumstances may be life saving.

(d) 'TIPS' stands for **'transjugular intrahepatic portocaval shunt'**, and it is an effective procedure for treating acute variceal bleeding. A guidewire is passed via the jugular vein to the liver, and an expandable metal shunt is forced over the guidewire into the substance of the liver to form a channel between the portal and the systemic venous systems. TIPS is only used when simpler methods for stemming variceal bleeding have failed.

(e) β-blockers are effective at reducing portal pressures in the stable situation. Their effect is two-fold. Blockade of β-1 receptors decreases cardiac output, whilst blockade of β-2 receptors effectively blocks splanchnic vasodilation. They have been shown to decrease the frequency of re-bleeding, and some studies suggest that they are as effective as sclerotherapy at doing so.

[22] (a) F (b) F (c) T (d) T (e) F

The various **causes of vitamin B12 deficiency** are listed below . . .

- *Impaired absorption*
  Stomach
  - Pernicious anaemia: *most common.* → **(c)**
  - Gastrectomy
  - Congenital deficiency of intrinsic factor
  Small intestine
  - Ileal disease/resection
  - Bacterial overgrowth
  - Tropical sprue → **(d)**
  - Fish tapeworm
- *Low dietary intake*
  - Vegan diet
- *Abnormal metabolism*
  - Nitrous oxide (inactivates B12)
  - Congenital transcobalamin II deficiency

Contrary to popular belief, malabsorption of vitamin B12 due to pancreatitis, coeliac disease or treatment with

metformin is mild and does not usually result in significant B12 deficiency. → **(a)**

Pernicious anaemia is an autoimmune condition in which there is atrophy of the gastric mucosa mediated by **parietal cell auto-antibodies**, with consequent **failure of intrinsic factor production**, and hence vitamin B12 malabsorption. It is common in elderly, blue-eyed, fair-skinned populations, affecting more females than males and being associated with a number of other autoimmune conditions. It is linked to the development of **gastric carcinoma**. Onset is with insidious development of anaemic symptoms. Patients are often said to be **lemon yellow** in colour (due to excess breakdown of Hb due to ineffective erythropoeisis in bone marrow), and may also have features of glossitis and angular stomatitis. Neurological changes are of the greatest significance; if untreated, these can be irreversible. Initially, a peripheral polyneuropathy predominates, but progression to involve the posterior and eventually the lateral columns of the spinal cord occurs, leading to '*subacute combined degeneration*'. Vitamin B12 absorbing ability can be measured using the **Schilling test** (measures urinary excretion of known oral dose of radioactively labelled B12). Treatment is with oral administration of cobalamin, because small amounts are still absorbed even in the complete absence of intrinsic factor.

Tropical sprue is a malabsorption disease of **unknown aetiology** (likely to be infective) affecting the jejunum. It occurs in inhabitants of and visitors to the tropics. Malabsorption has to be of at least two differing substances (usually fat and vitamin B12), and is usually accompanied by **diarrhoea and malnutrition**. The jejunal mucosa in abnormal, showing **partial villous atrophy** (less severe than that seen in coeliac disease). It is endemic in most of Asia, some Caribbean islands, Puerto Rico and parts of South America. Although the aetiology is unknown, many patients improve when they leave the area, take folic acid, and take antibiotics (usually tetracycline). It may be necessary to treat for up to 6 months. Prognosis is excellent.

[23] (a) F (b) F (c) F (d) T (e) T

(a) 'Skip lesions' are pathognomonic of CD: they reflect the underlying **non-continuous** pathology of Crohn's.

(b) Micro-abscesses occur commonly in UC: they form when the submucosa becomes involved in the inflammatory process.

(c) Sulphonylurea drugs are used in diabetes. **Sulphasalazine**, which sounds similar, is the anti-inflammatory agent of choice used in inflammatory bowel disease. It initially induces remission of disease in over 50% of patients. It is a mixture of sulphonamide and salicylic acid (aspirin related).

(d) UC is **curable**, but only by surgical resection of the entire colon (total colectomy)

(e) UC is **more common** than CD: 2–10 per 100 000 population compared with 1–6 per 100 000 population for Crohn's.

[24] (a) F (b)T (c)T (d) F (e) F

(a) Unlike UC, CD involves **transmural** inflammation of the entire gut wall: mucosa, submucosa and serosa.

(b) Non-caseating granulomas are seen in ~60% of patients with CD.

(c) Skip lesions reflect the non-contiguous nature of the inflammation seen in CD compared with the contiguous inflammation of UC.

(d) Very bloody diarrhoea is more representative of UC. The predominant symptom of CD is severe abdominal **pain**.

(e) Patients with chronic CD often have malabsorption of carbohydrate, fat, protein and the vitamins B12, A, D, E and K ($\rightarrow$ think *clotting problems!*)

EMQs

Answer 19

(1) Renal cell carcinoma

An unusual tumour in that there are many paraneoplastic features including . . .

- Fever
- Normochromic normocytic anaemia
- Polyneuropathy
- Myopathy
- Disseminated intravascular coagulation (DIC)
- Disordered liver function tests
- Raised plasma viscosity

Regression of these features and even metastatic disease following resection of the primary tumour means that nephrectomy is often performed. Haematuria and a mass may be late features as here. Renal cell carcinomas are more common in the elderly. The tumours are divided into clear cell (most common) and granular cell types. Spread is by direct invasion and metastatic spread, classically as the solitary (cannonball) lung secondary. Invasion along the left renal vein can produce a left-sided varicocoel as it obstructs the left testicular vein which drains here (the right testicular vein drains into the inferior vena cava).

(2) Autosomal dominant (adult) polycystic kidney disease (APKD)

A relatively common (1 in 1000) autosomal dominant condition, the gene being located on chromosome 16. Small cysts (which arise from all segments of the nephron) are present in childhood and gradually enlarge into adult life. Presentation at around 20 years of age is typical. There is compression of and progressive damage to intervening renal tissue. Presentation can be with a mass (discomfort), progressive renal failure, hypertension or haematuria.

There are various associations . . .

- Other cysts, e.g. hepatic, ovarian, pancreatic, spleen
- Berry aneurysms: subarachnoid haemorrhage
- Renal tumours
- Heart problems, e.g. mitral valve prolapse and aortic regurgitation

An inexorable decline in renal function occurs which ultimately requires renal replacement with dialysis and transplantation. Affected families can be offered antenatal screening. In this patient the presentation with features of severe (accelerated hypertension).

(3) Chronic myeloid leukaemia (CML)

A disease of middle age characterized by the production of very large numbers of mature-looking myeloid precursors. The presentation is frequently with constitutional symptoms of malaise, weight loss, night sweats and abdominal discomfort due to the massive enlargement of the liver and spleen that occurs. The total neutrophil count is often massively raised to over 100×10^9, leading to features of hyperviscosity. Typically the disease follows an indolent course for a few years until an accelerated phase (blastic transformation) occurs with the development of an acute leukaemia, which may be either acute myeloid leukaemia (in 80%) or acute lymphocytic leukaemia (in 20%). Ninety per cent of those with CML have the so-called Philadelphia chromosome, which consists of a balanced translocation between chromosome 9 and 22. It is also found in a smaller proportion of acute lymphocytic leukaemia (ALL) and acute myeloid leukaemia where its presence is associated with a poorer prognosis.

(4) Abdominal aortic aneurysm (AAA)

An aneurysm is an abnormal dilatation of an artery (or heart chamber) and may either be congenital (e.g. berry aneurysms) or more commonly acquired due to . . .

- **Trauma** (false aneurysms)
- **Inflammatory disease,** e.g. vasculitis, syphilis, subacute bacterial endocarditis.
- **Degenerative disease,** e.g. artheroma (as in AAAs).
- **Abnormal blood flow,** e.g. turbulence distil to a stenosis (post-stenotic dilatation).

A **true aneurysm** has all the three layers (adventitia, media and intima) of the vessel wall covering it, whereas a false aneurysm does not. **False aneurysms** are frequently due to trauma or infection (e.g. subacute bacterial endocarditis) causing a leak through the intima, forming a sac between it and the adventitia.

In this case the patient had presented previously with an episode of pain possibly due to a small leak, the so called 'herald bleed'. The current history suggests a larger leak or rupture. Most (95%) AAAs occur below the origin of the renal arteries. Most patients are asymptomatic and the aneurysm is noted incidentally as a pulsatile swelling of variable size. Although the aorta is dilated the internal lumen is frequently restricted in size due to arteriosclerosis and thrombus formation, hence the peripheral pulses may be diminished. Symptoms from an aneurysm indicate an immediate risk of rupture. Low back pain and renal angle pain are common presentations; however, they may present as an acute abdomen. The diagnosis can be made clinically; however, abdominal ultrasound is helpful and CT scanning is used for assessment before elective repair. Frequently calcification within the wall of the aneurysm can be seen on a plain radiograph.

Complications of aneurysms

- Embolization ('trash foot')
- Occlusion due to thrombosis
- Leak or rupture
- Fistula formation
- Pressure effect on surrounding structures
- Infection

AAAs greater than 5 cm in diameter have an enhanced risk of rupture in the short term and are generally repaired electively, which carries an operative mortality in the order of 2–3%, compared to around 50% for repair of a leaking AAA.

(5) Hereditary spherocytosis

Here a haemolytic anaemia is suggested by an elevated unconjugated (pre-hepatic) bilirubin, raised reticulocyte count and the enlargement of the spleen. The liver function tests would otherwise be expected to be normal in jaundice caused by haemolysis, rather than hepatic or post-hepatic disease. (See OSCE 44, p. 306)

Hereditary spherocytosis is an autosomal dominant disorder, but 25% of cases occur by spontaneous mutation. Abnormalities (various types described) in the red cell membrane protein structure lead to loss of red cell surface area such that they assume a spherical shape. Lysis occurs as these abnormal cells pass through the spleen. Splenic enlargement occurs due to increased activity. Patients present with anaemia, splenic enlargement and leg ulcers, but this may be delayed for many years. In common with most haemolytic anaemias, the course of the disease may be interrupted by aplastic (e.g. due to parvovirus infection), haemolytic or megaloblastic crises.

As the haemolysis is not immune mediated, the direct Coombs test will be negative. A blood film will reveal spherocytes, reticulocytes and red cell fragments. The fragility of the cells may be demonstrated by the relative ease in which they undergo lysis compared to normal red cells when placed in hypotonic solutions (red cell osmotic fragility test).

Splenectomy is performed to improve the symptoms unless the condition is very mild.

(6) Infectious mononucleosis

Caused by Epstein–Barr virus infecting B-lymphocytes. This results in an abnormal proliferation of T-lymphocytes (atypical mono-nuclear cells). Heterophil antibodies are produced, the detection of which is the basis of the monospot test. There are several causes of a false positive monospot test including . . .

- Lymphoma
- Hepatitis
- Leukaemia
- Rubella

- Malaria
- SLE

The typical presentation is with an acute tonsillitis with lymphadenopathy (which may be diffuse) in a young adult. Petechiae on the hard palate are characteristic. The illness may cause profound lassitude, which may persist for up to six months after an episode.

There are numerous potential complications . . .
- Gastrointestinal
  - Hepatitis (common)
  - Splenic enlargement and (rarely) rupture
- Haematological
  - Autoimmune haemolytic anaemia (Coombes positive)
  - Thromocytopenia
  - Agranulocytosis (rare)
  - Lymphoma (rare)
- Cardiovascular
  - Myocarditis
  - Pericarditis
- Nervous system
  - Encephalitis
  - Aspetic meningitis
  - Neuropathy
  - Guillain–Barré syndrome
- Skin rashes
  - Morbilliform due to infection
  - Temporary amoxicillin allergy rashes

The differential diagnosis includes CMV viral infection, toxoplasmosis, hepatitis, streptococcal infection and HIV conversion illness. The treatment is symptomatic. Steroids are occasional used for splenomegaly where there is concern about possible splenic rupture.

Answer 20

(1) Uraemic pericarditis

The patient who has poor glycaemic control is known to have impaired renal function when last seen in out patients. The clinical findings suggest uraemia is now present. Uraemic pericarditis is a well-recognized complication of advanced renal failure. The speed of accumulation of the pericardial fluid dictates the severity of the clinical picture. For example, 200 mL accumulating rapidly can cause acute cardiac tamponade, whereas 500–1000 mL can accumulate slowly in the pericardial

space with little effect on cardiac output. The pericardial effusion is typically haemorrhagic and can cause cardiac tamponade, as has happened here, with an elevated JVP that rises with inspiration (Kussmaul's sign), tachycardia and hypotension. In addition a fall in pulse volume occurs with inspiration (pulsus paradoxus).

Diabetic nephropathy can be predicted by the presence of diabetic retinopathy as the microvascular pathology is frequently co-existent. It is a risk factor for ESRF and cardiovascular mortality. Thickening and leakiness of the glomerular basement membrane occurs leading to **glomerular sclerosis** which may be diffuse or nodular (the so-called Kimmelstiel–Wilson lesion) on microscopy. Early in the process protein begins to be leaked in very small amounts (microalbuminuria) with smaller molecules being lost in preference. Microalbuminuria cannot be detected using normal dipsticks, so urine must be sent for radio-immunoassay. In practise, the selectivity of the leak is quantified by comparing the ratio of albumin (small molecule) lost to that of creatinine (large molecule). Initially the deterioration in renal function is clinically silent and the urea and electrolytes are normal but progression to renal failure will occur over approximately 10 years, with the proteinuria becoming heavier (detectable on dip testing) during this period. Once commenced there is an **inexorable decline in the renal function** which can only be slowed, but not prevented, by strict glycaemic (HbA1C target 6.5–7.5%) control and control of blood pressure (using ACE inhibitors to achieve BP below 135/75). Also remember diabetes as one of the causes of nephrotic syndrome.

(2) (Diabetic) Syndrome X

A poorly understood syndrome consisting of extreme insulin resistance, hypertension and ischaemic heart disease. It is hypothesized that insulin behaves as a growth factor acting to cause proliferation of the vascular endothelium, which results in increased peripheral vascular resistance and hypertension. Very large doses of insulin are required to achieve adequate control of the blood glucose.

Do not confuse this with the *cardiovascular* Syndrome X [see EMQ Answers Q17 (4), p. 127], which occurs in patients who experience ischaemic chest pain but have normal coronary arteries on angiography. The ischaemia is due to microvascular insufficiency.

The absence of skin findings (e.g. striae, acne, bruising) and the distribution of the obesity, count against

Cushing's disease, which would also cause hypertension and hyperglycaemia.

(3) Acanthosis nigricans

A typical description is given in the question. It may be associated with insulin resistance (diabetes and acromegaly), internal malignancy (carcinoma of the stomach), or may be idiopathic and associated with obesity. It may be found on the back of the neck or in the axilla.

Know the other classical skin conditions in diabetes . . .
- **Necrobiosis lipoidica:** 1% of diabetic patients. Atrophic (visible subcutaneous vessels), shiny brown plaques, frequently on the shins. No useful treatment is available
- **Granuloma annulare**: if extensive may be associated with diabetes. Ring-shaped intradermal nodules occur frequently over the dorsum of the hands. These lesions respond to local steroid injections (triamcinolone)
- **Diabetic dermopathy**: occurs in around 50% of diabetics. Recessed reddish scars often over the shins
- **Local infections:** *Candida*, staphylococcal
- **Vitiligo**: Type I diabetes only due to association with other autoimmune illnesses
- **Ulcers**: Vascular or neuropathic usually on the lower limbs
- **Iatrognic:** Lipo-atrophy at injection sites

(4) Autonomic neuropathy

The history of nocturnal diarrhoea is very suggestive. There are no pointers in the history or examination towards a serious cause (malignancy, inflammatory bowel disease or malabsorption). The polyps found are incidental. Other possible features which may occur in autonomic neuropathy . . .
- **Postural hypotension**: syncope episodes caused by failure of reflex increase in cardiac output and alteration in vascular tone on standing. Postural ischaemia may cause angina, and muscle pain in the back and shoulders. In normal people blood pressure should elevate on standing. A fall in systolic blood pressure by 15 mmHg or more is likely to be clinically significant. Unlike a vasovagal episode in normal individuals a person with autonomic failure will have warm peripheries and an absence of sweating during an episode.
- **Abnormal sweating** and vasomotor symptoms, e.g. after meals, heat intolerance

- **Sphincter disturbances**: urge incontinence
- **Nocturnal polyuria** due to loss of the predominant parasympathetic tone that occurs at night, which normally inhibits the urge to void urine
- **Impotence**
- **Dry mouth and eyes**
- **Horner's syndrome**

Other causes of autonomic failure
- **Acute autonomic failure**
  - Guillain–Barré syndrome: cardiac arrhythmias may be problematic
  - Drugs, e.g. tricyclic antidepressants
- **Chronic autonomic failure**
  - Age related
  - Shy-Drager syndrome (Parkinson's disease variant; multi system atrophy)
  - Alcoholism
  - Amyloidosis
  - Paraneoplastic disease

Patterns of diabetic neuropathy
- **Autonomic** (see above)
- **Symmetrical sensory polyneuropathy** in a glove and stocking distribution (ultimately). Early features are loss of vibration sensation and deep pain (squeeze the Achilles tendon). The patient may complain of numb feet and incur accidental trauma e.g. due to stones in the shoes or hot baths. Chacot's joints may develop in the ankle resulting in an anaesthetic grossly disorganized joint
- **Mononeuritis multiplex:** e.g. causing cranial nerve palsies; especially the third (sparing of the papillary reflexes due to sparing of the pupillomotor fibres; the so called 'medical third nerve palsy'). Also peripheral nerves, e.g. median nerve palsy or common peroneal nerve (foot drop)
- **Diabetic amyotrophy**: painful wasting of the quadriceps in older, often male diabetics with poor glycaemic control. Uniquely this may improve after a period of stricter control of blood glucose
- **Painful diabetic neuropathy**. Typically a neuropathic (clawing, tingling, shooting, burning) pain in the lower legs and feet. May occur acutely at the onset on diabetes due to elevated blood sugars, and may improve with treatment. The later onset type can be a difficult problem although drugs like gabapentin, amitriptyline and carbamazepine are often used.

ANSWERS 4

(5) Hyperosmolar non-ketotic coma (HONC)

A state of high plasma osmolarity and very high glucose levels, dehydration and predisposition to infections (e.g. pneumonia) and thrombotic episodes (e.g. stroke, myocardial infarction). The patient will be typically an elderly type II diabetic who is often previously undiagnosed. The onset is very gradual with thirst and polyuria. There is no evidence of acidosis (ketones, hyperventilation). The patient may be drowsy or unconscious. Plasma osmolarity can be roughly calculated using the formula

$$\text{Plasma osmolarity} = 2(\text{Na} + \text{K}) + \text{urea} + \text{glucose}.$$

Levels over 350 mosm/kg are consistent with the diagnosis.

The management involves insulin (sliding scale like DKA) and intravenous rehydration (monitor urine output and JVP/CVP) with gradual correction of the electrolyte imbalance over 48–72 h to avoid cerebral oedema. Treating associated infection and prophylactic heparin to avoid thrombotic events.

(6) The patient can be diagnosed as having diabetes

Patients can be **diagnosed** as having **diabetes if any of the following apply** . . .

- A **single fasting blood glucose** is greater than **7.0 mmol/L and** the patient has symptoms (e.g. thirst, polyuria, weight loss). **Two fasting samples greater than 7.0 mmol/L** are required if the patient does not have symptoms
- A **single random glucose** is greater than **11.1 mmol/L and** the patient has symptoms (as in this question). **Two random samples greater than 11.1 mmol/L** are required if the patient does not have symptoms
- If the **glucose is greater than 11.1 mmol/L 2 h following a glucose tolerance test** (patient given a oral load of 75 g of glucose taken in 300 mL of water following an overnight fast)

Glucose tolerance tests are required to diagnose diabetes where the above results are borderline or in gestational diabetes. **Impaired glucose tolerance** is said to exist if the glucose measured 2 h following a glucose tolerance test is between 7.8 and 11.1 mmol/L. This group comprises up to 5% of the population and has an increased risk of developing ischaemic heart disease but not the microvascular (retinopathy, neuropathy and nephropathy) com-

plications of diabetes. Weight reduction, lifestyle modifications (exercise and smoking cessation) along with evaluation and modification of other cardiovascular risk factors is required (hypertension and cholesterol).

(7) Diabetic maculopathy

Oedema of the macula may not be detectable clinically by direct inspection. Deterioration in visual acuity may be the only indication of the problem. It occurs in type II diabetics. Later there may be a ring of hard exudates around the macula that indicate the problem. Diabetic maculopathy causes an early marked loss in the visual acuity and left untreated will lead to blindness. Treatment is with laser photocoagulation.

Diabetic retinopathy consists of the following order of progression . . .

1. Background retinopathy

10–20 years of diabetes. Use the mnemonic **HAVOX** . . .

   H Haemorrhages: '*dot and blot*'
   A Aneurysms
   V Venous dilatation
   O Oedema
   X Exudates; hard exudates cause by leaked lipids

Action required:
- Strict glycaemic control
- Control of blood pressure
- Smoking cessation
- Annual retinal photography watching for encroachment of exudates onto the macular area

2. Diabetic maculopathy (as above)

3. Pre-proliferative retinopathy

- Cotton wool spots: oedema from infarcts of the retina. (NB Not specific for diabetes as may also be seen in hypertension and retinal vein occlusion)
- Venous loops
- Venous beading

Action required: ophthalmology referral in addition to strict control of blood pressure and glucose.

4. Proliferative retionopathy and advanced retinopathy

Frond-like growth of new vessels either along the retinal surface or forward into the vitreous, promoted by hyopoxia. The vessels are fragile leading to bleeding with sudden visual loss. Subsequent organization of the haemorrhage can lead to fibrosis and retinal detachment. New vessels may grow forward onto the iris and cause blockage of the drainage angle with a resultant secondary glaucoma. Urgent opthalmology referral for pan-retinal photocoagulation is required.

Answer 21

(1) Addison's disease

In this case due to tuberculosis causing destruction of the adrenal gland, which remains the second most common cause after autoimmune destruction.

The adrenal cortex consists of three layers from the exterior inwards: the zona **G**lomerulosa, zona **F**asciculata and zona **R**eticularis (remember **GFR**). The adrenal cortex produces both glucocorticoids and mineralocorticoids. Mineralocorticoids (aldosterone) are produced in the zona glomerulosa. Aldosterone production is regulated separately by the renin–angiotensin–aldosterone system and released is stimulated by the direct effect of angiotensin II.

Glucocorticoid production is under the control of the hypothalamus and anterior pituitary gland. Cortisol releasing hormone (CRH) is produced by the hypothalamus in response to stress and also the normal circadian rhythm (high cortisol levels in the morning and low levels during the night) causes the release of ACTH by the anterior pituitary leading to cortisol release from the adrenal cortex. Cortisol levels impose negative feedback on both the pituitary and hypothalamus. ACTH has a melanocyte stimulating hormone type action, leading to abnormal pigmentation if levels are elevated.

In **Addison's disease** there is failure of the adrenal gland affecting **all three layers (glucocorticoid and mineralocorticoid production)**. The resultant lack of negative feedback of cortisol on the hypothalamus and pituitary leads to **excess ACTH production**, which causes **pigmentation**. This is prominent particularly over areas of skin trauma e.g. scars or pressure points, e.g. elbows and buccal mucosa.

Only rarely is hypoadrenalism due to hypothalamic or pituitary failure. When this is the mechanism there is no rise in the levels of ACTH and therefore **pigmentation does not occur**. There is also **no effect on the pro-** duction of mineralocorticoid and therefore neither hyponatraemia nor hyperkalaemia occur.

Causes of Addison's disease (primary adrenal failure)

- **Autoimmune destruction** (associated with pernicious anaemia, vitiligo and type I diabetes): this accounts for 90% of cases. Autoantibodies can be measured
- **Tuberculosis**: previously the most common cause and remains so in certain communities. Accounts for approximately 10% of cases
- Surgery
- Haemorrhage, e.g. Waterhouse–Freidrichsen's syndrome due to meningococcal septicaemia
- Malignant infiltration
- Amyloidosis
- HIV infection

The symptoms of Addison's disease

- Weight loss
- Weakness (and muscle) pain
- Syncope due to postural hypotension
- Gastrointestinal symptoms
  - Nausea and vomiting
  - Abdominal pain
  - Diarrhoea and constipation

The signs of Addison's disease

Use mnemonic **PPP** . . .

    P pallor (anaemia and vitiligo)

    P pigmentation (elbows, scars, buccal mucosa, generalized)

    P postural hypotension (very useful sign)

Routine blood tests *may* point towards possible Addison's disease . . .

- **Anaemia**; **normochromic** due to chronic disease or **macrocytic** due to co-existent vitamin B12 deficiency
- **Hyperkalaemia and hyponatraemia** (metabolic acidosis) due to mineralocorticoid deficiency
- Hypercalcaemia
- Hypoglycaemia

If suspected, **the diagnosis of Addison's disease is urgent** as patients are vulnerable to cardiovascular collapse. Although frequently Addison's is a low-grade chronic illness waiting to be diagnosed (like hypothyroidism), it may present acutely with hypotension, hypo-glycaemia and coma.

Diagnosis
- **Failure of cortisol levels to rise adequately with a short (30 min) ACTH (synacthen) test confirms hypoadrenalism**
- **The long ACTH test** (prolonged stimulation) is then performed to differentiate primary adrenal failure from adrenal glands which have had prolonged inactivity due to:
  - Suppression with of exogenous steroids (recently withdrawn)
  - Pituitary or hypothalamic failure

In the acute situation glucocorticoid replacement should not be delayed by these investigations. The management involves intravenous fluid resuscitation and hydrocortisone (100 mg every 6 h). There is no requirement to replace mineralocorticoids (fludrocortisone) urgently as glucocorticoids have sufficient mineralocorticoid activity.

(2) Primary polydipsia

There is a normal response to a water deprivation test with good concentration of urine following a rise in plasma osmolality. The associated headaches are probably tension headaches.

The **differential diagnosis of thirst and polyuria include . . .**
- **Diabetes mellitus**
- **Diabetes insipidus**
  - *Cranial* **diabetes insipidus**: a failure of pituitary ADH production due to damage by . . .
    Malignancy (breast, lymphoma, leukaemia, primary pituitary)
    Infarction (Sheehan's syndrome)
    Infections (TB meningitis)
    Trauma (surgery)
    Rare congenital defects
  - *Nephrogenic* **diabetes insipidus**: renal insensitivity to ADH due to . . .
    Drugs (lithium, glibenclamide, demeclocycline)
    Hypokalaemia
    Hypercalcaemia
    Renal tubular damage (site of ADH action), e.g. sickle cell disease, renal tubular acidosis
- **Polydipsia**
  - **Primary** for psychological reasons

- **Dry mouth conditions**:
  Sjögren's syndrome
  Anticholinergic side effects of medications, e.g. amitriptyline, oxybutynin

First-line investigations for polydipsia include **urea and electrolytes** (normal potassium?), plasma **calcium** and a **random blood sugar**.

A **water deprivation test** can be used to differentiate between the cranial diabetes insipidus, nephrogenic diabetes insipidus and primary polydipsia. In the test the patient is deprived water whilst serial (hourly) measurements of plasma osmolality, urine osmolality and weight are made. The test is potentially dangerous if diabetes insipidus is present, as unabated polyuria and dehydration will continue; therefore, the test is stopped if more than 3% of body weight is lost. The patient must ideally be observed to prevent surreptitious fluids being taken by patients with the primary form of the disease.

The normal response (in individuals with a healthy ADH pituitary-renal axis) is a progressive rise in both plasma and urinary osmolality as progressive dehydration occurs. Urine osmolality would be expected to rise above 600 mOsm/kg. Plasma osmolality would be expected to remain within the normal range demonstrating normal water conservation measures (normal plasma osmolality is 275–295 mOsm/kg). An initial plasma osmolality in the low normal range (as in this case) suggests the diagnosis of primary polydipsia.

If during the test plasma osmolality rises whilst the urine remains unconcentrated then diabetes insipidus exists. If this pattern continues following the administration of ADH (desmopressin 2μg i.m.) then nephrogenic diabetes insipidus can be diagnosed, but if it corrects then cranial diabetes insipidus can be diagnosed.

(3) Ectopic ACTH production

Cushing's syndrome may be suggested by . . .
- **Clinical features**
  - Symptoms:
    Weight gain (central obesity)
    Weakness
    Acne
    Insomnia
    Loss of libido
    Back pain (osteoporotic crush fracture)
    Polyuria (steroid induced diabetes)
    Psychosis
  - Signs:
    Central obesity

Moon face

Striae

Bruising

Acne

Hypertension

- **Biochemical stigmata**
  - Metabolic alkalosis
  - Hypokalaemia
  - Raised plasma glucose (impaired glucose tolerance test)

Cushing's syndrome may be screened for using either . . .
- 24 h urinary free cortisol estimation *or*
- Looking for the loss of the normal 24 h diurnal variation in cortisol excretion by measuring midnight and 09.00 hours plasma cortisol levels

The **low dose dexamethazone suppression test** is used initially to confirm cortisol excess (Cushing's syndrome). However, the **differential diagnosis of Cushing's syndrome** is as follows . . .
- Cushing's disease
  - Raised pituitary ACTH
- Exogenous
  - Corticosteroids or ACTH
- Adrenal tumours
  - Producing excess cortisol
- Ectopic ACTH
  - Various tumours, e.g. bronchogenic small cell
- Ectopic CRH
  - Very rare

Pituitary dependent **Cushing's disease is subject to the normal negative feedback mechanisms such that CRH and ACTH will be suppressed** (in 90% of cases) with the **high dose dexamethazone suppression test**. Failure to suppress (as in this case) suggests either ectopic ACTH/CRH or cortisol production from an adrenal tumour, neither of which is subject to normal feedback mechanisms. However, only ACTH dependent disease will cause increased pigmentation, making ectopic ACTH the most likely option in this case.

Once Cushing's syndrome is confirmed biochemically, a search is commenced for the source of the problem. First-line investigations include a chest radiograph followed by bronchoscopy for suspected ectopic ACTH production from a pulmonary tumour. MRI scanning is helpful in localizing adrenal or pituitary lesions.

Definitive treatment is by **surgical removal** (transsphenoidal approach for pituitary lesions) of the tumour where possible. Radiotherapy is an alternative for failed surgery.

Medical therapy to reduce cortisol levels can be used for . . .
- Control of symptoms prior to surgery
- Inoperable lesions (age, co-morbity)
- Non-localized lesions
  Drugs used include metyrapone (11β-hydroxylase blocker) plus ketoconazone (synergistic with metyrapone).

Nelson's syndrome occurs where bilateral adrenalectomy (previously used for pituitary dependent Cushing's disease) results in excessive pigmentation and an enlarging pituitary adenoma, due to the loss of negative feedback (adrenal cortisol) on ACTH production from the pituitary lesion.

(4) Hypothyroidism
The combination of weakness, heart failure and dry skin are very suggestive. Remember hypothyroidism due to autoimmune thyroid failure (by far the most common cause) is a very common condition in the elderly, seen frequently in clinical practice and is regularly tested in examinations.

Key points regarding thyroid disease
- Hypothyroidism is a potent cause of the syndrome of inappropriate ADH (**SIADH**); hence volume retention with oedema, hypertension, pleural and pericardial effusions and ascites may occur. Low plasma sodium may occur
- Both hypothyroidism and hyperthyroidism can cause hypertension, muscle weakness, heart failure and confusion/psychosis.
- Pretibial myxoedema is a feature of hyperthyroidism and *not* hypothyroidism
- **Skin features** of hypothyroidism include pallor (anaemia), cold, puffy, dry skin with hair loss (noticeable on the eyebrows)
- Hypothyroidism (along with vitamin B12 deficiency, folate deficiency, pregnancy, alcoholism and liver disease) can cause a **macrocytic anaemia**
- Both **thyrotoxicosis and hypothyroidism** can cause mood change, psychosis and confusion. Hypothyroidism should never be forgotten (along with syphilis, vitamin B12 deficiency, uraemia, liver

failure, malignancy non-metastatic manifestation and hypercalcaemia) as a potentially reversible cause of dementia

- **Cardiovascular effects** of hypothyroidism include bradycardia, hypertension, heart failure and pericardial effusions. Hypercholesterolaemia occurs

Investigations and treatment
- **Ask about . . .**
  - Cold intolerance
  - Energy levels
  - Constipation
  - Weight change
  - Heavy periods
  - Skin/hair changes (? old photograph)
  - Family history of thyroid disorders
- **Examine for . . .**
  - Skin changes (general end of the bed appearance)
  - Pulse (bradycardia)
  - Carpel tunnel syndrome
  - Anaemia
  - BP
  - Goitre
  - Associated heart failure
  - CNS features:
    Confusion (mini-mental state examination)
    Cerebellar signs
    Slowly relaxing reflexes
    Hypotonia
    Weakness
- There is no diurnal variation in the secretion of thyroid stimulating hormone (TSH) and T4
- Hypothyroidism is easily diagnosed with a raised TSH and reduced T4
- **Antithyroid antibodies** can often be found but are not routinely measured. There is an association with other autoimmune illness, e.g. type I diabetes, Addison's disease, vitiligo and RA

Treatment requires lifelong thyroxine replacement. Start with a small dose, e.g. 25 µg once a day, especially in the elderly to avoid precipitating heart failure. Increase the dose gradually (25 µg increments every 4–6 weeks) over several months until the TSH is suppressed back into the normal range. A typical maintenance dose is around 150 µg/day.

In **hypothyroidism due to pituitary failure** replace corticosteroid *before* giving thyroxine. Once established on thyroxine, check thyroid function annually.

Sick euthyroid syndrome refers to a state of low T4 and normal (or low normal) TSH in patients debilitated by a systemic illness (e.g. chronic renal failure) and is due to various mechanisms, including reduced thyroid binding globulins, reduced TSH production and reduced peripheral conversion of T4 to T3.

(5) Acromegaly

An excess of growth hormone (GH). The vast majority of acromegaly is due to a pituitary tumour. It may rarely be due to ectopic production of gonadotrophin releasing hormone (GnRH) from a bronchial carcinoid tumour. The pituitary tumour produces headaches due to enlargement within the pituitary fossa and visual field defect due to pressure on the optic chiasm. Insidious onset occurs with bone and soft tissue overgrowth.

Ask about . . .
- Headaches
- Visual problems
- Tight rings
- Breathlessness (cardiomyopathy)
- Polyuria (diabetes mellitus)
- Change in appearance (ask for old photographs)
- Muscular weakness (myopathy)
- Excessive sweating
- Joint pains (arthritis)

Examine . . .
- Hands: 'spade like' enlargement, carpel tunnel syndrome
- Skin: sweaty, thickened, hirsute
- BP: hypertension.
- Jaw: enlargement, prognathic, dental malalignment and separation of teeth
- Large tongue
- Visual fields: confrontation testing for bi-temporal hemianopia
- For cardiac failure

The **diagnosis** is made by the failure of GH to suppress (below 2 mU/L) when a **standard glucose tolerance test** is performed. Plasma Insulin Like Growth factor (IGF-1) is raised and can allow the monitoring of treatment. The tumour can be imaged with a pituitary MRI scan. Frequently the enlarging tumour results in a degree of hypopituitarism (check thyroid function, prolactin, LH, FSH and testosterone), and hyperprolactinaemia is common (30% of tumours excrete prolactin also).

Treatment is required to prevent an excess of deaths due to cardiovascular events and tumours (especially large bowel). A trans-sphenoidal surgical approach for removal is usual. Radiotherapy can be used for patients unfit for surgery. Medical therapy with bromocriptine (dopamine agonist) or octreotide can be used to shrink the tumour prior to surgery. Following successful treatment the features of acromegaly unfortunately do not regress.

Answer 22

(1) Subacute bacterial endocarditis (see also OSCE 32, p. 285)

A chronic infection of the endocardium, more common where there is a structural abnormality (e.g. septal defects, previous rheumatic fever, prolapsing mitral valve) creating turbulent flow, although one third of cases have no structural abnormality. Infection typically occurs along the edges of the valves. Fibrin and platelets form aggregations around the infection and are known as vegetations. These vegetations attract further bacterial and further aggregations of fibrin and platelets and therefore grow in size.

Infection occurs more frequently on the left (high pressure) side of the heart and the aortic valve is the most commonly involved. Septal defects may produce 'jet lesions' on the opposite ventricular wall, e.g. right ventricle in ventricular septal defects. Drug addicts tend to produce right-sided endocarditis (and pulmonary abscesses) via injected venous bacteraemia (60% due to *Staphylococcus aureus*).

Predisposing factors
* Abnormal valves
* Prosthetic valves
* Septal defects (especially high pressure left to right shunts)
* Bacteraemia (IV drug abuse, intravenous lines, dental sepsis, colonic surgery)
* Debilitated patient (HIV, alcoholism, diabetes)

Organisms involved
* Streptococci: 50% of cases (especially *S. viridans*, a mouth and upper respiratory tract commensal)
* *Staphylococcus aureus*: 25%, skin commensal, hence more common following IV drug abuse, IV cannulation

* Enterococci: 10% (bowel, prostate and pelvic surgery)
* Others: Gram-negatives, fungal (*Candida* and aspergillus), mycobacteria, brucella, coxiella (Q fever)
* No organism cultured: 10%

The clinical picture
Depends on the virulence of the infecting organism and the immediate effect on cardiac function. Subacute presentation with fever, sweats and weight loss is the most common pattern. Acute presentation can occur with fever and valvular disruption and consequent heart failure can also be seen occur. Fever, splenomegaly (chronic infection) and the development of a new or changing murmur should arouse clinical suspicion. The clinical picture can be divided as follows . . .
* **Cardiac complications**
  * Acute valvular disruption (mitral regurgitation)
  * Heart failure and pulmonary oedema
  * Cardiac wall abscess
  * Conduction disturbances
* **Septic embolic events**
  * Brain
  * Limbs
  * Pulmonary (right-sided lesions)
* **Immune complex mediated vasculitis**
  * Hands:
    Splinter haemorrhages (nails and sclera)
    Clubbing
    Osler's nodes (tender pulp nodules)
    Janeway lesions (painless palmar vascular lesions)
  * Eyes:
    Roth spots (retinal haemorrhagic vasculitic lesions
  * Renal:
    Glomerulonephritis, haematuria (immune complex mediated)
  * Joints:
    Flitting large joint arthritis

Investigations
* **Blood cultures**: three sets of cultures from different sites at different times. Prolonged culture. 75% of cases give positive blood cultures
* FBC: normochromic anaemia of chronic disease, neutrophil leucocytosis
* Urea and electrolytes: possible renal failure
* Immunoglobulins: increased; reduced C3 complement due to immune complex formation
* Urine dip test: possible blood and protein.
* Chest radiograph: possible cardiac failure

ANSWERS 4

- **Echocardiogram**: extremely useful to identify vegetations and valve dysfunction

Management

- **Antibiotics**: discuss with microbiology. Start with penicillin V 1.2 g i.v. 4-hourly and gentamycin (monitor levels) 80 mg i.v. every 12 h. Adjust according to the cultures and sensitivities
- **Surgery:** possibly for . . .
  - Prosthetic valve infection
  - Critical valve dysfunction
  - Cardiac abscess
  - Large vegetation
  - Major embolization
  - No response to medical therapy (high mortality rate here)
- **Antibiotic prophylaxis**
  - For dental work and pelvic surgery
  - Look up the relevant procedure and current recommendations in the British National Formulary

(2) Mitral valve prolapse

A condition more common in younger females. Myxomatous degeneration and enlargement of the mitral valve occurs. During systole there is sudden prolapse of the valve producing and mid-systolic 'click' followed by a late-systolic or pan-systolic murmur radiating in the usual direction. On echocardiography there is posterior movement of one or both mitral valve leaflets into the left atrium during systole.

Associations

- Marfan's syndrome
- Thyrotoxicosis
- Rheumatic fever
- Atrial septal defects
- Hypertrophic obstructive cardiomyopathy

Complications

- Thromboembolic events
- Atypical chest pain (typified in the question)
- Ventricular arrhythmias
- Sudden cardiac death (rare)

Management

- Beta-blockers
- Anticoagulation
- Prophylaxis against endocarditis with antibiotics

(3) Rheumatic fever

A once common complication of group A streptococcal infection, acute rheumatic fever is now rare but does still occur. It is more common in Asia and South America. Antibodies raised against the streptococcal infection also target myosin and laminin on cardiac tissue.

The characteristic lesion is the **Aschoff nodule** (a grauloma), which can occur in any layer of the myocardium (a pan-carditis). Vegetations can occur on the heart valves. Acute valvular dysfunction affects the mitral valve in particular (regurgitation; in this question there is a diastolic flow murmur in addition).

Fifty per cent of cases go on to develop **chronic rheumatic heart disease** with stiffening and immobility of the mitral and aortic valves in particularl, frequently giving a picture of stenosis and incompetence occurring together.

Diagnosis of acute rheumatic fever

Based on the **Duckett Jones criteria** (five major and six minor) . . .

- *Major* criteria
  - **Carditis:** new murmur, pericardial rub
  - **Arthritis:** classically a flitting polyarthritis of large joints
  - **Nodules:** subcutaneous hard nodules over bony prominences, e.g. the elbows
  - **Erythema marginatum:** pink, raised, spreading, ring-like rash
  - **Sydenham's chorea:** St Vitus's dance; fidgeting movements. May re-occur years later (e.g., during pregnancy)
- *Minor* criteria
  - Fever
  - Previous rheumatic fever
  - Raised white cell count
  - Prolonged PR interval on ECG
  - Arthralgia
  - Raised ESR or CRP

Diagnosis relies on *two major criteria plus evidence of streptococcal infection*, or *one major and two minor criteria plus evidence of streptococcal infection*. Evidence of streptococcal infection includes culture, a raised ASO titre or clinical Scarlet fever.

Management

- Bed rest
- Aspirin (licensed for children with rheumatic fever)
- Penicillin V 500 mg four times a day then 250 mg/day

until aged 20 years or for five years to prevent recurrent episodes
- Prednisolone orally for carditis

(4) Systemic amyloidosis

A young man with heart failure, hepatosplenomegaly and heavy proteinuria. Systemic amyloidosis is a disease characterized by an abnormal accumulation, in various organs, of a fibrillary protein originating from the immune system. Amyloidosis may be primary or secondary to chronic inflammation (stimulation of the immune system). Primary amyloidosis (serum amyloid A) is very similar to myeloma. The diagnosis is made on staining of the amyloid material with Congo Red (actually stains green confusingly) on tissue biopsy (rectal biopsy often used).

Causes of secondary amyloidosis

(due to immunoglobulin light chains)
- Rheumatoid arthritis and sero-negative inflammatory arthritis
- Chronic osteomyelitis
- Malignancy, e.g. renal cell carcinoma.
- Familial Mediterranean fever

Clinical features of amyloidosis

- Hepatosplenomegaly
- Gingival hypertrophy and macroglossia (large tongue)

- Cardiomyopathy (restrictive) [see EMQ Answers Q5 (5), p. 74]
- Nephrotic syndrome
- Autonomic neuropathy
- Vessel fragility (easy bruising)
- Carpal tunnel syndrome

(5) Atrial myxoma

The most common (although still rare) cardiac tumour. It is benign and most commonly occurs in the left atrium. As it is pedunculated it acts like a 'ball valve' across the mitral valve producing a mid-diastolic murmur (like mitral stenosis) followed by loud first heart sound. The tumour can produce a 'plop' like prominent third heart sound (which is unlikely in mitral stenosis) as it halts against the mitral valve during atrial systole. Systemic symptoms of fever and embolization may occur. Clinically it may closely resemble bacterial endocarditis; however, it can be easily diagnosed on an echocardiogram. Surgical removal is required and is curative.

Answer 23

(1) Polymyalgia rheumatica

An interesting and reasonably common disease of unknown aetiology affecting elderly females. Giant Cell Arteritis (GCA) and polymyalgia are at either end of a spectrum where features of either may be prominent or any mixture occurs. The clinical features are . . .

Polymyalgia	GCA
Generalized muscle pain (especialy shoulders and pelvic girdle)	Temporal headache Tenderness and swelling of temporal artery Blindness (opthalmic artery) Scalp tenderness (e.g. combing hair)
Anaemia of chronic disease	Jaw claudication (fatigue and pain on chewing/talking)
Tiredness Weight loss Fever	Tirednesss Fever
Raised CRP/ESR Raised alkaline phosphatase	Raised CRP/ESR Raised alkaline phosphatase Biopsy of the temporal artery shows Giant Cells

The diagnosis is based on the clinical picture in polymyalgia, a raised ESR or CRP in combination with the usually excellent responce to oral steroids (prednisolone 30–60 mg o.d.). The differential diagnosis includes malignancy. Jaw claudication is a very specific symptom in polymyalgia but only occurs in about 20% of cases. Steroids are then very gradually reduced over 18–24 months. The last 5 mg is reduced in 1-mg decrements.

In suspected temporal arteitis high dose oral steroids (e.g. prednisolone 60 mg per day) should be commenced straight away because of the concern over blindness. These can always be stopped if a subsequent normal CRP or temporal artery biosy refutes the diagnosis. Colour duplex ultrasonography has proven a sensitive, non-invasive means of diagnosing temporal arteritis.

Side effects of steroids

Use the mnemonic '**IM SHAGED O**ut!' . . .

I	Infections	
M	Muscle wasting	
S	Skin	Bruising, striae
H	Habitus	Central obesity, proximal muscle wasting
A	Adrenal suppression	Doses of prednisolone over 5–7.5 mg/day; 6–12 months to return to normal production after withdrawal
G	GIT	Dyspepsia
E	Endocrine/metabolic	Na^{2+} retention leading to fluid retention and hypertension K^+ loss, hypergylcaemia (important in DM)
D	Depression/psychosis	
O	Osteoporosis/ occular cataracts	

(2) Felty's syndrome

A syndrome of rheumatoid arthritis, neutropenia and splenomegaly (pancytopenia). Skin pigmentation may also occur. There is predisposition to infections. Treatment is with splenectomy.

Other causes of neutropenia

Use the mnemonic '**EPIC HAT**' . . .

E Endocrine; hypothyroidism, hyperthyroidism or pituitary failure

P Pancytopenia (marrow failure; any cause):

    Aplastic anaemia

    Infiltration

    Drugs

    Hypersplenism

    Sepsis

    Paroxysmal nocturnal haemoglobinuria

I Infections

C Cyclical (episodes of neutropenia occuring over three weeks and then return to nonrmal. May present with skin infections. Is thought to be familial)

H Haemolysis; autoimmune destruction (e.g. Coombes positive haemolytic anaemia):

    Viral infections

    Severe bacterial in the elderly

A Alcohol and liver disease

T Toxins and drugs, e.g. carbimazole

(3) Reactive arthritis (see also EMQ 18, p. 132)

A variety of infective agents can result in acute joint inflammation. Usually large joints such as the knee are affected. The male to female ratio is 20:1. Responsible infective agents include . . .

- *Chlamydia* (non-specific urethritis)
- Gonococcal
- *Salmonella*
- *Shigella flexneri* and *Sh. dysenteriae* (not *Sh. sonnei*)
- *Yersinia enterocolitica*
- *Campylobacter*

A rash, **keratoderma blennorrhagica,** which is clinically and histologically indistinguishable from pustular psoriasis, occurs usually on the soles of the feet.

Reiter's syndrome consists of . . .

- A reactive arthritis that is asymmetrical and affects large joints, e.g. knee and hip
- Conjunctivitis
- Urethritis

Other features of Reiter's syndrome may include . . .

- Circinate balanitis
- Achilles tendonitis
- Mouth ulceration
- Anterior uveitis
- Pericarditis
- Aortitis
- Pulmonary infiltrates
- CNS involvement
- Peripheral neuropathy

It is presumed that shared antigens (predicted by HLA type B27 in 70%) occur on the infective agents and the synovium of affected joints. Antigenic material from the infection can be extracted from the synovial fluid of these patients. Seventy per cent make a complete recovery, 25% get occasional relapses and 5% of patients a chronic recurrent arthritis develops especially if HLA B27 positive.

(4) Psoriatic arthritis

Arthritis complicates psoriasis in 7% of cases. The arthritis and the psoriatic rash do not need to coexist. Here the presence of nail pitting, which is typical of psoriasis, indicates the diagnosis. Together with anklosing spondylitis, reactive arthritis and the inflammatory bowel arthritides, it comprises the seronegative arthritides. These have certain shared features, any of which may coexist to a variable extent (see EMQ 18, p. 132).

Patterns of psoriatic arthritis

- A form like **RA** affecting proximal inter-phalangeal joints (PIPJs)
- A form like **osteoarthritis** (but asymmetrical) affecting distil interphalangeal joints (DIPJs)
- A form like **ankylosing spondylitis** affecting the spine and sacroiliac joints
- A large joint oligoarthritis (like **Reiter's** syndrome)
- **Arthritis mutilans** (serve erosions leading to telescoping of the digits)

Differential diagnosis of a swollen large joint

(e.g. knee)
- Sepsis (the most urgent differential to exclude)
- Haemarthrosis (trauma/haemophilia)
- Reactive arthritis (including Reiter's syndrome)
- Acute gout or pseudogout
- Gonococcal arthritis
- Other sero-negative arthritis, e.g. inflammatory bowel disease associated, psoriatic arthritis, ankylosing spondylitis
- Pallindromic RA
- Rare
  - Tuberculous arthritis
  - Behçet's disease
  - SLE
  - Henoch–Schönlein purpura
  - Lyme disease
  - Bacterial endocarditis
  - Rheumatic fever

(5) Acute gout

The knee is the second most common joint to be affected after the first metatarsophalangeal joint (75%). Gout is caused by the crystallization of uric acid within joints, which provokes a very brisk inflammatory reaction. It is possible to have gout with the uric acid within the 'normal' range, although it is unlikely that the value would be in the bottom 50% of the normal range. For this reason the measurement of plasma uric acid is not very helpful in making the diagnosis. More useful is to identify (from a joint aspirate) the negatively birefringent crystals of uric acid under polarized light microscopy. This is only really needed (and possible) when the knee is involved as the diagnosis has a wider differential (see above).

Most gout is idiopathic, occurring in middle-aged males, and is related to a familial tendency to under excrete uric acid via the kidneys. Uric acid is formed from the breakdown of purines. Gout can be due to either under excretion or to over production of uric acid.

Causes of impaired uric acid excretion
- Renal disease (clinical gout however, unusual)
- Drugs: thiazide diuretics, low dose aspirin, cyclosporin
- Toxins: lead poisoning
- Acidosis
  - Lactic acidosis; alcohol, exercise
  - Ketoacidosis; diabetes, starvation

Causes of increased uric acid production
- Haematological malignancy
  - Myeloproliferative disease
  - Lymphoproliferative disease.
- Cell lysis: chemotherapy
  - Carcinomas
  - Psoriasis
  - Diet high in purines, e.g. beer
- Rare genetic disorders
  - Lesch–Nyhan syndrome (X-linked hypoxanthine guanine phosphoribosyl transferase deficiency)
  - Glucose-6-phoshatase deficiency (Von Gierke's disease)

Complications of gout
- **Tophaceous gout**; collection of urate crystals in soft tissue such as ear cartilage and periarticular skin
- **Joint erosions** like punched out lesions proximal to the joint.

ANSWERS 4

- **Nephropathy**: three patterns are seen . . .
  - Tubulo-interstitial disease
  - Acute tubular precipitation causing acute renal failure (post-chemotherapy)
  - Stone formation.
- **Side effects of treatment**
  - NSAIDS principally upper GI haemorrhage
  - Allupurinol (this commonly used drug has some important side effects):
    Hypersensitivity; rashes (Stevens–Johnson syndrome), malaise, muscle pain and fever
    Haematological; leukopenia, leukocytosis, eosinophilia, aplastic anaemia
    Peripheral neuropathy
    Hepatitis
    Renal impairment
    Cataracts
    Allopurinol should be reserved therefore for:
      Recurrent episodes (following discussion with the patient)
      Tophaceous gout
      Nephropathy
      Chemothepathy prophylaxis
      Lesch–Nyhan syndrome
    Note that allopurinol should not be started during an acute episode of gout.

(6) Pseudogout (calcium pyrophosphate deposition)

Various metabolic and endocrine conditions predispose to this condition, which is more common in elderly patients. These include (mnemonic **WIP A HOG**) . . .

  W Wilson's disease
  I Idiopathic
  P Primary hyperparathyroidism
  A Alkaptonuria
  H Haemachromatosis
  O Osteoarthritis
  G Gout

The clinical picture is one of osteoarthritis involving not only joints such as the hip and knees, but also unusual joints such as the MCPJs and the wrists. In addition, bouts of acute joint inflammation and pain can occur in pseudogout, typically affecting the knee. Pseudogout is differs from gout in that . . .
- Male : female ratio is approximately equal
- It is often polyarticular (except for exacerbations)

- **Brick shaped positively birefringent crystals** precipitate in the joint
- Calcification within the joint space (**chondrocalcinosis**) can occur

Answer 24

(1) Assessment of the cardiac rhythm followed by DC cardioversion

Only if the patient is in a suitable rhythm (VF or VT). It is vital that the candidate is familiar with the algorithm for both Basic Life Support and Advanced Life Support according to the latest guidance give by the European Resuscitation Council.

(2) Giving intravenous naloxone

The circumstances and the findings on initial survey suggest a probable opiate overdose and it is therefore the next appropriate step to give naloxone immediately to avoid a cardiorespiratory arrest. Boluses of 0.4 mg should be given repeatedly at 2-min intervals until the patient just becomes rousable and develops spontaneous respirations, and avoids precipitation of an acute withdrawal syndrome. This should not be delayed in order to question possibly unreliable associates about what has happened. For significant overdoses, patients will then require admission and an infusion of naloxone as the half-life of many opiates (especially methadone) is long.

Complications and associations of IV drug abuse
- Sepsis
  - Septicaemic shock due to injected bacteria
  - Endocarditis (right-sided)
  - Pulmonary septic emboli
  - Cellulitis at the injection sites
- Non-cardiogenic pulmonary oedema
- Rhabdomyolysis and renal failure due to prolonged stasis and muscle compression
- Secondary pulmonary hypertension (injected insoluble material, e.g. talc).
- Hypothermia
- HIV and Hepatitis B, C
- General ill health
  - Malnutrition
  - TB
  - Anaemia

Causes of unconsciousness
- **Raised intracranial pressure**
  - Mass lesion, e.g. tumour, haemorrhage
  - Oedema
  - Inflammation, e.g. meningitis/encephalitis
- **Metabolic abnormalities**
  - Hypoglycaemia
  - Hypoxia
  - Acidosis, e.g. DKA, hypoxia, sepsis
  - Alkalosis
  - Hepatic encephalopathy
  - Uraemia
  - Drugs (overdose) and toxins:
    Opiates
    Tricylic antidepressants
    Salicylates (severe/late)
    Benzodiazepines
    β-blockers
    Paracetamol (late)
  - Alcohol
  - Endocrine:
    Addisonian crisis (?pigmented, anaemic, hypotension, muscle wasting)
    Hypothyroidism (?pale, dry and puffy skin, hair loss)
    Diabetes (DKA, HONC, hypoglycaemia)
- **Cerebrovascular accidents** (central or brainstem infarctions)
- **Epilepsy**

The approach to the assessment of the unconscious patient
- **Assess and support the airway, breathing and circulation**
  - Give 100% oxygen unless the patient has COPD
  - Connect to ECG monitor and assess cardiac rhythm
  - Perform 12-lead ECG
  - Record temperature, pulse rate, blood pressure and peripheral oxygen saturation
  - Check a BM stix glucose level
  - Establish IV access and take blood for biochemistry, haematology, clotting screen, paracetamol and salicylate levels, random blood sugar, blood cultures
  - Commence IV volume expansion with colloid if hypotensive.
- **Give immediate treatment where indicated**
  - **Naloxone** for opiate overdose (or the possibility of). May require an infusion as the half-life is shorter

than most opiates
  - **Flumazanil** for benzodiazepine overdose (contraindicated in epilepsy)
  - **Glucagon** for hypoglycaemia and beta-blocker overdose
  - **Calcium gluconate followed by dextrose and insulin** for hyperkalaemia
- **Get brief history from any available source,** e.g. relatives, friends, ambulance crew, as to the events leading up to the episode and any relevant past medical history including medications
- **Examination**
  - **Perform Glasgow coma scale** rating and repeat every 30 min
  - Assess **pupils**:
    Pinpoint in opiate overdose
    Unequal in raised intracranial pressure
  - Assess **fundi** for papilloedema
  - Look for signs of **head injury**
  - Examine for **meningism** (provided no suspicion of cervical spine injury)
  - Examine the **skin**:
    Purpura in meningococcal septicaemia
    Scratch marks in uraemia
    Jaundice and other stigmata of chronic liver dysfunction
  - **Assess for brainstem** dysfunction as a sign of brain shift, metabolic toxicity or central cerebrovascular accident:
    Doll's eye movements (semicircular canals and CVIII to CIII, IV, and VI)
    Respiratory pattern
      Depressed in opiate or benzodiazepine toxicity
      Cheyne–Stokes (non-specific) and other breathing 'arrhythmias' may indicate brainstem damage
    Pupil reactivity
      Equal?
      Reactive to light both directly and consensually? (CII and III and internuclear connections via the Edinger-Westphal nucleus). Raised intracranial pressure causes herniation of the temporal lobe through the tentorial hiatus compressing (the contralateral) CIII at the edge of the tentorium. Further rises in pressure leads to compression of the cerebral peduncle on the side opposite to the mass lesion again against the tentorial edge. This produces an ipsilateral weakness as the pyramidal tracts decussate

below this level in the medulla.

Corneal reflex (CV)

Long tract signs

Limb tone

Reflexes

Plantar responses

- **Arrange an urgent CT scan** if raised intracranial pressure is suspected

(3) Blood glucose followed by intramuscular glucagon

A **measurement of the blood glucose** is an essential first step in any diabetic patient presenting with an acute illness. Here a BM stix reading would diagnose the hypoglycaemia that is suggested by the onset of unconsciousness in a previously well diabetic patient. Note that hypoglycaemia is more common in those diabetic patients who are well controlled. This should be followed by **administration of glucagon 1 mg i.m.** Remember that in diabetes sulphonylurias are also a cause of hypoglycaemia by causing a rise in endogenous insulin.

The presentation of hypoglycaemia includes symptoms of sympathetic nervous system drive (sweating, anxiety, tremor, pale skin and cold peripheries) together with features of low CNS glucose (confusion, tremor, aggressive behaviour, seizures and coma).

Note that hypoglycaemia can be physiological (normally corrected in part by gluconeogenesis so coma is rare) or pathological.

Causes of hypoglycaemia

- **Tumours**
  - **Insulinoma**: easily diagnosed by paradoxically high levels of insulin (with C peptide indicating endogenous origin) in the context of hypoglycaemia. Most are sporadic, but some form part of **multiple endocrine neoplasia type I.** 95% are benign. Present with multiple episodes of hypoglycaemia, sometimes over months or years
  - **Sarcomas** (glucose hungry)
- **Drugs**
  - Insulin
  - Sulphonylurias
  - β-blockers
  - Salicylates
  - Paracetamol
- **Liver disease**

- Alcohol (even in absence of cirrhosis due to inhibition of gluconeogenesis)
- Cirrhosis.
- **Renal failure**
- **Endocrine**
  - Hypothyroidism
  - Addison's disease
  - Hypopituitarism

(4) Get help, give salbutamol/ipratropium on oxygen, give intravenous hydrocortisone

The patient has ominous features consistent with **life-threatening asthma**. The British Thoracic Society Guide lines for this are clear.

Features of life-threatening asthma

- PEF < 33% of best or predicted
- $PaO_2 < 92\%$
- Silent chest, poor respiratory effort, cyanosis **(Chest)**
- Bradycardia, arrhythmia, hypotension **(Cardiovascular)**
- Exhaustion, confusion, coma **(CNS)**

Management of life-threatening asthma

If any of the above are present the initial action should be to . . .

- **Call for senior/ICU help**
- **Give salbutamol 5 mg and ipratropium via oxygen driven nebulizer**
- **Give IV hydrocortisone 100 mg** (or oral prednisolone 60 mg)

Followed by . . .

- Measure arterial blood gases
  - Severe asthma indicated by:
    $PaCO_2 > 4.6\,kPa$
    $PaO_2 < 8\,kPa$
    pH < 7.35
- Repeat the salbutamol and ipratropium nebulizer every 15 min
- Consider continuous salbutamol nebulizer 5–10 mg/h
- Consider magnesium sulphate 1.2–2.0 g i.v. given as a bolus over 20 min
- Correct electrolyte imbalances
- Arrange chest X-ray
- Admit to hospital

(5) Intravenous fluids followed by blood cultures

The patient probably has neutropenia and has septicaemic shock as a consequence. The first two steps in the management would be to commence **IV fluid resusitation** for the hypotension and to take **blood cultures**. In addition to blood cultures, cultures should also be taken from any long lines *in situ* (remove and send the line for investigation), sputum, throat, stool (*Clostridium difficile*). Antibiotics should be commenced immediately without waiting for the results of microbiological investigations. A typical regimen would be Vancomycin 1 g every 12 h and ceftazidime 2 g every 8 h. Serious infections do not usually occur until the neutrophil count is below 1×10^9.

Part 3 History and Examination Routines

Cardiovascular System

The cardiovascular system-based history is the bread-and-butter of history stations and it is almost guaranteed that you will be asked to take a cardiovascular history in your OSCE. You should be rubbing your hands together in glee as you walk into the OSCE station because you know you are onto a winner!

Typical past patient scenarios have included . . .

This patient has chest pain. Take his history.

This patient has presented with shortness of breath. Ask her some relevant questions. (Important early on to differentiate between respiratory and cardiovascular causes of breathlessness.)

This patient has a painful blue left foot. Take a cardiovascular focused history.

This lady has come to see you because of palpitations. Ask her some questions.

The history routine

The vital questions to ask in taking a cardiovascular system-based history are . . .

Chest pain

For *any pain* anywhere, use the **SOCRATES** mnemonic . . .

S Site
O Time of onset: exact or approximate? whilst eating/exerting?
   Nature of onset: sudden or gradual?
   Nature since onset: constantly present or periods free from pain since initial onset? If constantly present since onset, is it increasing, decreasing or staying the same?
C Character of pain: sharp, dull, heavy, stabbing, tight
R Radiation: interscapular, to jaw, neck or arm(s)?
A Associated features, specifically presence of dyspnoea, palpitations, nausea, loss of consciousness, sweating
T Timing: what were you doing when it came on?
E Exacerbating factors: inspiration, movement? Relieving factors: nitrates, leaning forward?
S Subjective severity: 1–10; worst ever pain/ worse than childbirth?
   Previous history of similar pain; any change in occurrence of patterns of pain?

Shortness of breath

- Time of onset
- Nature of onset: sudden or gradual?
- **Pattern** of occurrence: on exercising, at rest, at night, waking patient from sleep, on lying flat, with eating
- Nature since onset: constantly present or periods free from SOB? If constant, is it improving, deteriorating or staying the same?
- Previous history of similar?
- **Smoking** history
- Associated features: especially cough, expectoration, haemoptysis, wheeze, deterioration in **exercise tolerance** and ability to perform activities of daily living (ADLs)

Palpitations

- Time of onset: when did they come on? When do they come on normally?
- Nature of onset: what were you doing at the time? Were they sudden or gradual?
- Nature since onset: how long did they last? How have

they changed since coming on? Are they slow or fast, regular or irregular? Missed beats? Heavy beats?
- Pattern of occurrence: have you had it before? How many times over last week/month/year?
- Associated features, especially collapse, chest pain, loss of consciousness, sweating, vomiting

Episodes of loss of consciousness (witness history vital)

- Time of onset: when did the collapse occur?
- Nature of onset: did it come on suddenly or gradually? What were you doing at the time?
- Past history of similar: anything to suggest **amaurosis fugax** (temporary monocular blindness due to a clot of plaque in the carotid artery breaking off and travelling to the retinal artery in the eye. This blocks the artery for a time and causes loss of vision in that eye for as long as its blood supply is cut off)
- Features prior to collapse: did you feel strange? Did you get a warning of what was to come?
- Features during collapse, often taken from witness: any shaking, jerking, loss of continence, cyanosis, tongue biting
- Features after collapse: how quick did you 'come around'? Do you feel entirely back to normal now? Did you injure yourself anywhere or bang your head?

Orthopnoea

- Frequency: do you get short of breath on lying flat? Does it happen every night?
- How many pillows do you sleep with?
- Can you lay flat at all?
- Do you occasionally sleep in the armchair?

Paroxysmal nocturnal dyspnoea

- Is it true PND? Does the patient genuinely wake because of dyspnoea, or is it to pass urine or because they are coughing (COPD patients)?
- Actions before, during and after attack: is it resolved by standing at the window or outside whilst gasping for air?

Claudication

- True claudication, or cramp, or spinal stenosis? How quickly do you recover from the pain? Do you then recommence activity? How long is it before the pain returns?
- **Location** of pain: buttock, thigh, calf
- Other signs of arterial ischaemia: rest pain, paraesthesia, pallor, coldness of extremities

Peripheral oedema

- Onset: when did it start to be a problem? Is it worse at night, in the morning or is it constant?
- Nature since onset: has it got significantly worse recently?
- Progression: how far up the legs does it extend—ankle, mid-calf, knee, mid-thigh, hip, abdomen, sacrum?
- Is it pitting or tense? Do socks/shoes dig in to it?
- Does it improve on elevating the lower limbs?
- Are rings tight on fingers?
- Overlying dermatological changes: eczema or ulcers due to stasis
- NB Need to exclude lymphoedema in cardiac patients: take history of malignancy/lymph node removal, do not simply assume that oedema is cardiac in origin

Epigastric pain

- Can be due to cardiac ischaemia/infarction
- Can represent enlargement or rupture of abdominal aortic aneurysm

Exercise tolerance

- How far can patient walk on flat ground before symptoms occur/before they have to stop?
- Can they perform their activities of daily living?
- What symptom is it that eventually causes them to have to rest? Is it leg pain, chest pain or dyspnoea?

Symptoms of acute peripheral arterial ischaemia

- Pain
- Pallor
- Paraesthesia
- Perishingly cold
- Paralysis
- Pulselessness

Risk factors

- May be remembered with the mnemonic **SHIFT MAID**, what every junior doctor needs whilst on-call! . . .

S Smoking

H Hypertension

I Insulin dependent, or non-insulin dependent DM

F Family history of cardiovascular disease

T Triglycerides, fats, cholesterol

M Male sex

A Age

I Inactivity

D Diet, drink (alcohol)

As with all systems based histories, if you have time following elucidation of the presenting complaint and history of presenting complaint, you must go on to take . . .

- **Past medical history**
  - Specifically, a history of anaemia, diabetes, angina, MI, cardiac catheterization, coronary artery bypass grafting, carotid endarterectomy, rheumatic fever, high BP and high cholesterol are all vital to elucidate
  - A history of chronic pulmonary disease would give clues to right-sided heart failure
- **Drug history**
  - A full evaluation of all medications taken, including generic name, dose, frequency and length of time on medication is, as ever, vital
  - Expect the cardiac cripple to be on the usual recipe of nitrate, β-blocker, diuretic, calcium channel antagonist, ACE-inhibitor, statin and (often) antidiabetic drugs
  - Certain drugs should alert the historian to the fact that the patient's cardiovascular system is particularly frail, such as bumetanide, amiodarone, flecainide
- **Allergies**
  - Take details of all allergies, asking what happens with exposure to each of the proposed allergens
- **Family history**
  - A family history of myocardial infarction, ischaemic heart disease or cerebrovascular disease at early age effects a large amount of risk onto the patient, and all should be enquired into
  - Unexplained death of teenagers/young adults in the family should give warning of the possibility of hypertrophic obstructive cardiomyopathy
- **Social history**
  - Smoking history is vital: amount, type and length of time smoked (pack years). Many patients will say they don't smoke, but always ask these people if they have *ever* smoked. Many will tell you that '*Oh yes, I gave up 3 days ago doctor*', with an 80 packs per year history

- Dietary history may be relevant: excessive consumption of saturated fats
- Alcohol history is relevant: alcoholic cardiomyopathy
- Occupation is important: high levels of stress or inactivity predispose to cardiovascular disease
- **Systems review**

Cardiovascular disease affects all the systems of the body; hence a comprehensive screen of all major systems should be undertaken. Below is a brief example of questions that should be asked for each system as a screen. Obviously, further expansion should be undertaken in the presence of positive findings . . .

  - **Respiratory system**: shortness of breath, cough, expectoration, wheeze, inhalers, home nebulizers, home O_2
  - **Gastrointestinal system**: abdominal pain (ischaemic bowel), frequency of bowel opening, recent alteration in frequency of bowel opening, recent weight loss, blood PR
  - **Neurological system**: weakness, loss of sensation, loss of consciousness, headache, transient blindness (amaurosis fugax)

The examination routine

As with the cardiovascular history-taking station, the cardiovascular examination station is the bread-and-butter of the OSCE, and as such you are almost guaranteed that one will crop up in your OSCE. Common stations over the past few years have included . . .

Patients with murmurs, usually mitral regurgitation or aortic stenosis.

Patients with additional heart sounds.

Patients with chronic heart failure: raised JVP, hepatomegaly, bi-basal crepitations, peripheral oedema, cyanosis.

Patients with an abdominal aortic aneurysm (variously also included in GI system examination).

Patients with stigmata of subacute bacterial endocarditis.

Occasionally, actors may play out a more acute cardiovascular scenario in the OSCE situation, and you should be prepared to take a history and/or examine in the situation of . . .

Patients with acute coronary syndrome or myocardial infarction.

Patients with dissecting aortic aneurysm.

Patients having had a syncopal episode.

You will variously be instructed . . .

'Examine this patient's cardiovascular system.'
'Auscultate this patient's heart.'
'Palpate this patient's peripheral pulses.'
'Examine this patient for stigmata of bacterial endocarditis.'

Begin by introducing yourself to the patient, stating your full name and grade, and by explaining what you are proposing to do. Attempt to gain consent with a relatively closed statement: 'Are you happy with that?' Patients in OSCEs will always say that they are happy for you to proceed, so do so. Ensure that the patient is sat at an angle of 45°, that they are comfortable and that they are adequately but not overly or prematurely exposed.

Inspection from the end of the bed

- General body **habitus** (e.g. obesity, cardiac cachexia)
- **Dysmorphic features** are a clue to congenital cardiac anomalies in children
- Listen for **abnormal sounds** (mechanical artificial valves are audible from the end of the bed)
- **Level of comfort** at rest (e.g. any dyspnoea/obvious pain or distress)
- Face:
  - Malar flush (mitral stenosis)
  - Hypo- or hyperthyroid facies and habitus (expect AF + hypo- or hyperdynamic circulation)
  - Addisonian or Cushingoid appearance
  - Dyspnoea (heart failure)
  - Cyanosis (heart failure)
  - Polycythemic
  - Pallor (anaemia, shock)
  - Earlobe creases (looking for **Frank's sign**, which is a diagonal crease in the lobule of the auricle; deeper and more obvious creases are statistically associated

with an increased likelihood of death from coronary artery disease in younger patients)

- **Neck:**
  - **Corrigan's sign** is visible distension and collapse of the arterial pulse seen in the neck in **hyperdynamic conditions associated with a run-off of blood** from the arterial circulation (e.g. aortic regurgitation)
  - Vigorous carotid pulsation may be noted in coarctation of the aorta
  - Raised JVP may be noted in congestive cardiac failure, tricuspid regurgitation and pulmonary hypertension (e.g. due to mitral stenosis)
  - Thyroid gland goitre/thyroidectomy scar
- **Praecordium**
  - Thoracotomy scar (often for mitral stenosis)
  - Midline sternotomy scar (often for coronary artery bypass grafting, CABG)
  - Valvotomy scar
  - Obvious pulsation
  - Scars from pacemakers/AICDs (automatic implantable cardioverter-defibrillators—feel like big pacemakers)
- **Ascites**
- **Peripherals**
  - GTN spray, O_2, ECG machine, walking aids, personal cardiac record book

Hands

- Clubbing (congenital cyanotic cardiac disease, subacute bacterial endocarditis, atrial myxoma, axillary artery aneurysm, brachial and bronchial arteriovenous malformation; the latter three may cause unilateral clubbing)
- Peripheral cyanosis
- Pallor of palmar creases
- Splinter haemorrhages
- Osler's nodes (circumscribed *painful* erythematous swellings in the skin and subcutaneous tissues of the hands and feet; range in size from a pinhead to a pea)
- Janeway lesions (irregular erythematous flat *painless* macules on the palms, soles, thenar and hypothenar eminences of the hands, tips of fingers and plantar surfaces of the toes; may be haemorrhagic or purple in colour)
- Tar staining from cigarette smoking (don't say 'nicotine staining' as nicotine is a clear liquid)
- Koilonychia (spoon-shaped nails associated with iron-deficiency anaemia)

NB Be **fast yet thorough** through the hands during OSCE: examiners hate to see you getting bogged down at the hands when often the real pathology is in the chest/abdomen.

Palpation

- Radial pulse (check *rate* and *rhythm*; check for *radio-radial delay* as seen in subclavian artery stenosis; check for *radio-femoral delay* as seen in coarctation of the aorta)
- Watch out for slow AF, a rhythm that can easily appear regular, but is not. Try to concentrate on the length of pauses **between** beats when trying to tell whether a pulse is regular or irregular
- Brachial pulse (check *character* and *volume*; look for **scars** over brachial pulse from previous catheterization). The character of the pulse can be described as . . .
  - **Normal**
  - **Collapsing** ('water-hammer'): has a short, tall up-stroke and an abrupt down-stroke; it runs across all the fingers as the arm is lifted whilst palpating the brachial region; associated with *aortic regurgitation* or patent ductus arteriosus; never lift the arm to check for a collapsing pulse without first asking the patient if they have any pain in the relevant shoulder: examiners will commonly fail candidates for such an oversight
  - **Slow-rising**: also known as a plateau pulse for is slow yet sustained character; associated with *aortic stenosis*
  - **Jerky**: associated with hypertrophic obstructive cardiomyopathy and is due to the variable obstruction to left ventricular outflow

Non-invasive BP recording

Look at the arms/elbows . . .

. . . for evidence of tendon xanthomata, rheumatoid nodules, gouty tophi and nodules of rheumatic fever

Face (as above, plus on closer inspection . . .)

- Look around eyes for xanthelasma
- Look in eyes for arcus senilis
- Look at fundi for Roth spots (in bacterial endocarditis,

these are round, white retinal spots surrounded by haemorrhage)
- Look at conjunctivae for pallor
- Look under tongue for signs of central cyanosis
- Look for dental work as the potential cause of bacterial endocarditis

JVP

- Patient *must* be seated at 45° for examination of JVP
- Look for pulsation **between two heads of sternoclei-domastoid muscle** and the **mastoid process** of the skull
- Time any waves seen in the JVP by **palpating the carotid on the opposite side**
- Exacerbate by performing **hepato-jugular reflex** (momentary)
- Palpate to see if pulsations **palpable**
- Occlude with edge of finger and observe from which end it fills
- Formally assess the height of any raised JVP by measuring the *vertical distance above the sternal angle*

Apex beat

- Inspect for visible pulsation
- Palpate, and if apex beat is vigorous, stand one finger on it to localize the *point of maximal impulse*. The apex beat can be graded as . . .
  - **Impalpable**
  - **Just palpable**
  - **Lifting**: in diastolic overload, as in mitral or aortic regurgitation
  - **Thrusting**: stronger than lifting, in mitral or aortic regurgitation
  - **Heaving**: in outflow obstruction, as in aortic stenosis or hypertrophic obstructive cardiomyopathy
  - **Tapping**: easier to detect if hand is placed from left lower sternal edge to the apex, with fingers lifted off whilst feeling for the parasternal tap with the palm; characteristic of mitral stenosis. This manoeuvre will also detect thrills (palpable murmurs) in the mitral area, associated with mitral valve disease

Heaves and thrills

- Feel in the left parasternal region for right ventricular lift, a sign of right ventricular hypertrophy; usually due to pulmonary hypertension caused either by cor pulmonale or mitral stenosis

- Feel in the pulmonary and aortic areas separately for thrills of pulmonary and aortic stenosis, respectively

Auscultate the heart

- Whenever listening to the heart, always time the heart sounds by feeling a central pulse, preferably the carotid
- You are listening for **heart sounds 1 and 2** and for the presence of added sounds, which may include **murmurs**, a **third** heart sound, a **fourth** heart sound, the **ejection click** of aortic stenosis or the **opening snap** of mitral stenosis
- Remember that *left-sided murmurs are best heard with empty lungs* (i.e. on end-expiration), whereas *right-sided murmurs are best heard with full lungs* (i.e. on end-inspiration)
- Begin by listening at the apex with the bell. Ask the patient to roll over onto their left side, keeping the bell on the apex. You are listening for the low-pitched rumbling mid-diastolic murmur of mitral stenosis. Do not press too hard when listening with the bell otherwise you will simply turn it into a diaphragm, and this is not the point of using it to listen with
- Change to the diaphragm
- Listen at the apex and in the axilla
- Listen at the left parasternal edge
- Listen in the pulmonary (left 2nd intercostal space, parasternal edge) and aortic (right 2nd intercostal space, parasternal edge) areas
- Listen over the carotids for bruits of atherosclerosis and the radiation of aortic stenosis murmur.
- Deliberately sit the patient forward and listen with the diaphragm at the left parasternal edge in end-expiration for the murmur of aortic regurgitation
- If you hear a murmur anywhere, you must decide whether it is systolic or diastolic, where it is in systole or diastole, and grade it 1 to 6 (1 to 4 realistically for diastolic murmurs) based on the following criteria . . .

Grade	Description
1	Very faint, heard only after the listener has 'tuned in'; may not be heard in all positions
2	Quiet, but heard immediately after the examiner has placed the stethoscope on the chest
3	Moderately loud
4	Loud, with palpable thrill
5	Very loud, with thrill. May be heard when stethoscope is partially off the chest
6	Very loud, with thrill. May be heard with stethoscope entirely off the chest

If you hear a murmur in a young person, or in someone whom you are surprised to be able to hear a murmur, look for the **10 Ss** that will reassure you that it is an innocent murmur . . .

Symptom-free

Systolic

Short

Soft

Site (heard over small area only)

Split second sound

Sitting and standing cause murmur to vary

Sternal depression (pectus excavatum can cause innocent murmurs)

Signs (no other abnormal signs, all peripheral pulses normal)

Special tests (all normal, i.e. normal ECG/CXR/echo)

- Finish auscultation by listening at the lung bases (it's slick because you already have the patient sitting forward to listen for aortic regurgitation) for fine crepitations associated with left ventricular failure

Check for sacral and peripheral oedema

(Again, slick since you have the patient sitting forward)

Palpate the liver . . .

. . . to see if it is pulsatile, as would be the case in tricuspid regurgitation, or if it is enlarged, as would be the case in terminal cardiac failure. The patient must be laying flat for this

Dipstick the urine . . .

. . . to check for microscopic haematuria in bacterial endocarditis; it would also be necessary to palpate for splenomegaly

Palpate peripheral pulses

- Radial
- Ulnar
- Brachial
- Axillary
- Carotid
- Posterior tibial
- Dorsalis pedis
- Popliteal
- Femoral
- *Check for abdominal aortic aneurysm*

Auscultate the abdomen

Check for renal artery bruits or turbulent flow within an aneurysmal dilatation of the abdominal aorta

Now you have finished!

- **Cover** the patient up
- **Thank** them

Present your *positive findings* and *relevant negative findings* to the examiner

If required, postulate a diagnosis at the end, having listed all your evidence initially to make it clear how you have reached your conclusion. If postulating a diagnosis, also provide the examiner with a list of differentials.

Useful notes

The different murmurs
- **Systolic**
  Ejection systolic
  1 Aortic stenosis
  2 Pulmonary stenosis
  3 Atrial septal defect (ASD)
  4 Aortic sclerosis (just a murmur, no pressure drop across the valve)
  5 Physiological flow murmur
  Pan-systolic
  1 Mitral regurgitation
  2 Tricuspid regurgitation
  3 Ventricular septal defect (VSD)
  Late systolic
  1 Mitral valve prolapse (Barlow's syndrome)
  2 Hypertrophic obstructive cardiomyopathy (HOCM)
  3 Coarctation of the aorta
- **Diastolic**
  Early diastolic
  1 Aortic regurgitation
  2 Pulmonary regurgitation
  3 Graham–Steell murmur
  Mid-diastolic
  1 Mitral stenosis
  2 Tricuspid stenosis
  3 Austin–Flint murmur
- **Pan-systolic and diastolic**
  1 Patent ductus arteriosus
- **Murmurs radiating through to the back**
  1 Patent ductus arteriosus
  2 Coarctation of the aorta
  3 Pulmonary regurgitation

Where are murmurs heard best?
- **At the apex . . .**
  1 Mitral stenosis
  2 Mitral valve prolapse
  3 Austin–Flint murmur
- **At the apex, radiating to the axilla . . .**
  1 Mitral regurgitation
- **At the left sternal edge . . .**
  1 Aortic regurgitation
  2 Tricuspid stenosis
  3 Graham–Steell murmur
  4 Pulmonary stenosis
  5 ASD

Hx & Ex ROUTINES

6 Tricuspid regurgitation
7 VSD
8 Coarctation of the aorta
9 Patent ductus arteriosus
• **At the right sternal edge . . .**
  1 Pulmonary regurgitation

• **In the aortic area . . .**
  1 Aortic stenosis (radiating to the carotids)

Note that this is where these murmurs are heard **best**, *not heard exclusively.*

Respiratory System

The history routine

Q: **This patient has been experiencing some short-ness of breath, would you ask him some relevant questions.**

Q: **This patient has been experiencing some dif-ficulty breathing. Take a five-minute history and then summarize the findings.**

As with the cardiovascular history, the respiratory his-tory can be divided into direct questions regarding the **symptoms** of respiratory disease and **risk factor ques-tions** for respiratory history.

Shortness of breath

- Onset?
  - Suddenly? (PE, myocardial infarction, asthma, pneumothorax, cardiac arrhythmia)
  - Gradually? (Over how long)
- Exercise tolerance?
  - Ask about day-to-day activities
  - What has changed?
  - What can they no longer do?

Cough

- Onset and duration?
- Nocturnal? (asthma)
- Post-exertion? (asthma)

Sputum

- Colour (clear, creamy, yellow, green?)
- Volume (teaspoon, egg cup, cup?)

Haemoptysis

- Amount
- Frequency
- Causes of haemoptysis include . . .
  - Infections:
    Pneumonia (rusty coloured with *Streptococcus pneumoniae*)
    Tuberculosis
    Bronchiectasis (sometimes massive)
    Cystic fibrosis
  - Tumours; primary or secondary
  - Vascular:
    Pulmonary embolism
    Pulmonary oedema (frothy)
    Vasculitis (Wagener's, PAN, RA, SLE, Osler–Weber–Rendu)
    Pulmonary hypertension (primary or secondary, e.g. mitral stenosis)
    AV malformations
  - Trauma
  - Coagulation/platelet disorders/warfarin treatment

Chest pain

- Location, intensity, radiation, aggravating and reliev-ing factors
- Pleuritic pain is worse with deep inspiration and coughing
- Constant pain with neoplastic disease invading the chest wall.
- Respiratory causes of chest pain
  - Infections:
    Pneumonia (late)
    Tuberculosis
  - Pneumothorax (early symptom)
  - Tumours; chest wall involvement (especially mesothelioma)

- Pulmonary embolism (late feature)
- Trauma:
  Rib fracture with coughing

Wheeze

- Check the patients understanding what of wheeze (a musical whistle not feeling short of breath)
- Causes include
  - Asthma
  - COPD
  - Bronchiectasis
  - Cardiac failure
  - Infections (acute bronchitis/bronchiolitis in children)
  - A fixed obstruction causing a monophonic solitary wheeze (tumour, foreign body, lymph nodes)
  - Aspiration
- Ask about triggers (asthma)?
  - Pets (cats, dogs)?
  - Dust?
  - Pollen (seasonal)?
  - Cold?
  - Exertion?
  - Emotion?
  - Morning or evening? (Poorly controlled asthmatics have 'dips' in the morning peak flow compared to the evening)
  - Drugs? (Aspirin and β-blockers)

Other questions to assess asthma

- Days missed from work?
- Use of oral steroids?
- Admissions to hospital?
- Disturbed sleep?
- Home peak flow meter?
- Home nebulizer?
- Family history of atopy? (Asthma, hayfever, eczema, allergic rhinitis)

Weight loss

Especially in . . .
- Tumours
- Fibrosing alveolitis
- Tuberculosis
- Bronchiectasis
- Cystic fibrosis

Smoking history

- Cigarettes, cigars or a pipe?
- Duration?
- Amount? (pack years)
- Passive smoking? (home or work)

Occupational and environmental

- Occupation? (dust, irradiation, fumes, animals)

NB Exposure to asbestos was very common in many occupations up until the 1980s. Even brief exposure can lead to asbestos-related pulmonary disease in later life and smoking is synergistic with asbestos in the causation of bronchogenic carcinoma. **Any asbestos exposure no matter how brief is important.** Occupations particularly at risk include ship builders, heating engineers, and builders.

- Farmers (extrinsic allergic alveolitis; Farmer's lung)
- Hotels/factories; possible Legionella from organisms aerosolized from the air conditioning
- Pets (birds; *Chlamydia psittaci*)

Drugs

- Full **drug history** required; inhaler sizes and type of device used
- **Inhaler technique** checked?
- **Home oxygen** (concentrator or cylinders) and nebulizers
- **Other treatments** such as physiotherapy. This may be being performed by relatives/parents
- Many **drugs are can cause respiratory symptoms** by a variety of means . . .
  - Fibrosis: amiodarone, bleomycin
  - Asthma: β-blockers, aspirin
  - Cough: ACE-inhibitors
  - Eosinophilia: sulphasalazine, penicillin, NSAIDS
  - Vasculitis: hydralazine, isonizid, dapsone

General review of systems

Many respiratory illness are multisystem . . .
- Sarcoidosis (lung, eye, skin, bones, CNS)
- Tuberculosis (lung, bone, renal, skin, GIT)
- Tumours
- Atypical pneumonias (GIT, skin, renal, hepatic, haematological)

- Vasculitis (SLE, PAN, RA)
- COPD (cor pulmonale)

Social history

- Many patients with chronic pulmonary pathology will be severely incapacitated by dyspnoea. A full picture of their home life with adaptations and their support network is highly relevant.
- If there is time, a few simple brief questions regarding the impact of the disease upon a patient's mental well-being will earn merit for showing insight into the disease. For example, 'How do you find having . . . has affected your mood/happiness?'

The examination routine

Q: Examine this patient's respiratory system

Q: Auscultate this patient's lung fields

In general, there is only a limited number of different types of chest case (see the following cases) included in medical examinations. Remember (as always) that in an undergraduate the examiner is looking for good approach to the patient, orthodox examination technique and communication skills, rather than the actual diagnosis (although this will, of course, attract further marks).

Unless asked specifically to examine a particular area (e.g. the lung bases) go through the whole respiratory examination routine from start to finish. Many students ask if they should give 'a running commentary'. In general, unless the examiner asks for this, just keep quiet and go steadily through the examination. You will usually be interrupted at some stage, but don't panic if you are allowed to go all the way through to the end before being asked about your findings — it probably means you're doing well.

Remember the initial peripheral part of the chest examination routine, although important not to omit, should take less than a couple of minutes. You are going to get most of the information by listening to the chest and so should get onto this quickly before your examiner starts getting inpatient. Candidates most often forget to count the respiratory rate and listen to the apices in the supra-clavicular fossae (so do not!).

First of all . . .

- Introductions
- Request to examine

Exposure

- If required, undressed to the waist, reclined at 45°

Then stand at the end of the bed.

General inspection

- Peripheral
  - O_2 cylinder
  - Nebulizer
  - Sputum pots (look and comment)
- The patient
  - Respiratory rate (count over 15 s; normally <15/min in an adult, greater than 25/min in moderate severe asthma)
  - Short of breath or comfortable at rest?
  - Accessory usage
  - Intercostal recession
  - Pursed lipped respiration
  - Scars
  - Peripheral cyanosis
  - Chest symmetry

Hands

- **Clubbing**
  - Increased fluctuance of the nail on the nail bed followed by . . .
  - . . . progressive loss of the nail fold angle (examine nail profile)
  - Respiratory causes include:
    Carcinoma of the bronchus
    Bronchiectasis
    CF
    Fibrosing alveolitis
    Pulmonary abscess
- **Tar staining of the fingers**
- **Flap**
  - Arms outstretched, wrists back, eyes closed and fingers spread. Demonstrate this to the patient first
  - Occurs with CO_2 retention (usually due to COPD). (Performed in exactly the same way when examining the patient with liver disease)

- **Bounding pulse**
  - Another sign of CO_2 retention as above
- **Pulse rate**
  - Tachycardia common in hypoxic states
  - Rate >110 significant in asthma as a sign of moderately severe exacerbation

Head and neck

- **Eyes**
  - Anaemia (pallor of the conjunctiva)
- **JVP**
  - Raised in cor pulmonale/pulmonary hypertension/PE
- **Mouth**
  - Central cyanosis seen on examining the buccal mucosa
  - *Candida* with inhaled or oral steroids, or HIV infection
- **Trachea**
  - **Centrality**: palpate with the third digit whilst the second and forth rest on the sternocostal junctions. The trachea should be mid way between the latter two points. This may be uncomfortable so warn the patient in advance
  - Reduction of **suprasternal notch to cricoid cartilage distance**, indicating hyperinflation. This distance should normally admit three fingers
- **Lymph nodes**
  - **Virchow's node** behind insertion of the left sternocleidomastoid muscle. Feel specifically with a finger either side. This is Troisier's sign (from carcinoma of the bronchus or stomach)
  - Check quickly for other nodes in the anterior and posterior triangle of the neck

Chest

- **Inspection**
  - Movement symmetrical and normal?
  - Chest shape: AP diameter increased in COPD; examine from the side
- **Palpation**
  - **Apex beat**: this together with the trachea gives an indication of the position of the mediastinum which may be displaced (either pushed or pulled by pulmonary disease)

- **Expansion**: your technique will be watched here. Remember fingers and distil palms applied lightly to the lateral aspect of the chest wall with thumbs pointing to the midline but held *off* the chest. Ask the patient to take a deep breath and observe for symmetrical movement of the thumbs away from each other. Perform above and below the breast
- **Tactile vocal fremitus** (vocal resonance): ask the patient to say '99' whilst you hold the ulnar aspects of both your palms to the chest wall. Repeat in three positions from the infraclavicular area down. This will be increased over areas of consolidation and reduced over a pneumothorax or emphysematous lung
- **Percussion**. Remember the supraclavicular fossae. Compare left with right. Four or five areas each side. Finish by asking the patient to put his hands on his hip and percuss at two levels laterally. Do not percuss the clavicle directly; percuss you finger over the clavicle
- **Auscultation**: again, do not forget the supraclavicular fossae. Use the diaphragm unless the patient has a very hairy chest. Show the patient how you would like him/her to take regular deep breaths in and out through a wide mouth (to avoid transmitted sounds from the upper airway). Compare left with right. Again, four or five areas on each side should suffice. If you home in on something interesting, it is acceptable to give this some closer attention with a couple of extra listens around about its locality

Repeat the above chest examination routine for the back of the chest. Do not have the patient sitting backwards and forwards as you perform each component of the examination, first on the front and then the back of the chest!

Finishing off

- Thank the patient and help them to redress or cover up
- Say that you would like to ideally go on to examine for other features of cor pulmonale (peripheral oedema, an enlarged liver, etc.) in addition to the (possibly) raised JVP already found.
- Ask to look at the . . .
- Temperature chart
- Respiratory rate
- Peak flow charts
- Oxygen saturation recordings

The Chest Radiograph Routine

Q: Comment on the chest X-ray

If you can immediately spot the abnormality and, better still, know the diagnosis or a differential list, say so straight away. Then go through your list looking for anything else, if the examiner allows you to.

Otherwise work through the film in a methodical manner, giving the examiner a running commentary as you go. The 'art' of commenting on radiological material is having the vocabulary to describe what you can see, and applying your knowledge of what is normal.

Initial comments

- Refer to the image as a **'chest radiograph'** not an 'X-ray' to avoid a pointless and pedantic discussion with the examiner
- Comment on the **whether the film is PA or AP**. PA (Posterior to Anterior) is usual allowing the scapulae to be rotated as far as possible out of the film. AP views general occur in the acute setting with the film placed behind the patient (lying on a trolley or in bed). The heart appears slightly enlarged on an AP view (0.5–1.0 cm) compared to the PA view
- Check the **orientation**. There should be marker either 'L' or 'R' on the *patient's* left or right side. Patients with dextrocardia occur regularly in medical examinations, look for associated bronchiectasis ('ring shadows', air-fluid levels, 'tramline' thickening of airway walls, interstitial shadowing) in possible Kartagener's syndrome. Typically the radiograph will have been deliberately orientated the wrong way round to try and mislead you
- Check the **inflation** of the chest. Count six ribs anteriorly. If less than six can be counted it is under-inflated (? debilitated patient). If you can count seven or eight ribs there may be hyperinflation with asthma or COPD
- Check the **centrality** of the view. The ends of the clavicles should be equidistant from the spinous processes. If this is not the case, say which way the patient is rotated

Trachea

- Check the **trachea is central** and not pushed (tension pneumothorax) or pulled (fibrosis, pneumonectomy) to one side. The right border of the trachea can normally be traced down to the right bronchus
- There is a line down the right border of the trachea known as the **paratracheal stripe** which is normally 5 mm or less, but widened by mediastinal lesions such as tumour, lymphadenopathy and sepsis (mediastinitis)
- Check the **carinal angle**: this is the inferior angle between the left and right main bronchus. It is normally 60–75° but widened by an enlarged right atrium or mediastinal lymphadenopathy

Cardiac silhouette

Cardiac silhouette

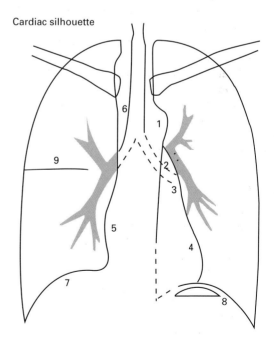

1   **Aortic knuckle**
2   **Left main bronchus**
3   **Left atrium**
4   **Left ventricle**
5   **Right ventricle**
6   **Superior vena cava**
7   **Right hemi-diaphragm**
8   **Left hemi-diaphragm**
9   **Horizontal fissure**

- Check the **cardio-thoracic ratio** is less than 1:2. Otherwise suggest cardiac failure. If there is 'globular' (like a bag of fluid) enlargement suggest a possible pericardial effusion
- Check that the **borders of the heart are sharp and distinct**
- Look a the various **chambers of the heart** to see if enlarged e.g. enlarged left atrium with mitral stenosis
- **Look into the heart** silhouette for calcification (aortic or valvular) and the rings of prosthetic heart valves
- **Look behind the heart** for fluid levels (hiatus hernia or achalasia)

The hilar areas

Note that the left hilum is normally slightly higher than the right side. They are normally approximately the same size, and are concave outwards in shape.

The hilar areas are composed of . . .
- The main bronchi
- Pulmonary arteries and veins
- Lymph nodes; which contribute little to the bulk unless enlarged

Enlargement is usually due to lymphadenopathy. The most common causes are malignancy, TB, lymphoma and sarcoidosis.

The lung fields

Normally there is a relative lack of vascular markings (oligaemia) in the upper zones due to gravity. The horizontal fissure can usually be seen in the right lung field. The costophrenic angles should be sharp. Total lung volume should be symmetrical.
- **Effusions**: look for loss of the sharp costophrenic angle as an early sign. Look for the meniscus of the effusion creeping up the chest wall laterally. Look for associated coin (malignancy) lesions (you may be shown an intentionally over penetrated film to look *into* the effusion) indicating malignancy as a possible cause
- **Coin lesions** (large round lesions)
  - Tumour (primary or secondary); most frequently
  - Abscess
  - TB
  - Rheumatoid nodule
  - Cyst
  - Hydatid disease
  - Infarction
  - AV malformation
- **Cavitating lesions**: remember **CAVIT**: Carcinoma (especially squamous cell tumours), Autoimmune (Wegener's granulomatosis, rheumatoid nodules, sarcoidosis), Vascular (infarctions and septic emboli), Infections (especially Staphylococcal, *Klebsiella* and TB), Traumatic. Note the appearance of a mycetoma, which is that of a ball of fungus (aspergillosis) within a previous TB cavity. The ball appears to move about if the patient is X-rayed in different positions.
- **Nodular lesions** (small round lesions; 0.5–1.0 cm); causes include . . .
  - Metastatic lung disease
  - Septic emboli
  - Wegener's ganulomatosis
  - Rheumatoid nodules
  - Caplan's syndrome
  - Progressive massive fibrosis
  - AV malformations
- **Miliary shadowing** (very small round lesions; 1 mm, diffuse); causes include . . .
  - Miliary TB
  - Metastatic disease
  - Sarcoidosis
  - Dust (pneumoconiosis, silicosis)
  - Extrinsic allergic alveolitis
  - Fungal disease (histoplasmosis, coccidiomycosis)
- **Alveolar (fluffy) shadowing**: soft, fluid-containing shadows; causes include . . .
  - Infection
  - ARDS
    Sepsis
    Trauma, head injury
    Embolism; especially fat or amniotic fluid
    Aspiration, inhalation
    Multisystem disease; DIC, liver failure, pancreatitis, eclampsia, vasculitis
  - Pulmonary oedema

- Pulmonary haemorrhage
- Drug reactions, e.g. amiodarone alveolitis
- Reticular shadowing (fibrosis): lace-like hard lines; pulmonary fibrosis

The bones

Look for . . .
- Metastatic disease (discrete lucent areas)
- Fractures
- Cervical ribs
- Absent clavicles (congenital); easy to miss if bilateral
- Rib notching: due to enlarged collaterals in aortic coarctation forming notches on the inferior edge of the anterior rib surfaces
- Looser's zones: linear areas of bone demineralization (so-called pseudo-fractures) seen in osteomalacia
- Brown tumours: cyst-like areas of demineralization seen in advanced hyperparathyroidism
- Paget's disease: localized irregularity and thickening of bone

The soft tissues

- Check there are two breast shadows in females.
- Surgical emphysema: dark, gas-containing defects within the soft tissues. Easiest to see in the soft tissue lateral to the lung fields or in the cervical soft tissue. Gas may outline normally invisible structures (e.g. pectoral muscles) due to the interface of a different density

If the chest radiograph appears normal . . .

- Check the **left right orientation**, i.e. no dextrocardia
- Look for **small pneumothorax** at the apex.
- Look for **small apical pulmonary lesion** (Pancoast tumour, TB, apical fibrosis, mycetoma)
- Look at the apex for a **cervical rib**
- **Retrosternal goitres and thymoma** (?myasthenia gravis) are easy to ignore. Look for a soft tissue shadow extending inferiorly in the upper part of the chest
- Look **behind the heart for a fluid level** (?hiatus hernia, achalasia, oesophageal tumour)
- Look **in the heart shadow** for the ring bases of prosthetic heart valves
- Look again at the **bones**
- In a female check there are both **breast shadows**

- Check for air under the diagphram (?air under the diagphram, liver cyst)
- It may be normal!

Some example radiographs

1   Dextrocardia
The film may be put up the wrong way round

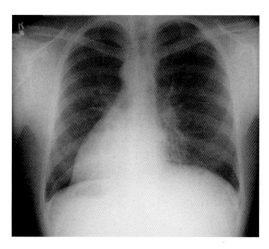

2   Hilar lymphadenopathy

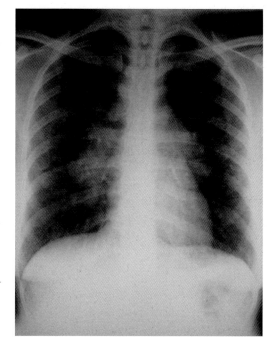

3   Right apical Pancoast tumour

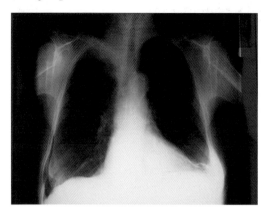

5   Large hiatus hernia

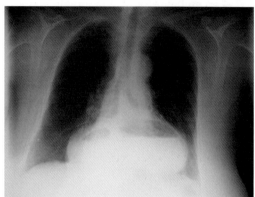

4   Mesothelioma

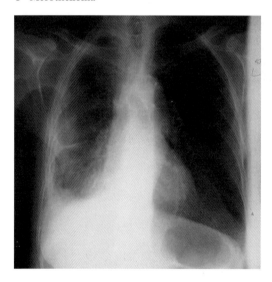

6   Mitral stenosis with gross resultant cardiomegaly
Note the bulge over the left atrium.

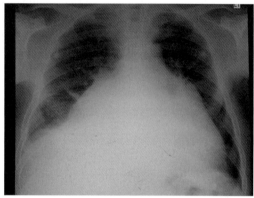

Gastrointestinal System

The history routine

Ask about . . .

Appetite

Weight

- Any change (loss or gain) and over how long? Ask about the fit of clothes if the patient is uncertain of figures

Tiredness

- lethargy (malabsorption, anaemia)

Nausea

Vomiting

- Duration
- Frequency

Haematemesis

- Frank blood or coffee grounds
- Volume and frequency

Regurgitation

- Recognizable undigested foods (physical obstruction, pharyngeal pouch)

Swallowing (dysphagia)

- Solids or liquids or both?
- Is food sticking? If so ask the patient to point where

- Duration
- Episodes of choking
- Progressive or intermittent
- Hot or cold foods

Heartburn symptoms

- Retrosternal burning pain
- Frequency
- Aggravating factors (alcohol, lying down, and recent weight gain)
- Relieving factors (antacids)
- Nocturnal symptoms

Waterbrash

- A bitter tasting fluid coming into the throat or mouth
- Associated with reflux

Abdominal pain

- Location
- Onset
- Radiation; e.g.
  - Biliary pain radiates to the back
  - Renal colic radiates to the groin
  - Gynaecological pain often radiates to the legs
  - Abdominal aortic aneurysm pain radiates to the buttocks and legs
- Constant (somatic) or colicky (visceral)
- Change in nature
- Previous episodes
- Aggravating and relieving factors

Abdominal bloating symptoms

- Obstruction
- Constipation
- IBS

Alteration in bowel habit

- Duration
  - Carcinoma of the rectum often has a relatively short 6–8-week history
  - Irritable bowel syndrome typically occurs in bouts lasting a few days or weeks; the patient (or medical records) often reporting similar previous episodes in the past
- Intermittent problem or a definite change
- Ask about their usual bowel habit (wide normal range)
- Bleeding per rectum
  - Colour of the stools? (melaena is black, tar-like and has an offensive smell)
  - Duration
  - Every time the bowels are opened
  - Before, during or after the stools
  - Mixed in with the motions or surrounding
  - Amount
- Mucus? (ask about oily discharge with the stool)
- Pain on opening the bowels
  - Anal fissure
  - Thrombosed haemorrhoids
  - Constipation
- Diarrhoea
  - Watery or just loose motions
  - Ask about travel, takeaway food, drugs, contacts, affected family or friends, bloody diarrhoea (bacterial infection, tumour, colitis)?
  - Offensive, bulky, floating diarrhoea suggests small bowel malabsorption and steatorrhoea
- Incontinence
  - Frequency
  - Need to use pads
  - Take a social history as often elderly

Associated risk factors for GI disease

- Liver disease risk factors (see OSCE 44, p. 304)
- Alcohol intake
- Smoking (upper GI cancers)
- Diet
  - Poor, unusual or food exclusion diets
  - Fibre intake (ask the patient if they know what foods contain fibre)
- Current medications
  - NSAIDS (melaena/dyspepsia)
  - Antibiotics (diarrhoea, pseudomembranous colitis)
  - Most drugs have non-specific GI side effects, e.g. nausea, vomiting and diarrhoea

- Specific GI treatments
- Drugs for dyspepsia and *H. pylori* eradication therapy
- Inflammatory bowel disease
- Previous investigations or interventions
  - Upper or lower GI endoscopy
  - Barium studies
  - CT scans
  - Surgery
- Social history
  - Impact of illness on their life, work, home, ability to cope, carers

---

The examination routine

First of all . . .

- Introductions
- Request to examine the patient

Exposure and position

- Ask the patient to expose the upper torso to the hips for a man or from the bra to the bikini line for a woman, allow one pillow. Be aware many patients, especially the elderly, find it unpleasant or painful (osteoarthritis of the cervical spine?) to lie flat so be flexible if this is the case.

Inspection from the end of the bed

- Surrounding evidence? All of which are unlikely in an exam, e.g. vomit bowl, nutrient drink supplements, weight chart, IV lines, etc.
- Distressed or comfortable?
- Evidence of weight loss? (skin folds, loose clothing)
- Patient appears underweight?
- Patient appears obese? ('the patient appears to have a raised BMI')
- Abdominal distension?
- Obvious scars? (say where)
- Stigmata of chronic liver disease?
- Jaundice?
- Abdominal distension? (Fluid, Flatus, Fat, Faeces or Foetus)

Hands

- Clubbing (increased fluctuance of the nail bed, loss of the nail fold angle and increased nail curvature)
- Liver flap (asterixis)
- Dupuytren's contracture (liver disease, epilepsy, Peyronie's disease, trauma)
- Leuconychia (hypoalbuminaemia)
- Palmar erythema (liver disease, RA, working outdoors, pregnancy)

Eyes

- Jaundice in the sclera: ask the patient to look up whilst gently retracting the lower eye lid
- Anaemia at the same time in the retracted conjuctival sac
- Xanthelasmata (white/yellow lipid deposits around the eyes)
- Corneal arcus

Mouth and lips

- Dentition
- Fetor hepaticus
- Apthous ulceration
- Angular stomatitis
- Glossitis
- Chelitis: inflamed fissured lips (CD)

Neck

- Virchow's node behind insertion of the L sternocleido-mastoid muscle. Feel specifically with a finger either side. This is Troisier's sign (carcinoma of the bronchus or stomach)

Chest

- Spider naevi
- Gynaecomastia (palpate for glandular tissue)

Abdomen

- **Inspect for . . .**
  - Visible peristalsis, (obstruction) normal movement of the abdomen with respiration
  - Caput medusae (collateral veins radiating out from the umbilicus in portal hypertension. Check which

way the blood is flowing by occluding the vessel with two separated fingers, removing each one in turn)
  - Scars
  - Obvious herniae
- **Palpation for tenderness and masses**
  - Remember the examiner is looking to be reassured by an absolutely orthodox routine here in addition to deference and due consideration being given to the patient
  - Ask the patient to put his arms beside himself and to relax. Warm your hands by rubbing them. Ask about any tender areas first and avoid deep palpation of these
  - Lower yourself until your head is level with the abdomen and watch the patients *face* whist you gently proceed through **superficial and then deep palpation.** Come to any tender area last
  - Remember to put your hand flat on the abdomen and flex at the metacarpophalangeal joints keeping the fingers straight
  - If tenderness is discovered say so and avoid further palpation of that area
  - If a mass is discovered describe the usual features:
    Size?
    Shape?
    Consistency/surface?
    Tenderness?
    Moves with respiration?
    Can get above it?
    Pulsatile?
    Bruit?
    Associated lymph nodes and scars?
- **Liver enlargement**
  - Start palpating and in the **right iliac fossa**, ask the patient to take repeated deep breaths, and move the palpating hand up between each breath
  - Feel for the **sharp edge of an enlarged liver coming down** with respiration to meet (flick underneath) the lateral border of the index finger
  - Say how many **finger breaths** below the right costal margin the liver is enlarged to, whether it is tender (hepatitis), smooth (hepatitis), hard and craggy (malignancy) or composed of nodules (alcoholic liver disease)
  - Then **percuss the liver** from below, moving over the liver onto the right anterior chest wall. Normally the hepatic dullness extends up to the fifth rib level

- **Enlargement of the spleen**
  - It is normally not possible to palpate the spleen
  - Starting again in the right iliac fossa feel for an enlarged spleen with the lateral border of the index finger
  - The patient is asked to take repeated deep breaths through an open mouth
  - A bimanual technique is employed with the left hand placed gently behind the lower left lateral ribs and applying a gentle pulling force
  - Feel for the notch of the spleen. It is not possible to feel the upper border of the spleen as it is under the ribs
  - Then percuss for the spleen in a similar direction from the right iliac fossa. Unlike the kidney the spleen is dull to percussion
- **Palpation for the kidneys**
  - In slim people it may just be possible to palpate the kidneys
  - A bimanual technique is again employed
  - The right hand is placed over the anterior abdominal wall over the central area lateral to the rectus muscles. The left hand is placed posteriorly just inferiorly to the renal angle
  - Again the patient is asked to take repeated deep breaths
  - With each inspiration the kidney moves inferiorly; it is balloted with the inferior hand pulling up and the abdominal hand dipping down
  - On percussion the kidney is resonant due to overlying bowel. The kidney enlarges inferiorly and the upper border can be palpated (get above it). This contrasts with enlargement of the spleen
- **Ascites** (see p. 246)
  - Examine for ascites only if the abdomen appears distended
  - Elicit fluid thrill and shifting dullness
- **Abdominal aortic aneurysm** (see p. 287)
  - Examine for specifically by palpating in the central area gently using a bimanual technique
  - If found, gradually separate the palpating fingers until the pulsations can no longer be felt to approximate its size

To finish . . .

Say you would like to . . .
- Listen for bowel sounds and bruits (renal artery stenosis)

- Examine for hernias
- Check for the femoral pulses
- Perform a rectal examination
- Examine the external genitalia

Then cover and thank the patient.

Radiology of the GI tract
Barium studies

Likely diagnoses include . . .
- **Crohn's disease**: skip lesions, small bowel strictures (string sign of Kantor), fistulas, 'cobblestoning' and thickening of the valvulae conniventes suggest CD (see p. 282)
- **Ulcerative colitis**: continuous featureless (loss of haustrations) 'hosepiping', pseudopoylps (mucosal oedema) and megacolon suggests UC (see p. 283)
- **Diverticular disease of the sigmoid colon**
- **Polyps of the small or large bowel**
  - All need removal for histology
  - May form the apex of an intussusception
  - Speculate about familial polyposis coli and Gardener's syndrome (autosomal dominant; GI polyps, dermoid abdominal tumours, osteomas of the skull and skin soft tissue tumours)
- **Carcinoma of the large bowel**: an 'apple core' lesion (shown below)

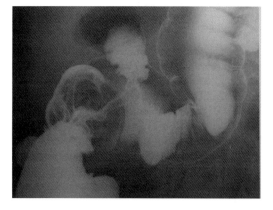

- **Pneumatosis coli:** gas (nitrogen) filled cysts within the bowel wall. It is associated with COPD
- **Intussusception**
- **Gastric lesions**
  - Ulcers/malignancy
  - Linitis plastica (shown below)

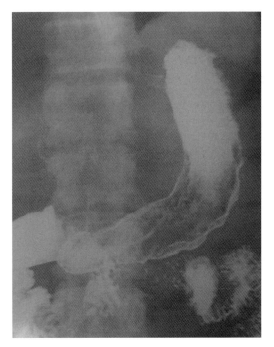

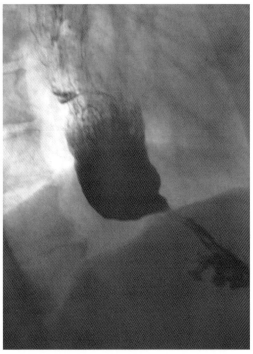

- **Carcinoma of the oesophagus:** an abrupt and irregular stricture

- Hiatus hernia

The barium swallow

Likely diagnoses . . .
- **Achalasia:** tapering of the lower oesophagus variously described as like a 'rat's tail' or 'bird's beak'

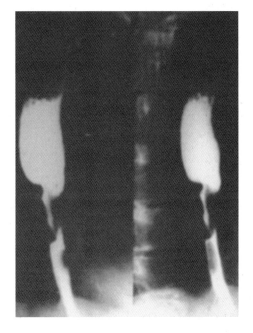

- **Oesophageal candidiasis**: furry appearance of the oesophagus. Suggest immunosuppression due to HIV, steroids, alcohol abuse, diabetes or malignancy as possible causes

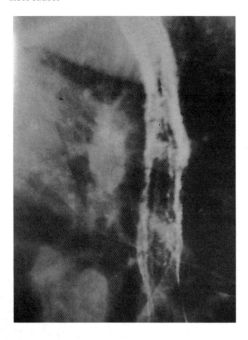

- **Plummer–Vinson syndrome**: ring like narrowing in the postcricoid region. Associated with iron deficiency, the patient may have koilonychias, angular stomatitis and glossitis

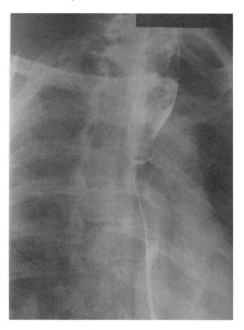

- **Oesophageal varices**: serpiginous lower oesophageal filling defects

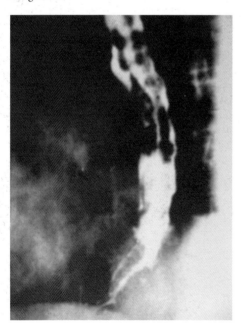

The plain abdominal radiograph

Check for
- Air fluid levels (? obstruction if frequent)
- Free air (? perforation)
- Bowel wall diameter. Large bowel upper limit of normal 5.5 cm. Small bowel upper limit of normal 2.5 cm
- Normal bowel markings. Large bowel haustrations extend partially across the diameter of the large bowel. Small bowel valvulae conniventes extend fully across the diameter of the small bowel
- Abnormal calcification of pancreas, gallbladder and an abdominal aortic aneurysm
- Bone abnormalities. Sacroiliitis, spinal metastases, femoral heads and pelvis (e.g. Pagets disease, Looser's zones, fractures)

Likely diagnoses . . .
- **Obstruction of the small or large bowel**: multiple air fluid levels. Note that small bowel lesions tend to be more central. Also small bowel transverse markings

(valvulae conniventes) extend fully across the diameter of the bowel, whereas large bowel haustral lines extend only partially across the bowel
- *Large bowel obstruction*

- **Stones:** 10% of gallstones but 90% of kidney stones are visible on a plain radiograph. Consider gallstone ileus if small bowel obstruction is also present in the same film

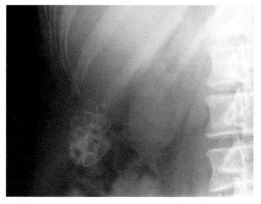

- **Calcification of the gallbladder (porcelain gallbladder):** a premalignant condition

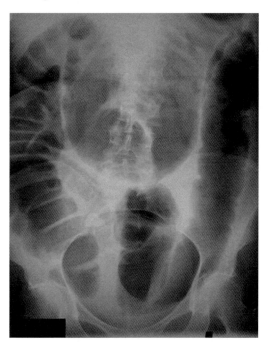

- *Small bowel obstruction*

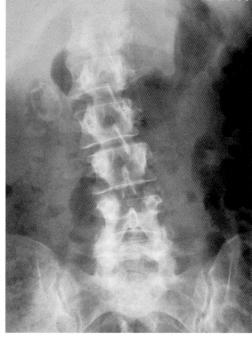

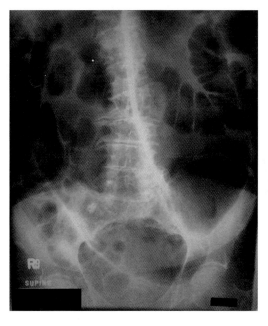

- **Calcification of the pancreas** in chronic pancreatitis

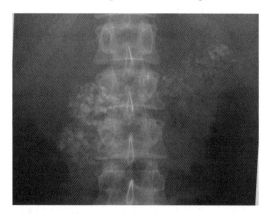

- **Air under the diaphragm** (perforation/recent laparotomy)

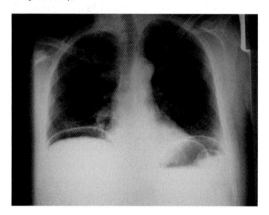

- **Large bowel volvulus**: horseshoe-shaped segment of dilated (most commonly) large bowel, having its axis in the left (caecal volvulus; shown below) or right iliac fossa (sigmoid volvulus)

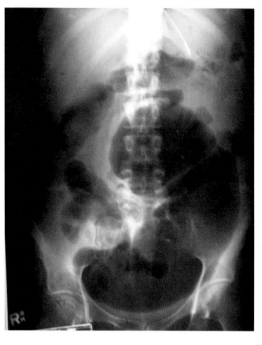

Endoscopic retrograde cholangiopancreatogram (ERCP)

You may see the head of the endoscope and contract out-lining the biliary tree. Look for . . .

- **Strictures** due to cholangiocarcinoma or sclerosing cholangitis (as a complication of inflammatory bowel disease; shown below)

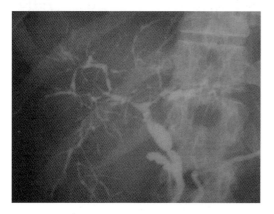

- **Gallstones**: single or multiple filling defects with a dilated common bile duct above

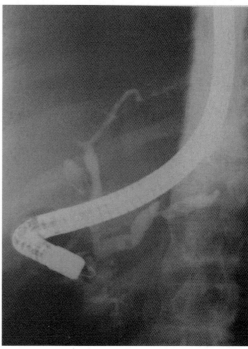

Neurological System

The neurological history is commonly the **most difficult to take** for myriad reasons . . .
- Symptoms are **complicated** and not as well 'packaged' as with other systems
- Patients are often **difficult to communicate with** through no fault of their own
- You often find yourself taking a **history from relatives/friends/observers**
- Certain terms can mean something different to the patient than that which they mean to the examiner, e.g. dizziness requires clarification as the patient may mean vertigo, ataxia, light-headedness, transient impairment of consciousness or minor seizure activity

Typical patient scenarios include . . .

This patient has been experiencing headache. Ask him some questions.

This patient has presented due to a collapse. Take a relevant history.

This patient has been brought to A&E following a seizure. Ask her some relevant questions.

This patient has been sent to A&E with sudden onset of right-sided weakness. Take her history.

The history routine

The vital questions to ask in taking a neurological-system based history are . . .

Headache

It's a pain, so **SOCRATES** . . .

S Site: frontal, occipital, temporal, generalized, supra-orbital (cluster headache)

O Time of onset: exact or approximate?
Nature of onset: sudden or gradual? Like being hit over back of head with a brick, presence of aura or warning symptoms, history of trauma, flashing lights (migraine)
Nature since onset: constantly present or periods free from pain since initial onset? If constantly present since onset, is it increasing, decreasing or staying the same?

C Character of pain: sharp, dull, pressured?

R Radiation: back of eyes, neck, face (temporal arteritis)?

A Associated features: specifically presence of focal neurological symptoms (such as weakness or numbness), neck stiffness, vomiting, loss of consciousness, earache, dizziness, fever, drowsiness, blurred vision, rash

E Exacerbating factors: bright light, coughing, head movement
Relieving factors: any analgesia taken? Darkened environment, lying still?

S Subjective severity: 1–10; worst ever pain/ worse than childbirth?
Previous history of similar pain: first ever, worsening of a chronic headache, previous migraine history?

Loss of consciousness

- Circumstances **preceding** LOC: presence of any aura or warning, stressed, standing for protracted period, flashing/strobing lights, rising from seated/lying position, sweating, weakness, confusion?
- Events occurring **during** LOC: (witness history) colour of patient, jerking of extremities, foaming at mouth, tongue biting, loss of continence, injury?

189

- Associated focal neurology (TIA)
- Time to recover, post-ictal phase?
- History of similar event(s)

Seizures/fits

- Circumstances **surrounding** seizure: location of patient, mood of patient, presence of strobing light?
- Events **during** seizure: shaking of extremities, tongue biting, foaming at mouth, rigidity, absence, loss of urinary/faecal continence?
- Events **post**-seizure: speed of recovery, presence of Todd's paresis, post-ictal period, confusion?
- Associated injuries consequent on seizure
- History of similar: **frequency increasing or decreasing?**
- Family history
- History of head trauma

Loss of power/weakness

- Onset: sudden or gradual, new or longstanding?
- Location: unilateral, bilateral, arms or legs, proximal or distal?
- Progression: improving, deteriorating, staying the same, improves with exercise, fatigues quickly?
- Associated neurology: focal neurology, facial weakness, slurring of speech, choking on swallowed food/drink, difficulty in walking, numbness?
- History of viral illness (important in Guillain–Barré syndrome)

Loss of sensation/numbness

- Onset: sudden or gradual, new or longstanding, preceeded by **paraesthesia**
- Area affected: uni- or bilateral, legs or arms or head, proximal or distal, glove-and-stocking, sensory level, mononeuropathy?
- Progression: improving, deteriorating, remaining same, moving from distal to proximal, jumping from one region to another (mononeuritis multiplex)?
- Presence of associated neurology: slurring of speech, choking, weakness?

Tremor

- Difficulty with writing and fine finger movements
- Frequency (fine or coarse?)
- When first noticed?

- Getting better/getting worse/staying the same?
- Exacerbated by movement (intention tremors are worse at extremes of movement: cerebellar disease), alleviated by alcohol (→ benign essential tremor)?
- Worse at rest (Parkinson's pill-rolling tremor)?

Visual symptoms

- Diplopia: double vision
- Flashing (migraine or cluster headache—teichoplasia, fortification spectra)
- Photophobia
- Dizziness
- Vertigo
- Floaters in visual axis
- Blindness or visual field defect: scotoma, hemianopia, quadrantanopia, total blindness? Denial of blindness (Anton's syndrome)
- Transient visual loss (amaurosis fugax)

Auditary symptoms

- Deafness: presbyacusis, ototoxic medications (e.g. gentamycin)?
- Tinnitus: if associated with deafness and vertigo, consider Menière's disease

Balance and falls

- Recent falls: increased frequency?
- Social support network, adequacy of home for patient, occupational therapy input?
- When does loss of balance occur: in the morning, on standing, at night, all the time, only with eyes closed?
- Associated vertigo: spinning of self or environment?
- Associated focal neurology?
- Great care required to differentiate between neurological loss of balance and simple trip: patients often very keen to ascribe worrying neurological symptoms as a simple trip: do not be cajoled!

Olfactory symptoms

- Strange smells
- Anosmia: unilateral or bilateral

Taste symptoms

- Strange tastes

- Loss of taste sensation: anterior or posterior tongue, particular aspects of taste

Speech

- Ask the patient if they have subjectively been having problems with their speech
- If so, for how long
- Did it come on suddenly or gradually
- Is there any associated focal neurology: facial palsy, unilateral upper motor neurone signs
- If there is a speech problem, you should ask questions to decide between the following . . .
  - **Dysphonia**: difficulty producing speech of audible volume; ask patient to maintain a note, such as 'eeee'; if it is barely audible then dysphonia is likely, and is a clue toward local vocal cord or laryngeal paralysis
  - **Dysarthria**: difficulty producing speech of good pronunciation and quality due to mechanical difficulty, usually in oral cavity or upper pharynx; ask the patient to say something complicated like '*west register street*'; may be spastic, extrapyramidal or cerebellar (see section on examining speech)
  - **Receptive dysphasia**: difficulty understanding the spoken word, though production of meaningless, normal words is easy for the patient; ask the patient a question—if you get a fluent though totally meaningless answer then it is likely receptive dysphasia is present
  - **Expressive dysphasia**: difficulty finding appropriate words, even though understanding of the spoken word remains intact; ask the patient to name some common items like a button, a pen, a book; if they appear to have great difficulty in getting the words out despite great frustration, then it is likely that an expressive dysphasia is present

Memory

- Recent difficulty with memory?
- Short-term memory
- Long-term memory
- Writing **lists**
- Over-reliance on friends/family
- Becoming frustrated with self
- Bills remaining unpaid
- Memory mistakes being noted by family

- History of head injury, repeated head trauma (boxer, footballer)
- Family history of dementia
- Chorea

Further history

As with all systems based histories, if you have time following elucidation of the presenting complaint and history of presenting complaint, you must go on to take . . .

Past medical history

- Of special relevance is the presence of **systemic disease** such as hypertension, diabetes or heart disease, as this gives clues towards the presence of any atherosclerotic disease within the CNS/PNS
- Past history of meningitis, encephalitis and spinal injury are all relevant
- Presence of **autoimmune conditions** in the past is also important: cerebral vasculitis
- Recent history of **viral infection** may be relevant in cases of progressive ascending weakness (Guillain–Barré syndrome)

Drug history

- Many drugs can cause or relieve neurological symptoms, and a full drug history is as ever vital
- Be aware of special cases of drugs causing **toxic neuropathies**, such as those caused by chloramphenicol, disulfiram, isoniazid, nitrofurantoin and phenytoin
- **Neuroleptic drugs** (phenothiazines, butyrophenones, thioxanthines, clozapine and risperidone) can produce a variety of neurological consequences, including **acute dystonic reactions, Parkinsonism, akathisia and tardive dyskinesia**

Allergies

Family history

- Of relevance due to the presence of the numerous inherited neurological conditions (e.g. Huntington's) and also because a family history of stroke, hypertension, diabetes and ischaemic heart disease can predict cerebrovascular disease in a given patient
- Take care to ask the approximate age at which the family member was affected by the relevant condition ('anticipation' in triplet repeat disorders)

Social history

- **Occupation** is important as it reveals exposure to certain chemicals or toxins which may act on the neurological system (e.g. heavy metals)
- **Smoking** history is important because it is thought protective in Alzheimer's disease, but deleterious in cerebrovascular disease, brain cancer and other neurodegenerative diseases
- **Alcohol** history is also vital: it predicts peripheral neuropathy and neurodegeneration/dementia, and the Wernicke–Korsakoff syndrome

Review of systems

- Don't forget that many neurological diseases are multisystem conditions and questions should be addressed towards these other systems appropriately, e.g. cerebrovascular disease, or presentation with stroke should prompt questions concerning the history of cardiovascular disease, peripheral arterial disease, diabetes and smoking, if these have not been already asked elsewhere
- Also, dysphagia is a common symptom of neurological disease, and it may be so severe that it leads to malnutrition in the poorly followed up patient

Useful notes

The typical characteristics of different headaches

- **Classical migraine**: unilateral, photophobia, flashing lights, nausea, vomiting
- **Meningitis**: photophobia, nuchal rigidity, fever, rash
- **Cluster headache**: supraorbital, come in bouts, associated rhinorrhoea and lacrimation, flushing
- **Spondylosis**: occipital headache, nuchal rigidity
- **Raised intracranial pressure**: drowsiness, vomiting, worse in mornings
- **Subarachnoid haemorrhage**: first ever/worst ever headache, thunderclap, like being hit in the back of the head with a brick
- **Tension headache**: bilateral tightness, recur frequently
- **Sinusitis**: ache over cheeks and forehead
- **Temporal arteritis**: pain and tenderness over temple, disturbance of vision

The examination routine

More than any other examination, it is easy for the experienced examiner to tell if a candidate is well practiced in performing neurological examination. It is vital in the months prior to final examinations that you practise giving instructions to genuine patients to facilitate a fruitful, brisk neurological examination. It is surprisingly difficult to get patients to do what you want them to and this is painfully obvious in the OSCE situation. Practice, practice, practice!

Common stations over the past few years have included . . .

Patients with previous dense strokes, with residual unilateral upper motor neurone signs

Patients with Huntington's chorea

Patients with Parkinson's disease

Patients with multiple sclerosis and optic neuritis

Diabetic patients with glove and stocking sensory loss

Patients with Brown–Sequard syndrome

Patients with Wernicke's or Broca's aphasia

You will variously be instructed . . .

'Examine this patient's arms/legs'
'Examine the tone/power/reflexes/co-ordination/ sensation in this patient's arms/legs'
'Examine this patient's gait'
'Examine this patient's speech'
'Examine this patient's higher mental functioning'
'Examine this patient's cranial nerves'
'Examine this patient's second cranial nerve'
'Examine this patient's vision/hearing'

Take a deep breath, and begin . . .

- Introduce yourself to the patient, stating your full name and grade
- Explain what you are about to do, and gain consent for this

- Split your examination thought-processes into **five sections** as outlined below; each section is long, complicated and difficult to perform, so it is unlikely you will complete any single part, never mind multiple parts in one OSCE station.

1 Central nervous system (CNS) examination

- Approach **in the order that the nerves are numbered**
- Be prepared to jump to the next nerve, as examiners quickly get bored if you are labouring at any single point during the exam

Cranial nerve I: the Olfactory Nerve

- Screen: '*any recent change in sense of smell?*'
- Use a **'smell box'**: four differing, readily recognizable odours (e.g. coffee, oil of clove, oil of lavender, oil of lemon)
- Cover the contralateral nostril, close patient's eyes
- Unilateral anosmia more worrying than bilateral

Cranial nerve II: the Optic Nerve

Acuity
- Tested with **Snellen chart** from **6 m**
- Allow **visual correctors** (e.g. spectacles) to be worn
- Test eyes independently
- Produces a measure of acuity in the form x/y, where
  . . .
  - x = distance of the patient from the chart
  - y = the number of the line at which the patient could no longer continue
- Normal acuity is **6/6**

- If patient cannot read the largest print from a distance of 6 m, allow them to move closer and adjust the produced figure accordingly, e.g. $3/y$
- If the patient cannot see the chart at all, then gauge their ability to **count fingers** or **perceive light and dark**

Fields
- Tested by **direct confrontation**
- Face the patient at arm's length away
- The patient covers an eye with the palm of their own hand
- The examiner covers the contralateral eye to the patient
- With the patient looking directly into the examiner's uncovered eye, the examiner, starting in the lateral portion of the visual field, brings in their hand whilst wiggling the first two fingers into the line of vision of the patient
- Repeat in the other three quadrants of vision
- Expect to see the wiggling fingers at the same time as the patient
- If there is a significant delay between examiner and patient seeing the wiggling fingers, then the patient has a visual field defect in that region: estimate its size by approaching the defect from other angles
- If a field defect is detected, then you need to decide what it is (see diagram overleaf)
- If the field defect appears to be very small, central or affecting the blind spot, then this can be assessed using a **red-topped pin** and moving it horizontally and vertically through and within the blind spot of each of the patient's eyes, from a position where it goes from being seen, to being unseen, to being seen again out the other side (the normal blind spot resides 15° temporal to the line of gaze).

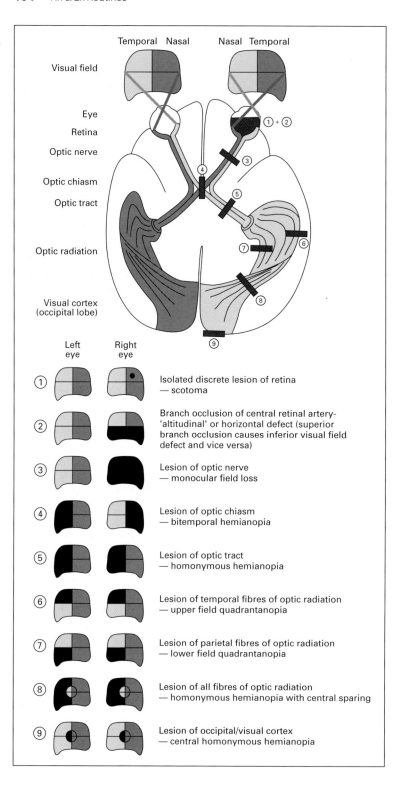

Visual inattention
- Position yourself in front of the patient
- Have the patient look directly into your eyes
- Holding both your hands laterally to the side of the patient on a level with their eye line hold the forefinger of each hand upwards and ask the patient to **point at which finger moves without losing your gaze**
- Move one finger in isolation, then the contralateral finger in isolation, then move both fingers together
- Failure to notice that both fingers are being moved together suggests a **parietal lobe lesion**

Fundoscopy
- Be familiar with the workings of the ophthalmoscope!
- Look at the patient's eye through the ophthalmoscope at arms length with the normal white light setting, looking for **normal light reflection**, any **floaters** or anything affecting the normal light reflection
- Advance on the patient's eye whilst continuing to look through the ophthalmoscope until you are close enough to view the fundus
- Find the **optic disc** (visible termination of the optic nerve): the origin of all the retinal vessels
- Comment on the disc's . . .
  - **Cup**
  - **Colour**
  - **Contour**
- Then move on to looking at the **fovea**, a darkened circular area temporal and slightly inferior to the optic disc. It marks the **point of central vision**, and is **surrounded by the roughly circular macula**
- Split the remaining fundus into **four separate regions** and examine each in turn, evaluating the colour and consistency of the retina, the blood vessels and any intervening foreign body between the ophthalmoscope and the fundus
- For completeness, rack through the lenses of the ophthalmoscope focusing from the back to the very front of the eye
- Consider topical **mydriatic** if examination restricted
- Repeat entire examination in the other eye

Pupillary light reflexes
- Afferent arm: **optic nerve**
- Efferent arm: **oculomotor nerve**
- Ensuring conditions are dark, shine a bright light into one of the patient's eyes
- Look for pupillary constriction in the ipsilateral pupil (*direct* **pupillary light reflex**)

- Shine the light into the same eye as before, but observe the contralateral pupil; this should constrict concomitantly due to crossing over of afferent fibres at the optic chiasm (*consensual* **pupillary light reflex**)
- Have a general look at the pupils: observe size, shape and symmetry; remember, 20% of the population have a benign difference in pupillary size of <0.5 mm— **'aniscoria'**

Pupillary accommodation reflexes
- Afferent arm: **optic nerve**
- Efferent arm: **oculomotor nerve**
- Only possible with a co-operative patient
- Ask the patient to stare into the distance at a point at least 5–10 m away
- Place your finger ~10 cm in front of their eyes but instruct patient **not to look at it until instructed to do so**
- Instruct patient to look at your finger: expect to see **convergence of the visual axis** and **miosis** of both pupils
- Remember that **the Argylle–Robertson (neurosyphillis) pupil accommodates but does not react to light**

Cranial nerve III: the Oculomotor Nerve
- Tested with CN IV and CN VI
- Innervates . . .
  - **Inferior oblique**: moves pupil superomedially
  - **Medial rectus:** moves pupil medially
  - **Superior rectus**: moves pupil superiorly
  - **Inferior rectus**: moves pupil inferiorly
- An object should be placed directly in the visual axis of the patient, approximately 1 m away
- The patient should be clearly instructed to follow the movements of the desired object by moving their eyes only, *not* **by moving their head**
- Move the object deliberately and slowly in a pattern that tests all of the movements precipitated by the extraocular muscles, e.g. the **lines of the Union Jack flag**, or an imaginary **'W' on top of an 'M'**
- Look for **loss of conjugate gaze** in any of the tested directions
- The pupil of a patient with a CN III lesion points **downwards and laterally**
- CN III also supplies **sphincter pupillae muscle** (efferent arm of pupillary reflexes)
- Note the presence of **nystagmus** at extremes of gaze; if present, deduce the **direction** of gaze in which it appears and the **plane** in which movements occur (e.g.

horizontal, vertical, rotary or mixed); also deduce the direction of the quick and the slow components

Cranial nerve IV: the Trochlear Nerve

- Tested with CN III
- Innervates **superior oblique** muscle: inferomedial movement of the globe

Cranial nerve V: the Trigeminal Nerve

- Has sensory and motor components . . .

Facial sensation

- Trigeminal sensation is supplied to the face in **three discrete divisions** . . .
  - V_1: ophthalmic
  - V_2: maxillary
  - V_3: mandibular
- It is sufficient to test only light touch sensation in each of these three regions bilaterally using a cotton bud/cotton wool pinched to a tip
- Always perform a **'control' test** of sensation in a distant region of the body, e.g. the back of the hand or the sternum
- Ask the patient to close their eyes and say 'yes' when they feel you touching them
- Lightly dab: do not brush the stimulus as this introduces neurological 'noise' and is not a true test of light touch
- Ask the patient **'does it feel normal?'**
- Ask the patient **'does it feel the same on both sides?'**

The corneal reflex

- Afferent arm: **trigeminal nerve**
- Efferent arm: **facial nerve**
- Using a pointed piece of cotton wool, ask the patient to look to their left side, fully adducting the right eye
- Without giving warning and attempting to avoid showing the patient the impending stimulus, bring the cotton wool in slowly from the lateral aspect of the right eye and lightly touch the lateral aspect of the cornea, well away from the visual axis
- Expect the patient to blink and withdraw
- If the patient does not react, do not persist because you will likely cause corneal abrasion; take as a negative corneal reflex
- Repeat in the left eye

The muscles of mastication

- Trigeminal motor fibres innervate mastication mus-

cles: **temporalis**, **masseter** and **medial and lateral pterygoids**

- Ask the patient to relax and palpate the angles of the mandible bilaterally
- Ask the patient to clench their teeth and relax (tests temporalis and masseter)
- Then ask the patient to open their mouth and keep it open whilst, with light pressure, you attempt to close the patient's jaw (tests medial and lateral pterygoids)

The jaw jerk

- Place a finger across the anterior chin, asking the patient to relax their jaw completely
- Lightly strike the carefully positioned finger with tendon hammer
- Expect reflex closure of the jaw upon striking

Cranial nerve VI: the Abducens Nerve

- Tested with CN III
- Supplies the **lateral rectus** muscle: lateral movement of the globe

Cranial nerve VII: the Facial Nerve

- Numerous functions . . .
  - Motor to muscles of facial expression
  - Taste fibres to anterior two-thirds of tongue
  - Nerve to stapedius
  - Sensory to small area of skin around the external auditary meatus
- Usually only muscles of facial expression are tested
- Begin with inspection: loss of the nasolabial fold, drooping of the eyelid or loss of forehead creases suggests facial weakness
- Instruct: **'screw up your eyes tightly'**; make an attempt to open the eyes with the tips of the fingers whilst instructing the patient **'don't let me open them'** (tests **orbicularis oculi**)
- Instruct: **'bare your teeth'** or **'smile'** (tests risorius)
- Instruct: **'puff out your cheeks'**; make an attempt to break the seal with light pressure on the outside of the inflated cheeks (tests **orbicularis oris**)
- Instruct: **'raise your eyebrows'** (tests occipitofrontalis)
- Be aware that UMN lesions of the facial nerve have differing effects to LMN lesions due to hemispheric decussation of motor fibres (see diagram opposite)

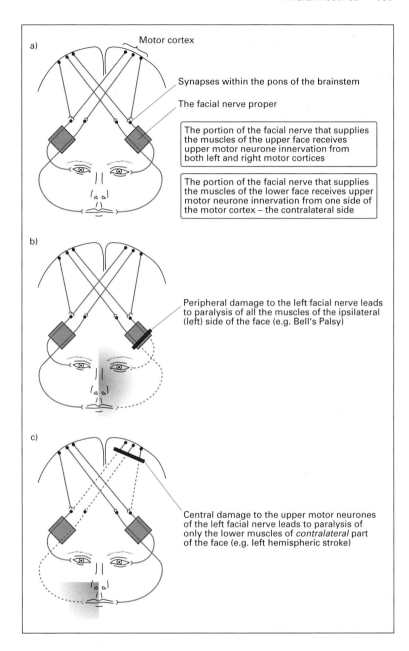

a)

Motor cortex

Synapses within the pons of the brainstem

The facial nerve proper

The portion of the facial nerve that supplies the muscles of the upper face receives upper motor neurone innervation from both left and right motor cortices

The portion of the facial nerve that supplies the muscles of the lower face receives upper motor neurone innervation from one side of the motor cortex – the contralateral side

b)

Peripheral damage to the left facial nerve leads to paralysis of all the muscles of the ipsilateral (left) side of the face (e.g. Bell's Palsy)

c)

Central damage to the upper motor neurones of the left facial nerve leads to paralysis of only the lower muscles of *contralateral* part of the face (e.g. left hemispheric stroke)

Cranial nerve VIII: the Vestibulocochlear Nerve

- The vestibulocochlear nerve supplies **hearing and balance sensation**; usually only hearing is tested
- Remember that nystagmus may be a sign of vestibular dysfunction, and that this may have been picked up on examination of CN III, CN IV and CN VI

Coarse tests of hearing

- Coarse methods for testing hearing include **whispering a number** in the ear of the patient and asking them to repeat what is said
- Alternatively, the examiner's **fingers and thumb are rubbed together**, starting at arm's length from the pa-

tient's ear; if you can hear the noise made at arm's length, so should the patient be able to
- More formal tests of hearing utilize a **512-Hz** (short) tuning fork to differentiate between **conductive (ossicle)**, **sensorineural (cochlear or central)** or **no hearing loss at all** . . .

Weber's test
- 'The **test for lateralization**': place vibrating tuning fork in the midline of the patient's forehead
- Ask the patient where they hear the note: is it louder on the right, the left or is it the same on both sides?
- The findings in different sorts of deafness are shown in table below

Rinne's test
- Allows **comparison of air and bone conduction**

- Place the base of vibrating tuning fork on mastoid process of temporal bone
- Ask the patient to tell you **when they are no longer able to hear the note**
- As soon as this happens, remove the fork from the mastoid and relocate the ends to the opening of the external auditary meatus
- Expect the patient to be **able to hear the sound when placed at the auditary meatus even though they cannot hear it any longer with the fork on the bone**, i.e. that air conduction is better than bone conduction (AC > BC)
- The findings in different sorts of deafness are shown in the table below
- To label the patient with conductive or sensorineural hearing loss or neither, you have to put the results of all the above tests together . . .

| | No hearing problem | Unilateral hearing loss | |
		Conductive	Sensorineural
Coarse tests of hearing	Hears and repeats whispered numbers; hears fingers and thumb rubbing together at arms length	Decreased ability to hear and repeat whispered numbers, or hear fingers and thumb rubbing together	Decreased ability to hear and repeat whispered numbers, or hear fingers and thumb rubbing together
Weber's test	Hears note equally in both ears	Hears note preferentially in affected ear	Hears note preferentially in unaffected ear
Rinne's test	AC > BC	BC > AC	AC > BC

Cranial nerve IX: the Glossopharyngeal Nerve
- Supplies **taste sensation to posterior third of tongue**: not usually tested
- Also responsible for **gag reflex**
  - Warn patient about the unpleasant nature of the test
  - Ask patient to open their mouth wide
  - With a **long blunt instrument (e.g. tongue depressor)** lightly stimulate the soft palate on one side
  - Expect the patient to gag immediately
  - Test contralateral side
  - Unilateral absence of gag reflex is more suggestive of a glossopharyngeal nerve lesion than a vagus lesion, though it may occur in either circumstance

Cranial nerve X: the Vagus Nerve
- Supplies **motor fibres to pharynx and larynx**: responsible for vocalization and lifting of soft palate
- Listen to patient's voice: **hoarseness** suggests a problem
- Ask patient to say '**ah**' with their mouth wide open; expect the **soft palate to rise symmetrically**, the posterior pharynx to move medially like a curtain, and the **uvula to remain in the midline** if there is no lesion of the glossopharyngeal or vagus nerves
- If there is a unilateral vagus lesion, the soft palate of the affected side fails to move, and **the uvula is pulled upward on the contralateral side to the lesion** by the

normally ascending soft palate, the uvula pointing *away* from the affected side

Cranial nerve XI: the Accessory Nerve
- Innervates **trapezius** and **sternocleidomastoid** muscles
- Inspect shoulders from behind for signs of trapezius **wasting** or **fasciculation**
- Ask patient to shrug shoulders and keep them shrugged, whilst exerting light downward force — patient should be able to resist this easily
- Test sternocleidomastoid muscle by placing your hand on the side of the patient's face, asking them to **turn their head against your hand**
- NB When patient is turning head to left, this is testing the *right* sternocleidomastoid, and vice versa

Cranial nerve XII: the Hypoglossal Nerve
- Supplies **tongue musculature**
- **Inspect** tongue *in-situ* on the floor of the mouth for **fasciculation** (protruding the tongue abolishes mild fasciculation), **wasting**, **scars**, **tumours** or **ulceration**
- Ask patient to protrude tongue, looking for deviation from the midline
- Tongue **deviates towards the affected side** in unilateral hypoglossal nerve lesion
- Request patient to move tongue from side to side, looking for symmetry and co-ordination of movement
- Ask patient to push tongue through the cheek in the lateral side of the mouth, and with external pressure, attempt to push the tongue back into the oral cavity
- Difficulty with speech articulation (dysarthria) may be a clue that there is a problem with CN XII

2 Peripheral nervous system (PNS) examination

Upper limbs
Inspection
- Observe . . .
  - Wasting
  - Fasciculation
  - Spasticity
  - Scars
  - Specific postures (e.g. waiter's tip, claw hand)
  - Tremor

Following this, the PNS examination of arms or legs may be split into **five parts:** tone, power, reflexes, co-ordination and sensation . . .

(i) Tone
- Take the weight of a single arm with both your hands by grasping the hand and cupping the elbow
- Emphasize to the patient that you want them to **relax**
- Whilst **supinating** and **pronating** the forearm in a **random** fashion, add in the extra movement of **flexion** and **extension** at the elbow
- Decide if the examined arm has **normal** tone, or is **hypertonic/rigid**, or **hypotonic/flaccid**
- Repeat in the contralateral upper limb

(ii) Power
- Test all major movements at all major joints . . .

Abduction of the arm at the shoulder	→C5
Flexion of the forearm at the elbow	→C6
Extension of the forearm at the elbow	→C7
Flexion of the hand at the wrist	→C8
Extension of the hand at the wrist	→C6, C7
Flexion of the fingers	→C8
Abduction of fingers	→T1
Abduction and flexion of the thumb	→T1

- Clinically, the three peripheral nerves of greatest importance in the upper limb are . . .
  - The **radial** nerve: supplies all the extensor muscles in the forearm
  - The **ulnar** nerve: supplies all the intrinsic hand muscles, except LOAF (see below)
  - The **median** nerve: supplies small muscles in hand; remembered by the mnemonic **LOAF** . . .
    L Lateral two lumbrical muscles
    O Opponens pollicis
    A Abductor pollicis brevis
    F Flexor pollicis brevis
- All movements should initially be performed **independently**, and if successful, each movement should be **resisted** by the examiner exerting opposite force
- If the movement cannot be performed independently, an attempt should be made to **eliminate gravity**, e.g. by having the patient lay flat on a bed and attempting the movements in the plane of the bed
- Power should be graded based on the **MRC scale**, 5 to 0 . . .
  5 **Normal power vs. resistance**
  4 **Diminished power vs. resistance**

3 **No movement vs. resistance, but movement against gravity**

2 **Movement only with gravity eliminated**

1 **Fasciculations only**

0 **No movement at all**

- If a motor deficit is noted whilst testing power, then a 'motor level' should be given, which is described as 'the most caudal segment of the spinal cord that supplies a key muscle with a power of at least 3/5 on MRC grading'. In complete injuries when some motor function is found below the lowest normal segment, this is described as a 'zone of partial preservation'.

(iii) Reflexes

- There are three major reflexes to test in the upper limb . . .
  1 **Biceps tendon reflex** (tests spinal level C5)
  2 **Supinator tendon reflex** (tests spinal level C6)
  3 **Triceps tendon reflex** (tests spinal level C7)
- If the response is poor, attempt to **'reinforce'** the reflex by distracting the patient's attention, e.g. have the patient **clench their teeth** immediately prior to striking the tendon
- Decide whether the tested reflex is **present** or **absent** (e.g. LMN lesion, spinal root damage by disc prolapse, peripheral nerve trauma or entrapment)
- If the reflex is present, then decide: is it **normal**, **increased** (hyperreflexic) or **decreased** (hyporeflexic)?
- Hyperreflexia is almost always a sign of an **UMN lesion** (e.g. previous stroke)
- Hyporeflexia suggests either **old age** or an **incomplete LMN lesion** (e.g. cervical or lumbar disc protrusion causing incomplete nerve entrapment)

(iv) Co-ordination

Co-ordination is mainly a test of **cerebellar** function . . .

- *The nose-finger test*: ask the patient to move directly from their nose to your stationary finger, held at arms length away, and repeat in multiple positions. Decide if movement is **imprecise in direction, force or distance**—'dysmetria'. Also try to decide if there is any 'intention tremor' (action tremor with past-pointing). Both dysmetria and intention tremor are signs of a **lateral cerebellar lobe lesion**
- *The test for dysdiadochokinesis*: ask the patient to repeatedly pronate and supinate a hand held above their other stationary supinated hand. Decide whether the patient's movements are **clumsier** or **more disorganized** than expected (**lateral cerebellar lobe** lesion)
- *The test for arm drift*: ask the patient to extend their arms fully out in front of them, with forearms and hands in full supination. Ask the patient to close their eyes and maintain the arms in the same position, noting . . .
  - **Slow pronation and gradual descent**: occurs due to weakness (e.g. that which occurs post-stroke) or due to impairment of proprioception
  - **Downward or medial drifting of one or both limbs**: signifies an UMN lesion
  - **Upward or lateral drifting of one or both limbs**: signifies cerebellar disease

You should also test **'rebound' drift**: firmly push down on one of the outstretched arms and sharply release, observing the result. Normal individuals quickly restore the position of the tested arm; patients with cerebellar disease will make **several oscillations of slowly declining amplitude before the arm restitutes itself to the original position**.

(v) Sensation

- As a screening test of sensation, **light touch** may be used as the stimulus, e.g. using the pinched up edge of a piece of cotton-wool, and **dabbing** it onto the arm; compare each side, and include a reference point
- Although dermatomes appear to be well-demarcated on text-book diagrams, there is **much crossover** between the boundary lines
- There are, however, **key regions** of each dermatome that are constant, and it is here that sensation should be checked
- The dermatomes that require checking in the **upper limb** are . . .
  - (C4: region over acromioclavicular joint of shoulder)
  - **C5**: lower region of deltoid, lateral aspect of arm in regimental badge region
  - **C6**: dorsal aspect of thumb
  - **C7**: dorsal aspect of middle finger
  - **C8**: dorsal aspect of little finger
  - **T1**: medial aspect of arm, just proximal to elbow joint
  - (T2: anterior aspect of axilla)
- The dermatomes that require checking in the **lower limb** are . . .

- (L1: region just inferior to groin creases)
- **L2**: medial aspect of mid thigh
- **L3**: medial aspect of knee
- **L4**: medial malleolus

- **L5**: dorsal aspect base of great toe
- **S1**: lateral aspect of calcaneus
- **S2**: posterior aspect of knee
- (S3: medial aspect of gluteal crease)

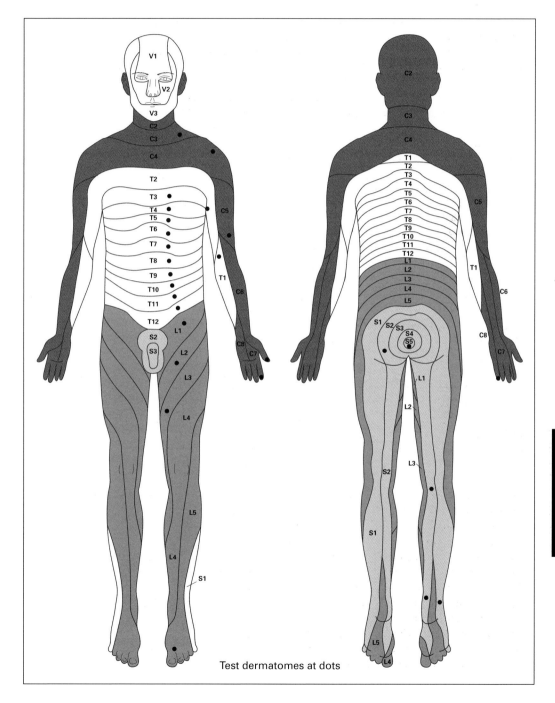

Test dermatomes at dots

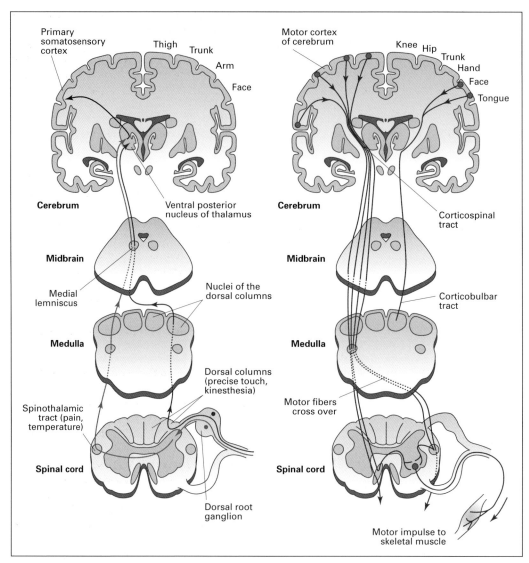

The key ascending and descending sensory and motor pathways.

- Aspects of the sensation of light touch are carried in both of the main tracts that carry afferent sensory impulses, so detecting an abnormality in light touch does not tell you which tract is affected
- Therefore, detection of a sensory abnormality should precipitate testing of multiple sensory modalities
- The two main tracts that carry sensory impulses centrally are (see diagram above) . . .

  The dorsal columns
  - Enter spinal cord through dorsal horn
  - **Ascend ipsilaterally** through spinal cord
  - Cross in brainstem
  - Synapse in thalamic nuclei before projection to cerebral cortex
  - Carry the sensory modalities of *vibration and proprioception*

  The spinothalamic tracts
  - Enter spinal cord through dorsal horn
  - Cross over immediately
  - **Ascend contralaterally** through spinal cord
  - Synapse in thalamic nuclei before projection to cerebral cortex

- Carry the sensory modalities of *pain* and *temperature*
- When a sensory deficit is detected, it is important to give a 'sensory level', which is defined as 'the most caudal segment of the spinal cord with normal sensory function on both sides of the body'
- In complete injuries when some sensory function is found below the lowest normal segment, this is described as a **'zone of partial preservation'**

Lower limbs
Inspection
- Look for . . .
  - Wasting
  - Obvious weakness or difficulty with movements
  - Fasciculations
  - Muscle contractures
  - Spasticity
  - Trophic changes in skin and nails
  - Tremor
  - Gait

As for upper limbs, after inspection there are five parts to the PNS examination . . .

(i) Tone
Tone in the lower limb is generally assessed by three manoeuvres . . .
1. **The leg roll**
   - Position the patient sitting or laying with their legs held straight in front of them
   - With the patient's leg relaxed, roll it from side to side
   - Suddenly and without warning, stop and note how long it takes the leg to come to rest
   - If movement ceases immediately, it is likely the leg is hypertonic; if the leg carries on moving for longer than expected, it is likely the leg is hypotonic
2. **The leg drop**
   - Grasp the relaxed leg behind the knee and lift the knee up and down off the bed in a random fashion
   - Without warning, drop the leg onto the bed
   - If the leg remains bent, it is likely to be hypertonic; if the leg drops onto the bed with a thud and immediately becomes flaccid-looking, it is likely to be hypotonic
3. **Clonus**
   - Grasp the relaxed foot in the palm of the hand and **randomly dorsi- and plantarflex** at the ankle

- **Suddenly and without warning, fully dorsiflex** the foot at the ankle
- The characteristic **coarse flapping tremor** of clonus should become apparent within a couple of seconds of holding the foot in dorsiflexion, and is characteristic of an **UMN lesion**

(ii) Power
- Test all movements at all major joints . . .
  - Flexion of the thigh at the hip   →L1, **L2**
  - Flexion of the leg at the knee   →**S1**
  - Extension of the leg at the knee   →L3, **L4**
  - Dorsiflexion of the foot at the ankle   →L4, **L5**
  - Plantarflexion of the foot at the ankle   →**S1**, S2
  - Extension of great toe   →**S1**
- All movements should be initially performed **independently**, then **against force** if successful
- Failure to perform movement independently should precipitate attempt to **eliminate gravity**, for example performing the relevant movement in the horizontal plane, along the surface of the couch or bed
- Grade the power **0–5** based on the **MRC criteria**

(iii) Reflexes
- Like the upper limb, there are three major reflexes that should be tested in the lower limb . . .
  1. **Patellar tendon or knee jerk reflex** (tests spinal levels L2–L4)
  2. **Achilles tendon or ankle jerk reflex** (tests spinal level S1)
  3. **Plantar or Babinski reflex** (tests for **UMN lesion**): take an unpleasant stimulus and trace a line from the heel, up the lateral aspect of the sole and across the base of the toes. Expect to see flexing of all the toes of the foot, termed a 'flexor plantar response'. An abnormal plantar response occurs when there is extension of the great toe, with fanning (abduction) and extension of all the other toes of the foot. This 'extensor plantar response' is a classical sign of an UMN lesion
- Reinforcement of reflexes in the lower limb can be performed either by **teeth clenching**, or by **reverse interlocking of the fingers** of the hands and asking the patient to pull the hands apart against each other immediately prior to striking the tendon (the Jendrassik manoeuvre)

(iv) Co-ordination
- The **'heel-shin test'**
  - Ask patient to place the heel of one leg on the anterior aspect of the ankle of the other

- Ask them to slowly trace up the shin of the leg with the heel until they reach the knee, at which point you want them to remove the heel from the leg, and with a semicircular motion, return the heel to the ankle, as if in the shape of a 'D'; repeat the movement
- **Intention tremor** and **dysmetria** are again signs to look out for which will suggest a lesion within the lateral cerebellar lobe

(v) Sensation
- Description of how to test sensation in the lower limb is given above in the section on checking sensation in the upper limb

3 Gait

- Stand the patient up **carefully**: the safest way to avoid falls is to ask the examiner if you may stand the patient
- Perform Romberg's test . . .
  - Ask the patient to close their eyes whilst standing freely (be ready to prevent falling)
  - If the patient is able to balance normally when standing freely, but becomes unsteady on closing the eyes, then this is Romberg's positive, and suggests **abnormal proprioception**
  - However, if the patient cannot even balance with the eyes open upon standing, then this suggests a degree of **cerebellar ataxia**, but this is *not* Romberg's positive
- Ask the patient to walk **5–10 m** away from you, turn on the spot and then walk back towards you
- Observe the **hip movement, leg swing** and **fluidity of movements and turning**
- Repeat, with patient walking . . .
  - Heel-to-toe steps
  - Only on tiptoes
  - On heels
- The common gait problems and their causes are outlined below . . .
  - *Antalgic gait*: **limping, painful** walking style caused by skeletal or muscular problems, e.g. osteoarthritis
  - *Festinating gait* (**extrapyramidal, propulsive or shuffling** gait): **stooped, rigid posturing**. There is shifting forward of the centre of gravity, causing a near loss of balance that results in necessarily increasingly rapid, short, shuffling steps and involuntary acceleration: 'festination'. Generalized lack of control over forward and backward movement. Cardinal sign of Parkinson's disease

- *Scissoring gait*: results from **bilateral spastic paresis of the lower limbs** (little effect on the arms). Typical **partial crouching stance**. On walking, **thighs adduct with each step and the knees cross anterior to each other** in a scissor-like movement. Usually seen in **cerebral palsy**
- *Spastic gait* (paretic, weak or hemiplegic gait): **stiff, foot-dragging walk caused by increased tone of one of the legs**. It indicates focal damage to the **corticospinal tract**. There is a **lack of normal leg swing** causing the foot to drag; to compensate for this, the ipsilateral pelvis tilts upward to lift the toes, leading to the **classical circumduction and abduction of the leg**. Commonly caused by **stroke**, MS, head trauma or space-occupying lesion in the brain (e.g. brain tumour or abscess)
- *High stepping gait* (prancing, equine or steppage gait): results from **foot drop** caused by weakness or paralysis of the pretibial/peroneal musculature. The toes scrape along the floor during ambulation. In an attempt to compensate, the hip externally rotates and the **hip and knee flex in an exaggerated fashion**. The foot is thrown forward and the toes hit the ground first, producing the characteristic **slap**. Commonly caused by **peroneal nerve trauma**
- *Waddling gait*: distinctive **duck-like** walk of paediatric patients, due to **deterioration of the pelvic girdle muscles** leading to inability to stabilize the weight-bearing hip during walking. This causes the non-weight bearing hip to sag, and the **trunk to lean to the contralateral side in an attempt to maintain balance**. Commonly caused by **muscular dystrophy**
- *Frontal lobe gait*: patients **shuffle** and appear to have great problems lifting their feet from the floor, as if they were **magnetized**. Typical of **normal pressure hydrocephalus**
- *Cerebellar gait* (ataxic gait): **very wide based, unstable and prone to falling**. Cannot walk heel to toe. Causes include alcohol, MS, posterior fossa tumour and phenytoin toxicity
- *Sensory gait*: wide-based gait, grossly worse in poor light. There is demonstrable **loss of vibration and proprioception** sensory modalities (carried in the dorsal columns). Causes include cervical spondylosis and **syphilitic tabes dorsalis**

4 Higher mental functioning

For the undergraduate OSCE, it will suffice to be able to perform the abbreviated mental test score, or AMTS. This gives a score out of 10, where 8–10 suggests normality, 7 suggests probably abnormal higher mental functioning, and 6 or less suggests definitely abnormal higher mental functioning. Questions on the AMTS vary slightly, but the original test as devised by Hodgkinson is given below, and exact details of how to score are given at www.jr2.ox.ac.uk/geratol/docamts.

Q1: **Age**

Q2: **Time**

Q3: **Short-term memory recall**, e.g. give address such as 42 West Street

Q4: **Recognition of two people**, e.g. doctor and nurse

Q5: **Year**

Q6: **Name of place they are in**

Q7: **Date of birth**

Q8: **Start of World War I or II**

Q9: **Name of monarch**

Q10: **Count backwards from 20→1**

Q3: **Short-term memory recall:** ask patient to remember address

If the patient performs badly, then you can suggest more formal investigation in the form of a **mini-mental state examination** (MMSE), which gives a score out of 30.

5 Assessment of speech

Engage the patient in a **normal conversation**, perhaps by asking their name, where they live and what they do for a living. This will immediately give clues as to the problem. The key to successful examination of the speech of a patient is to distinguish between . . .

- **Dysphonia**
  - **Paucity of voice production**
  - Local vocal cord or laryngeal pathology, damage to the recurrent laryngeal nerve
  - **Whispering or husky quality**
  - Unable to produce the normal volume of speech
  - Inability to maintain a note, such as '*eeeeee*', is a clue that myasthenia gravis is the cause of the dysphonia
- **Dysarthria**
  - **Mechanical disorder of articulation**
  - **Slurring** or difficulty in pronunciation of words
  - Accentuated by complicated phrases: '*west register street*'
- **Dysphasia**
  - **Language and communication disorder**
  - *Two* main types . . .

  (a) **Expressive dysphasia**: a frustrating defect of **expressive language, speech repetition, naming and reading aloud**. Speech can be produced, but it is **non-fluent** and takes great effort for the patient. Ask the patient to name a simple object, like a watch, a pen or a tie. A patient with expressive dysphasia will be unable to do so (nominal dysphasia). You can confirm that the problem is expressive by giving the patient a range of options: for example, when asked '*Is it a watch? Is it a car? Is it a dog?*', the patient with a true isolated expressive dysphasia will nod at the appropriate moment. A total inability to express language is expressive aphasia, or **Broca's aphasia**

  (b) **Receptive dysphasia**: the patient does not understand what is said to them, though they freely produce **fluent, meaningless speech**, with neologisms. Ask the patient to perform a simple command, such as '*Touch your nose*' or '*Open your mouth*'. The patient with receptive dysphasia will be unable to do this, not due to physical limitation but instead due to inability to comprehend the spoken word. A total inability to understand language is known as receptive aphasia, or **Wernicke's aphasia**

Last part

Phew! You will now have completed your neurological examination. Thank the patient, cover them up if they are exposed and present your findings to the examiner, attempting (if you can) to hang them around a diagnosis, giving sensible differentials.

Dermatological System

The examination routine

Q: Examine this rash.

When discussing skin findings it is more important than with any other system to imagine that your examiner is blind! **Your response should be as descriptive as possible using as few words as possible. Tell the examiner your diagnosis or differential diagnosis.**

For example, your examiner shows you a car. By responding '*this is a car*' you have given the correct diagnosis but given your examiner no clues as to any further information that will add to your exam marks. It is far better to give a concise, accurate, detailed description of the car, e.g. '*this is a five door, diesel, Volvo hatchback with a Y registration plate and alloy wheels*' This immediately tells your examiner that you have noticed far more detail and have demonstrated a greater knowledge about cars — get the point?

Even if you are unsure of the diagnosis, if you give a full, concise, detailed description of the rash, e.g. '*the patient has a florid, generalized, violaceous, papular rash with areas of superficial scaling and excoriation. I would like to exclude x, y or z . . .*', you are unlikely to fail and will still get significant marks.

For maximum marks describe the features of the rash, what features are associated (see below) **and present and what features are associated but absent**. For example, if shown a case of psoriasis your reply should include '*This patient rash is typical for psoriasis with salmon pink plaques over the extensor aspects, scalp, lower back, etc. There are associated features of nail dystrophy with onycholysis, subungual hyperkeratosis and pitting, but there is no evidence of psoriatic arthritis of the hands. I would like to ask the patient about his/her family history, drugs, etc.*'.

Observing and describing the most obvious abnormality

Detail to include
- **Rash**
  - Distribution/site
  - Colour
  - Lesion morphology
- **Associated features/problems**

Distribution
Is there a particular pattern to the rash?
- **Generalized**
  - Eczema (see later)
  - Psoriasis (see later)
  - Drug rash
  - Erythema multiforme (target lesions, mucous membrane involvement, Herpes simplex virus cold sore, streptococcal sore throat infection)
- **Flexural aspects**
  - Eczema
  - Flexural psoriasis
- **Extensor aspects**
  - Psoriasis
  - Dermatomyositis (Gottron's pads)
- **Photosensitive areas**
  - Lupus erythematosis (butterfly, photosensitive rash, with nail fold capillary changes,?alopecia)
  - Dermatomyositis (peri-ocular heliotrope rash, nail fold changes, Gottron's papules and pads, proximal muscle weakness)
  - Drug rash (thiazide diuretic, quinine, tetracyclines, sulphonamides, amiodarone, oral contraceptives, chlorpropamide)
  - Porphyria cutanea tarda (sun-exposed sites, milia, scarring, hypertrichosis,?alcohol/drug intake)
- **Dependent areas**

- Vasculitis (painful, palpable purpura)
- Venous hypertensive changes (varicose veins, eczema, gaiter ulceration, atrophy blanche, lipodermatosclerosis)
- **In scars**
  - Sarcoidosis
  - Minocycline pigmentation (also face, nails, teeth, palate)
  - Köebnerization: psoriasis, lichen planus, viral warts, molluscum contagiosum, vitiligo

Colour

- **Erythematous (red/pink)**
  - Eczema
  - Psoriasis
  - LE (butterfly distribution, nail fold changes ± alopecia, oral ulceration, arthropathy)
  - Erythema multiforme
- **Violaceous (purple)**
  - Dermatomyositis
  - Vasculitis (painful, palpable, purpura)
  - Lichen planus (papular, Wickham's striae on skin lesions and mucous membranes, pitted and ridged nails, occasional scarring alopecia, ?drugs/hepatitis C)
- **Grey**
  - Drug rash (Amiodarone, Minocycline, topical silver-containing agents)
- **Brown pigmentation**
  - Addison's disease
  - Post-inflammatory hyperpigmentation
  - Pityriasis versicolor
  - Malignant melanoma
- **Depigmentation**
  - Vitiligo
  - Post-inflammatory hypopigmentation
  - Pityriasis versicolor
  - Morphoea (erythematous edge, central sclerosis/scar like change, loss of appendages)
- **Haemorrhagic**
  - Vasculitis
  - Herpes zoster

Lesion morphology

- **Macular (flat)**
  - e.g. vitiligo
- **Papular (≤5 mm raised)**
  - Lichen planus

- Vasculitis
- Eczema
- Drugs
- Acne vulgaris (open and closed comedones, pustules, and nodules)
- Sarcoidosis
- **Nodular (>5 mm)**
  - Eczema
  - Tumour (primary or secondary)
  - Acne
  - Rheumatoid nodule (ulnar aspect forarm/elbow)
  - Sarcoidosis
- **Pustular**
  - Infection, e.g. *Staphylococcus aureus*
  - Pustular psoriasis
  - Reiter's syndrome (identical clinically and histologically to pustular psoriasis of the soles)
  - Drugs
  - Acne vulgaris or rosacea
- **Plaques (>2 cm diameter)**
  - Psoriasis
  - Cutaneous T-cell lymphoma
- **Vesicular (fluid blisters <5 mm)**
  - Eczema (often hands and/or feet)
  - Drug rash
  - Herpes simplex and zoster
- **Bullae (fluid blisters >5 mm)**
  - Bullous pemphigoid
  - Drug rash: diuretics, fixed drug eruption
  - Bullous impetigo
  - Bullous erythema multiforme
  - Porphyria cutanea tarda
- **Annular**
  - Erythema multiforme
  - Granuloma annulare
  - Tinea corporis
  - Lupus erythematosis
  - Psoriasis
  - Discoid eczema
  - Sarcoidosis
  - Morphoea
  - Alopecia areata (no inflammation, exclamation mark hairs, nail changes)
- **Scaley**
  - Eczema
  - Psoriasis
  - Infection: e.g. tinea
  - Discoid lupus erythematosis
  - Squamous cell carcinoma (nodule, sun exposed site)

- **Ulcerated**
  - Leg ulcer (venous, arterial, vasculitic, traumatic)
  - Basal cell carcinoma (sun exposed site, pearly skin coloured nodule with telangiectasia)
  - Necrobiosis lipoidica diabeticorum
- **Atrophic (thinned, tissue paper texture)**
  - Necrobiosis lipoidica diabeticorum (diabetic, shins, violaceous erythema ± ulceration)
  - Discoid LE
  - Morphoea
  - Lichen sclerosis
  - Cutaneous T-cell lymphoma
- **Other**
  - Urticarial (wheal):
    Urticaria
    LE
    Drug rash
  - Papillomatous (warty):
    Viral warts
    Pigmented naevus

Looking for associated problems

- **Nails**
  - Vasculitis: nail folds ragged with dilated capillaries
  - Psoriasis: pitting, onycholysis, subungual hyperkeratosis
  - Eczema: ridging, splitting
  - Lichen planus: pitting, longitudinal ridges, ptery-gium, nail loss
  - Alopecia areata: pitting, longitudinal ridging
  - Tinea infection: yellowing, hyperkeratosis, onycholysis
- **Joints**
  - Psoriasis: psoriatic arthritis (?mutilans)
  - Connective tissue disease
  - Reiter's syndrome
- **Alopecia (hair loss)**
  - Non-scarring: alopecia areata, telogen effluvium, connective tissue disease, drugs, psoriasis
  - Scarring: infection (e.g. tinea), discoid lupus, lichen planus
- **Mucous membranes**
  - Erythema multiforme
  - Pemphigoid
  - Connective tissue disease (ulcers)
  - Addisons (pigmentation)
  - Lichen planus (Wickham's striae, mercury amalgams)

- **Lymphadenopathy**
  - Tumours
  - Infection

The history routine

Q. What questions would you like to ask this patient?

Presenting complaint

- **Onset**
- **Duration**
  - Acute (<6 weeks) or chronic, persistent or intermittent?
- **Site(s) and spread**
- **Symptoms**
  - *Itch*: eczema, lichen planus, bullous pemphigoid, psoriasis (sometimes), infection (tinea, scabies), drugs
  - *Pain*: vasculitis, infection, arterial leg ulcer
  - *Asymptomatic*
- **Treatment**
  - Topical, oral, other (e.g. phototherapy—psoriasis or eczema; bandages—eczema, leg ulcers)?
  - Currently and in the past?
  - Beneficial or not?
- **Triggers**
  - Stress: psoriasis, eczema, lichen planus, alopecia areata
  - Sun exposure: (see photosensitive areas, above)
- **Relieving factors**
- **Associated factors**
  - Psoriasis: sore throats, drugs (lithium, β-blockers, antimalarials), alcohol intake, nail or joint problems
  - Lupus erythematosis: systemic symptoms, drugs, miscarriages, etc.
  - Dermatomyositis: muscle weakness, weight loss, etc.
  - Reiter's: arthropathy, GU or GIT symptoms
  - Eczema: asthma or hayfever, contact allergies, pets, family history
  - Necrobiosis or granuloma annulare: diabetes
  - Skin cancer: sun exposure, family history, immunosuppression
  - Vasculitis: drugs, sore throat, joint, urinary and gastrointestinal symptoms
  - Leg ulcers: DVT, PE, smoking, diabetes, ischaemic heart disease, hypertension, varicose vein surgery, cellulitis

Previous medical history

If relevant, e.g. eczema: asthma, hay fever, allergy (contact, dietary, airborne). Also see associated problems, above

Drugs

Always ask a full drug history

Allergies

Always ask

Family history

- Atopy
- Psoriasis
- Autoimmune disorders (RA, vitiligo, alopecia areata, pernicious anaemia, insulin dependent diabetes)

Social and occupational history

- Eczema: ?contact or airborne allergic element
- Leg ulcers (mobility, etc.)
- Impact on quality of life (school, work, home)

Part 4 OSCEs

Introduction

How will you be marked and assessed in the OSCE?

The first thing to say is that the way medical schools mark OSCEs varies with geographical location. However, this variability is decreasing greatly over time as the General Medical Council and the Council for the Heads of Medical Schools in the United Kingdom attempt to instil a degree of validity and reproducibility into what has the potential to be a very *subjective* rather than an objective test. Medical schools go to great lengths in an attempt to educate the examiners of the OSCE so that the test that you get is fair, reliable, reproducible and valid, and this should reassure you in the nervous days leading up to the examination.

Medical schools stress to their examiners that **the OSCE is *a test of clinical skills*,** not purely and simply a test of medical knowledge. Examiners are usually given specific instructions that the OSCE . . .

- Is *not* a viva voce
- Is *not* a time for them to devise their own station or marking scheme
- Is *not* a time to interfere with the role of the simulated patient
- Is *not* an opportunity for teaching

As a rule, there are only four types of OSCE station, and these will be discussed through the course of the book . . .

1. History taking
2. Clinical examination
3. Explanation and counselling
4. Clinical skills

There should be two examiners at each of the stations that you attend, and each will mark you independently. There will also be an additional examiner at some of the stations you undergo, but he/she will be examining the examiners, and not you. Try to imagine they are not there. Typically, and unlike OSCEs in your more formative years of medical school, the **examiners will not want you to talk your way through the station** that you are doing (especially if it is a clinical examination station); instead, perform the station and then present your findings at the end. This is a very difficult skill to master, commonly more difficult than performing the examination itself, and it is one you should practice so that when you do present on the day, your presentation will flow, be coherent and contain all the important positive and negative findings, and none of the superfluous things that get up examiners' noses. Saving your findings until you have completed the examination does allow you to concentrate on the patient and the signs, without your train of thought and examination routine being constantly interrupted.

The examiners will mark you by two main techniques . . .

- Marking schedules
- Global performance indicators

Marking schedules

This is the way that OSCEs have traditionally been marked. Examiners are given a list of criteria that you should fulfil during a particular OSCE station. Depending on the criterion, you will be judged to either fulfil that criterion (1 point) or not fulfil that criterion (0 points). With other criteria, you will be judged to have performed it completely (2 points), partially (1 point) or not at all/inadequately (0 points). The points available for each marking schedule also varies widely (see upcoming examples), as does the 'pass-mark', and ultimately whether you pass or not will also take into account your 'global performance' (see later in this section).

The good things about marking schedules are . . .
- They allow the examiner to know what the station-setter is looking for
- They reassure the candidate that the examiner has somewhat fixed, objective criteria to look for
- They allow the use of non-specialist examiners
- It is easy to pick up plenty of marks by doing simple things: make sure that you get these 'cheap' marks!

The bad things about marking schedules are . . .
- They may just reward robotic-like regurgitation of processes
- They may not satisfactorily reward candidates whose clinical skills and acumen are excellent
- They do not take into account the examiners expertise in the field examined

However, love them or hate them, marking schedules are here to stay in the assessment of OSCEs because, after all, they are supposed to be objective! There now follows three examples of typical OSCE marking schedules for different history-taking stations, like the ones you can expect examiners in your OSCE to be holding in their hands.

Example 1: chest pain history

Give these instructions to the candidate: '*Please take a focused history from this subject who represents a 50-year-old man who complains of an episode of chest pain yesterday. You will be given marks for taking a relevant history*'.

This marking schedule gives a mark out of a possible 20.

Criterion	Performed completely	Performed partially or adequately	Not performed adequately or at all
Duration of symptoms	1	0	0
Site of pain	1	0	0
Nature of pain	2	1	0
Associated symptoms	2	1	0
Previous episodes	1	0	0
Aggravating factors	1	0	0
Relieving factors	1	0	0
Past medical history	2	1	0
Family history	1	0	0
Smoking/drinking	1	0	0
Occupation	1	0	0
Medication	2	1	0
Attitude, approach, professionalism	2	1	0
Logical, well-constructed history	2	1	0

Example 2: sore throat history

'*Please take a history from this patient . . .*'

Criterion	Performed completely	Performed partially or adequately	Not performed adequately or at all
Appropriate introduction	2	1	0
Establishes what the interview is about	2	1	0

Continued

Criterion	Performed completely	Performed partially or adequately	Not performed adequately or at all
History aspects			
Time course of symptoms	–	1	0
Amount of pain	–	1	0
Swallowing difficulty	–	1	0
Fever	–	1	0
Vomiting	–	1	0
Malaise	–	1	0
Past history of similar	–	1	0
Appropriate questioning technique	2	1	0
Management			
Informs patient of likely viral nature of illness	–	1	0
Checks understanding of this point	–	1	0
Explains self-limiting nature of condition	–	1	0
Explains that antibiotics are not appropriate	2	1	0
Advise antipyretic	–	1	0
Advise gargling with paracetamol	–	1	0
Advise clear fluid intake	–	1	0
Express empathy with patient's concerns	2	1	0
Do not agree to patient request for antibiotics	2	1	0
Re-checks understanding	2	1	0
Systematic and organized manner	2	1	0

This marking schedule gives a mark out of a possible 29.

Example 3: temporal arteritis

'Please take a history from this patient . . .'

Criterion	Performed completely	Performed partially or adequately	Not performed adequately or at all
Appropriate introduction	2	1	0
Explain what interview is about	2	1	0
Appropriate style	2	1	0
Obtain consent	–	1	0
Regarding the headaches			
Onset/frequency	2	1	0
Duration	–	1	0
Site/radiation	2	1	0
Character	–	1	0
Exacerbating factors	2	1	0
Relieving factors	–	1	0

Continued on p. 216

Criterion	Performed completely	Performed partially or adequately	Not performed adequately or at all
Associated symptoms			
Scalp tenderness	–	1	0
Jaw claudication	–	1	0
Nausea	–	1	0
Visual disturbance	–	1	0
Photophobia	–	1	0
Supplementary questions			
Recent head trauma	–	1	0
Previous headaches/migraine	2	1	0
Summarizes history to patient	2	1	0
Elicits concerns	–	1	0
Responds appropriately to concerns	–	1	0
Systematic approach	2	1	0
Patient to evaluate			
'The candidate made it easy for me to talk'	2	1	0

This marking schedule gives a total out of 32 marks.

As you can see from the above, the marking schedules occasionally give credit for things that you might not expect them to. Nevertheless, these examples are based on genuine past OSCEs, so beware!

Global performance indicators

These have only recently been introduced alongside marking schedules, mainly **to utilize the experience of the examiner** in the marking of a particular OCSE station. This is because it was felt that marking schedules did not allow the examiner to utilize their clinical expertise sufficiently in marking the candidate. It was also felt that some superb candidates could finish the OSCE with the same marks as per marking schedule as some lesser can-

didates, and it was felt important that these candidates be credited for their superior clinical technique and acumen, even though the marking schedules could not separate them from the lesser skilled examinees.

Essentially, the examiner gives you one of five subjective grades . . .
1. **Excellent pass**
2. **Very good pass**
3. **Clear pass**
4. **Borderline pass/fail**
5. **Clear fail**

This mark is then taken into account alongside the marking schedule, but the weighting given to this differs depending on the station in question, and occasionally on the examiner marking the station, before a final mark on the station is calculated.

The OSCE Communication Skills Station

These stations are the newest type of station to be drafted into the OSCE setting. Some 5–6 years ago, communication skills was a topic rarely even taught to medical students, much less examined. However, with the advent of new curricula, communication skills have taken up a position of unprecedented importance, with lengthy lecture/practical courses for medical students, and comprehensive assessment, both during the course and in the final examination OSCE. The increasing inclusion of GPs into the setting of OSCEs over recent years has seen these stations become ever more popular, because this is a common form of assessment in postgraduate General Practice examinations. Indeed, over the last 2–3 years, the number of these stations in a given OSCE has risen from only one, to three or four, often at the expense of the more traditional history and examination stations. There follows a complete example of a communication skills OSCE station, along with a list of popular topics that have been shown to come up year-on-year.

Example: explaining the pathology report

Instructions to examiner

The aim of this station is to test the ability of the examinee to interpret information from a histopathology report and ensure that the patient understands the information contained within it, and it's implications. Ask the candidate to read the instructions, and start the interview when they have done so.

Instructions to candidate

You are a medical student attached to a surgical firm. You have a patient called Vera Black who had a wide local excision for breast cancer 4 days ago and is recovering on the ward. Your firm is now in possession of the histopathology report, which reads . . .

'The tumour is a moderately differentiated adenocarcinoma measuring 3 cm in maximum dimension. The resection margins are clear, but 3 out the 12 axillary lymph nodes sampled are involved with the malignant process. Oestrogen receptor immunohistochemistry is positive.'

The consultant surgeon (Mr Collins) has already spoken to Vera about the results, but she has asked one of the other doctors if you would be kind enough to go over things again, as she did not catch everything the first time around. You know from some previous reading that Vera has stage $T_2N_1M_0$ disease, or Manchester stage II disease, giving her an approximately 65% 5-year survival rate, with the correct follow-up chemotherapy.

Criterion	Performed completely	Performed partially/adequately	Not performed adequately or at all
Appropriate introduction	2	1	0
Checks what the patient wants to discuss	–	1	0
Checks what the patient knows already	2	1	0

Continued on p. 218

Criterion	Performed completely	Performed partially/adequately	Not performed adequately or at all
Explains . . .			
This is cancer/malignant	–	1	0
The original cancer is all out	2	1	0
Lymph nodes contain cancer	2	1	0
This is relatively advanced, with moderate prognosis	2	1	0
Elicits concerns	2	1	0
Avoids falsely reassuring patient	2	1	0
Checks new level of understanding	2	1	0
Invites further questions	–	1	0
Discusses potential benefit of chemotherapy	2	1	0
Responds to concerns	2	1	0
Patient marks . . .			
'I felt the candidate would make a good doctor'	2	1	0
'I understood everything that was said to me'	2	1	0

This gives a potential mark out of 27, with a global performance score to be taken into account before a final mark is reached.

Previous counselling stations with similar marking schemes have included . . .
- Explaining to angry relatives of a stroke patient why their loved one is 'nil-by-mouth'
- Explaining to an inquisitive mother the need for the MMR triple vaccine
- Explaining the disease implications to a newly diagnosed type I diabetic, especially the need for lifelong insulin therapy
- Explaining the need for lifelong treatment in a patient with heart failure/ ischaemic heart disease/ hypercholesterolaemia/ peripheral vascular disease
- Discussing genetic counselling in a patient with a family history of Huntington's chorea
- Breaking bad news: the death of a family member, the finding of terminal disease
- Explaining the need for per rectal examination in a trauma patient on a spinal board

The Top 50 OSCEs

OSCE station 1

Q. Examine this patient's respiratory system.
A.
A middle-aged or old-aged patient sat up in bed. There may be a sputum pot (inspect contents) next to the bed, along with a nebulizer and oxygen.

1. The patient appears **cyanosed** from the end of the bed. The respiratory rate is normal or reduced. There is a **flap of CO_2 retention** and the pulse is full and '**bounding**'. The **anterior-posterior diameter of the chest is increased** and there is loss of the usual bucket handle respiratory movement of the ribs. The **JVP is elevated** (cor pulmonale). There is **central cyanosis**. The cricosternal distance is reduced. The apex maybe displaced (cor pulmonale). **Expansion is symmetrically reduced**, but the percussion note is normal all round. Auscultation reveals bilaterally **poor air entry** (air trapping) with **scattered wheezes** and fine **crepitations**. There may be **ankle oedema** (cor pulmonale).

2. The patient appears **pink and breathless** from the end of the bed. There is **pursing of lips** (maintains end expiratory pressure, 'stenting' open airways that would otherwise collapse due to loss of elastic recoil). There is usage of the **accessory muscles** of respiration with sternocleidomastoid prominence in these frequently thin patients. The chest is **hyperinflated** with **increased anterior-posterior diameter**. The **JVP may be elevated** (cor pulmonale). **Expansion is symmetrically reduced**, but the percussion note is normal all round. There is generally **poor air entry** bilaterally and scattered expiratory wheezing. There **may be ankle oedema** (cor pulmonale).

Diagnosis is chronic obstructive airways disease (COPD).

These patients are very common in exams reflecting their abundance in practise. Candidates should be familiar with the aetiology (smoking), pathology and clinical features as well the acute and chronic management. In short, COPD is a core topic.

Q. What is the definition of chronic obstructive pulmonary disease?
A.
- **The NICE guidelines (2004) state . . .**
  - Chronic obstructive pulmonary disease (COPD) is characterized by airflow obstruction which is:
    Not fully reversible
    Not markedly changing over several months
    Predominantly caused by smoking
  - Airflow obstruction is defined as:
    FEV1 < 80% of predicted
    FEV1/FVC < 0.7
- The **terms chronic bronchitis and emphysema are now considered obsolete**. The so-called 'pink puffer' with **emphysema** and the so-called 'blue bloater' with **chronic bronchitis**, are at either end of a spectrum. Many patients have features of both these extremes, both clinically and pathologically. **These terms are avoided and the phrase 'COPD' used**
- The essential **pathological process** in both emphysema and chronic bronchitis involves progressive damage caused by chronic inflammation to the airway and parenchymal architecture of the lungs. This particularly affects the elastic recoil, with resultant premature collapse of the airway on expiration, leading to air trapping. There is reversal of the normal respiratory cycle pattern with expiration becoming longer than the inspiration phase, especially in emphysema. There is hyperinflation of the chest
- Significant airflow limitation can be present before the patient is aware of it

- There is much overlap with the management of asthma during an acute exacerbation of the disease
- Patients have central respiratory centres that are **desensitized to chronically raised CO_2 levels** (the normal stimulus to respiration); therefore, they rely on **hypoxia** for their respiratory drive. **Type II respiratory failure** (failure to ventilate the lungs) is characteristic particularly during exacerbations
- **Inappropriate administration of high concentrations (>24%) of oxygen leads to a loss of the hypoxic respiratory drive**. Gradual CO_2 accumulation (CO_2 narcosis) occurs with hypoxia and acidosis
- Chronic lung damage and hypoxia lead to **pulmonary hypertension** (one cause of secondary pulmonary hypertension) and consequent predominantly right-sided cardiac failure (cor pulmonale) with an elevated JVP and oedema

Q. Take a history from this patient with COPD.
A.

Key areas to cover include . . .
- Smoking status (plus any attempts or help to quit)
- Exercise tolerance levels (exact details of what they can and cannot do)
- Sputum production (volume and colour)
- Current medications (especially steroid usage, home nebulizers)
- Home oxygen therapy
- Recent exacerbations, hospital admissions, etc.
- Social situation (get an exact picture in your mind of this person, and how they live and manage from day to day, e.g. type of accommodation, stairs at home, outside support from family or social services, who does shopping, cleaning, etc.)
- Effect of the condition on the patient's mental state, e.g. symptoms of depression or anxiety are common

Q. How is the diagnosis of COPD made?
A.

There is no single test. The diagnosis relies upon a combination of . . .
- Typical features in the clinical **history**
  - Over 35 years of age
  - Smokers or ex-smokers
  - Frequent winter bronchitis
  - Symptoms of cough, sputum production, wheeze and breathlessness
- Typical findings on clinical **examination** (as above)

- **Airflow limitation** as demonstrated by spirometry (as above)

Treatment is commenced if there is reasonable clinical suspicion based on the above criteria.

Q. What grading do you know for breathlessness?
A.

The **Medical Research Council (MRC) grading for dyspnoea** is:
1. Breathless only on **strenuous exercise**
2. Breathless with hurrying or **slight hills**
3. Breathless **walking on the flat** and may have to stop
4. Has to **stop for breath after 100 m on level ground**
5. **Too breathless to leave home**; breathless when dressing

Q. What is the management of stable COPD?
A.
- **Stopping smoking**
  - Pharmacotherapy, e.g. nicotine replacement or bupropion (avoid in epilepsy and bipolar disorders)
- **Treat obese or underweight patients**
  - Dietetic advice
  - Nutritional supplements
- **Drug treatment**
  - Bronchodilation therapy; the following stepwise progression:
    Short-acting β_2 agonist plus short-acting anticholinergic therapy
    Long-acting bronchodilator (long-acting β_2 agonist or long-acting anticholinergic)
    Long-acting bronchodilator and inhaled corticosteroid (stop if no benefit after 4 weeks)
    Consider a theophylline
  - Treatment of cor pulmonale with diuretics
  - Mucolytic therapy for chronic productive cough
  - Influenza and pneumococcal vaccination should be offered
  - Treat associated anxiety or depression with conventional drugs
- **Long-term oxygen therapy (LTOT)**
  - The following patients should be assessed:
    FEV1 < 30% of predicted
    Oxygen saturations < 92% on air
    Cyanosis
    Polycythemia
    Cor pulmonale (peripheral oedema, elevated JVP)

- Patients are selected for long-term O_2 therapy by complying **with all the following criteria:**
  $PaO_2 < 7.3$ kPa (or 7.3–8 kPa with cor pulmonale, nocturnal hypoxaemia or secondary polycythemia)
  FEV1 < 1.5 L
  Normal or increased $PaCO_2$
- The **MRC trial** found that by giving O_2 (via nasal cannulae) for 15 h or more per day, such as to raise the PaO_2 to 8 kPa, improved the 3-year survival by 50%. Oxygen is delivered by a home oxygen concentrator
- **Surgery**
  - Bullectomy
  - Lung volume reduction
  - Transplantation

Q. *What are the typical chest radiological findings in COPD?*

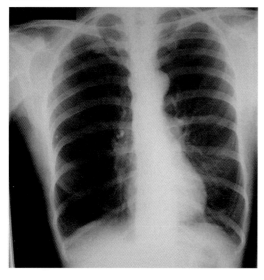

A.
The radiographic features of COPD include . . .
- **Hyperinflation** with more than five ribs visible anteriorly
- **Bullae:** air trapping resulting in sacs, which may be very large (as above)
- Areas of **consolidation** or features of intercurrent infection (fluffy shadowing)
- **Cardiomegaly (if cor pulmonale)**, pulmonary plethora, pleural effusions if cor pulmonale has occurred

- **Check for evidence of associated malignancy (coin lesion, effusion, hilar lymphadopathy)**

Q. *What are the available treatment options or interventions with an **evidence basis** of benefit in COPD?*
A.
- **In the acute management** . . .
  - Inhaled short-acting β_2 agonists, e.g. salbutamol, terbulaline
  - Inhaled anticholinergics, e.g. ipratropium bromide
  - Evidence exists for the combination of two drugs being more effective than either alone
  - Oral corticosteroids (no evidence exists in favour of the use of inhaled corticosteroids in either the acute or long-term management of COPD)
  - Theophyllines (e.g. aminophylline) are of marginal benefit but the adverse effects must be weighed against their side effects (nausea, diarrhoea, headache, seizures, arrhythmias)
  - Antibiotics
  - Physiotherapy
- **In the chronic management** . . .
  - Stopping smoking improves the outlook no matter how severe the disease

Q. *Describe the management of acute exacerbations of COPD.*
A.
- Sit the patient up
- Give 24 % oxygen to keep oxygen saturations above 92%
- Nebulized salbutamol 5 mg followed by ipratropium bromide 500 mcg
- Insert IV cannula and take routine bloods. (FBC, urea and electrolytes, blood sugar, blood cultures and theophylline levels)
- Arrange
  - EGC (possible evidence or right ventricular strain; right axis deviation, RBBB or atrial fibrillation)
  - Chest X-ray to exclude pneumothorax and pneumonia
  - Arterial blood gases; all are hypoxic, watch for acidosis indicating need for respiratory support (see below)
  - Sputum culture if purulent (*Haemophyllus influenzae, Streptococcus pneumoniae*)
- Give 100 mg hydrocortisone i.v.

- Give Prednisolone 30 mg orally continued for 14 days
- IV antibiotics, e.g. 500 mg amoxycillin, for purulent sputum
- Arrange physiotherapy
- Non-invasive positive pressure ventilation for ventilatory (type II) respiratory failure if . . .
  - $pH < 7.25$
  - Rising CO_2 despite above treatment

Q. What is the prognosis in COPD?
A.

- 26 000 deaths per year in the UK
- Overall there is a 50% 5-year survival for severe disease

OSCE station 2

Station 2a

A 78-year-old female presents with symptoms of **influenza** against a background of a more **chronic increase in shortness of breath** that has come to affect even the least taxing of her activities of daily living. On examination, you observe a **very thin, frail-looking** woman with an **irregularly irregular pulse** and a blood pressure of **110/68**. You note that she has a laterally **displaced apex**. Auscultation of her heart reveals a **systolic murmur**, loudest at the apex but also audible in the axilla with the diaphragm. There is also a third heart sound present. There is mild pitting ankle oedema.

Q. What valve lesion does this patient most likely have from the description given?
A.

She has *mitral regurgitation* (**MR**), the most common murmur to come up in medical undergraduate final examinations. As a consequence of the regurgitant valve, she has developed atrial fibrillation and a degree of left and right (congestive) cardiac failure.

Q. What three investigations would you perform to investigate the valve lesion?
A.

1. **CXR**: would be expected to show cardiomegaly, batswing peri-hilar oedema, upper lobe venous diversion, Kerley-B lines and bi-basal effusions due to the MR-mediated cardiac failure. You may also see some calcification of the mitral valve

2. **ECG**: would be expected to show left atrial delay (P *mitrale*, bifid P waves), signs of left ventricular hypertrophy and atrial fibrillation

3. **Echocardiography**: would show dilated left atrium and ventricle; Doppler studies would show the regurgitant jet of blood into the left atrium

Q. What is the treatment of chronic mitral regurgitation?
A.

Once symptoms develop in patients with mitral stenosis, surgery to replace the valve is mandatory. Because progressive and irreversible left ventricular dysfunction commonly develops before symptoms of mitral regurgitation manifest, prophylactic surgery should be considered in all patients who have this valve defect *and* a decreased ejection fraction (<60%) or marked left ventricular dilatation.

Station 2b

A 59-year-old female of African origin presents to her GP with a long history of lethargy and dyspnoea. Over the last few weeks she has noticed increased difficulty in performing her activities of daily living due to worsening **dyspnoea**. Worse than this, she has developed **swollen, puffy ankles**, causing social embarrassment. On examination, she is short of breath climbing onto the examination couch, respiratory rate **23 b.p.m.** She has **mild pitting ankle oedema**. Her heart rate is **90/min and is regular**. Her blood pressure is **160/65** (BP on her last visit to the surgery 6 weeks ago was 165/80). Her JVP is **4cm**. She has a **thrusting** apex which is **inferolaterally displaced**. Auscultation of the heart reveals a **high-pitched early diastolic murmur** that is only audible with the diaphragm at the left sternal edge when the patient is sitting forward holding her breath in end-expiration. There are mild fine crepitations at both lung bases.

Q. What valve lesion does this patient most likely have from the description given?
A.

She has *aortic regurgitation* (AR), a murmur you **must specifically look for**. The history of fatigue, symptoms of heart failure, lack of atrial fibrillation, wide pulse pressure and hyperdynamic, displaced apex beat are all clues for the diagnosis.

Q. What three investigations would you perform to investigate the valve lesion?

A.

1. **CXR**: would be expected to show cardiomegaly, bats-wing peri-hilar oedema, upper lobe venous diversion, Kerley-B lines and bi-basal effusions due to the AR-mediated cardiac failure. May also show some dilatation of the aortic root

2. **ECG**: would be expected to show left ventricular hy-pertrophy (tall Rs in V4–6; deep Ss in V1–3); patient would be expected to be in sinus rhythm unless the di-latation of the left ventricle caused by the regurgitation of blood had dilated the mitral annulus causing mitral re-gurgitation and subsequently atrial fibrillation

3. **Echocardiography**: would show vigorous cardiac contraction, a dilated left ventricle and an enlarged aortic root; colour Doppler studies would reveal the regurgi-tant jet traveling from the aorta into the left ventricle; it may also show mid-diastolic fluttering of the mitral valve leaflets caused by the regurgitant jet of blood — the cause of **the 'Austin–Flint' murmur**

Q. What further signs would you look for to confirm your diagnosis?

A.

There are four unusual signs associated with aortic re-gurgitation that are difficult to elicit, but important to know about . . .

(a) **Quincke's sign**: capillary pulsation in the nail beds

(b) **DeMusset's sign**: rhythmical head-nodding in time with cardiac systole

(c) **Duroziez's sign**: 'to-and-fro' or 'double' murmur over the femoral artery when pressure is applied distal to the site of auscultation in the groin

(d) **Pistol-shot femorals**: a sharp bang heard over the femoral arteries with each heart beat

Station 2c

A 54-year-old Zimbabwean asylum seeker presents to A&E complaining of a **single episode of unexplained loss of consciousness** whilst running around in the local park with his nephew. He states that there was **no warn-ing**, and although he was a little out of breath he did not feel that anything was amiss. The episode of loss of con-sciousness lasted only a few seconds and recovery was spontaneous and rapid. Past medical history reveals a **heart murmur as a child following a long feverish illness**.

On examination the patient is **tachycardic**, heart rate being 105/min and regular. Blood pressure is **110/97**. You think that the brachial arterial pulsation is **more sus-tained than usual**. The JVP is **4cm**. The apex beat is **heav-ing and undisplaced**. On auscultation of the heart there is a **systolic murmur** loudest in the second right inter-space. A murmur is **also audible in the carotids**. There is also an **audible click** that occurs consistently, just after the first heart sound. There are fine crepitations audible at both lung bases.

Q. What valve lesion does this patient most likely have from the description given?

A.

He has *aortic stenosis* (AS). Clues are the episode of exer-cise-related syncope, possible history of rheumatic fever, slow-rising plateau pulse, narrow pulse pressure, ejec-tion systolic murmur loudest in the aortic area, radiating to the carotids, with ejection click and signs of left and right heart failure.

Q. What three investigations would you perform to investigate the valve lesion?

A.

1. **CXR**: shows a small-normal sized heart with dilated ascending aorta (due to turbulent blood flow above the stenosed valve) and potentially a calcified aortic valve. The heart will only look large if cardiac failure has supervened

2. **ECG**: would be expected to show left ventricular hy-pertrophy, left atrial delay (P *mitrale*) and ventricular strain pattern due to pressure overload (depressed ST-segments/inverted T-waves in the leads looking at the left ventricle, i.e. I, aVL, V5 and V6). Usually the patient is in sinus rhythm, but ventricular dysrhythmias may be present

3. **Echocardiography**: would show thickened, calcified, immobile aortic cusps and left ventricular hypertrophy; colour Doppler imaging would demonstrate the steep pressure gradient across the valve

Q. What three clinical syndromes are commonly confused with aortic stenosis due to their similar examination findings?

A.

1. **Supravalvular obstruction**, for example in William's syndrome, where a congenital fibrous diaphragm develops above the aortic valve, leading to left ventricular

outflow tract obstruction. The syndrome is also associated with hypercalcaemia and mental retardation

2. Infravalvular obstruction, caused by congenital fibrous ridges or diaphragms immediately below the aortic valve

3. Hypertrophic obstructive cardiomyopathy (HOCM) causes septal thickening sufficient to obstruct outflow from the left ventricle

There are two important manoeuvres to perform during examination to differentiate between aortic stenosis and HOCM . . .

(a) Get the patient to *stand and squat*. **Standing decreases venous return to the heart and also decreases total peripheral resistance** (TPR). As a consequence, arterial BP, stroke volume (SV) and volume of blood in the left ventricle all also decrease. On squatting, these physiological parameters move in the opposite direction. The differing effects of standing and squatting on the murmurs of HOCM and aortic stenosis are outlined in the table below

(b) Get the patient to perform the *Valsalva manoeuvre*. **Straining against a closed glottis causes a decrease in the venous return to the right side of the heart**, akin to standing. There will shortly follow a decrease in left ventricular blood volume and arterial BP. Release of the Valsalva has the opposite physiological effect. The differing effects that the strain and release phases of the Valsalva have on the murmurs of HOCM and aortic stenosis are also shown in the table below

		Effect on murmur	
Manoeuvre	*Cardiovascular effect*	*HOCM*	*Aortic stenosis*
Standing / strain phase of Valsalva	↓ Left ventricular volume due to ↓ venous return; ↓ Vascular tone causing ↓ BP and ↓ TPR	↑ *Outflow obstruction causing* ↑ *intensity of murmur*	↓ *Blood volume ejected into aorta causing* ↓ *intensity of murmur*
Squatting / release phase of Valsalva	↑ Left ventricular volume due to ↑ venous return; ↑ Vascular tone causing ↑ BP and ↑ TPR	↓ *Outflow obstruction causing* ↓ *intensity of murmur*	↑ *Blood volume ejected into aorta causing* ↑ *intensity of murmur*

Station 2d

A 79-year-old female presents with a 2-week history of being increasingly unable to cope at home due to **shortness of breath**. She has a long history of **cough productive of fluffy white sputum** that has also worsened recently. She has presented acutely because she developed **sudden dense right-sided weakness** whilst sitting in her chair at home. Her family found her and brought her to A&E. By her own admission, the weakness has **now almost entirely resolved**. She admits to having had **St Vitus' dance** as a child.

On examination, you observe a well-nourished, **flushed-looking** woman with **clear bilateral pitting oedema** to her mid-thigh. She is **tachypnoeic**, respiratory rate 25 b.p.m. There is no clubbing or cyanosis. Her heart rate is 99/min, **irregularly irregular** and the volume of the brachial pulse appears weak. Blood pressure is **110/83**. JVP is at the earlobes. Apex beat is impalpable. Auscultation of the heart with the bell at the apex reveals a **rumbling mid-diastolic murmur** with *no* pre-systolic accentuation. There are florid fine crepitations throughout both lung fields. Full neurological examination **fails to find any focal neurological signs**. Gait, speech and higher mental functioning all appear normal. Chest radiograph shows Kerley B-lines, 'bat's wing' peri-hilar oedema, bilateral effusions and upper lobe venous diversion, as well as moderate cardiomegaly. Her ECG is shown opposite . . .

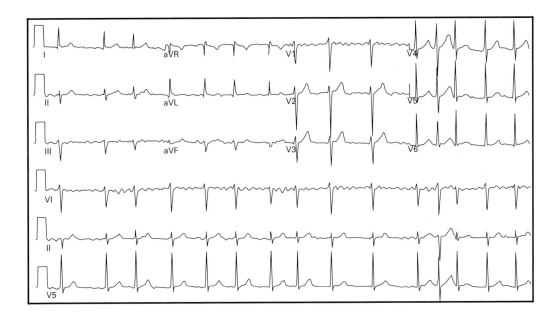

Q. What valve lesion does this woman most likely have?

A.

She has ***mitral stenosis***, as evidenced by: signs of congestive cardiac failure, history of transient ischaemic attack, history of rheumatic fever, malar flush, atrial fibrillation, peripheral oedema and the classical murmur of mitral stenosis.

Q. Is the history of St Vitus' dance relevant?

A.

Definitely. St Vitus' dance is the old term for **Sydenham's chorea**, the late developing chorea that occurs in association with rheumatic fever. Sufferers fidget, displaying spasmodic unintentional movements, and speech is often affected.

Rheumatic fever is an inflammatory disease affecting children and young adults secondary to infection with Lancefield group A β-haemolytic **streptococci**. The condition mainly affects heart, skin, joints and the CNS. Manifestations do not occur as a result of infection with the bacterium directly, but instead as a consequence of the autoimmune reaction that develops. Over half of all patients developing acute rheumatic carditis will go on to develop chronic valvular disease, predominantly of the mitral and aortic valves. The *Duckett–Jones criteria* are used to diagnose rheumatic fever, and are shown below. The diagnosis can be made when either two major *or* one major plus two minor criteria are present.

Major criteria . . .	*Minor criteria . . .*	*. . . Plus!*
Carditis	Fever	Evidence of antecedent streptococcal infection (i.e. positive throat swab, elevated ASO titre or recent history of scarlet fever)
Polyarthritis	Arthralgia	
Chorea	Past history of rheumatic fever	
Erythema marginatum	Raised ESR/CRP	
Subcutaneous nodules	Leukocytosis	
	First-degree heart block on ECG	

The following pages give a summary of the findings in all four of the valve lesions discussed above, and is the great majority of what you should know regarding valve lesions for undergraduate medical finals in the UK.

OSCEs

	Mitral stenosis	Mitral regurgitation	Aortic stenosis	Aortic regurgitation
Causes	Almost all due to rheumatic fever. Commoner in females	50% due to rheumatic fever. Also caused by prolapsing mitral valve, any condition causing left ventricular enlargement, bacterial endocarditis, HOCM, connective tissue or collagen disease, and MI	Three causes: rheumatic fever, congenitally bicuspid valve, and old age (causing wear-and-tear and calcification)	Usually rheumatic fever or bacterial endocarditis. Rarely, aortic dissection, syphilis, arthritides, hypertension and connective tissue disorders
Pathophysiology	Valve orifice shrinks→ ↑left atrial pressure→ hypertrophy and dilation of left atrium→ ↑pulmonary venous pressure→ pulmonary oedema→ ↑pulmonary arterial pressure→ ↑right heart pressure→ right heart hypertrophy, dilatation and failure	Chronic regurgitation into left atrium→ left atrial dilatation→ ↓left ventricular stroke volume→ left ventricular dilatation	Obstructed left ventricular outflow→ ↑left ventricular pressure→ left ventricular hypertrophy→ ischaemia of left ventricular myocardium→ angina, arrhythmias and left ventricular failure	Regurgitation into left ventricle during diastole→ left ventricular dilatation → ↓coronary perfusion due to diastolic run-off and less mechanically efficient left ventricle → cardiac ischaemia and dysrhythmias
Complications	Tricuspid regurgitation, atrial fibrillation, systemic embolization, pulmonary hypertension, lower respiratory tract infection, endocarditis	Atrial fibrillation, pulmonary hypertension, left- and right-sided cardiac failure	Angina, dysrhythmias, left-sided heart failure	Angina, dysrhythmias, left-sided heart failure
Symptoms	None until valve orifice markedly stenosed. Dyspnoea earliest symptom. Cough productive of blood-tinged sputum. Frank haemoptysis. Right-sided failure→ ↑JVP, oedema, ascites, hepatomegaly common	Often takes years to develop symptoms. Increased stroke volume may be sensed as palpitation. Dyspnoea develops as left heart fails. Fatigue, lethargy and cachexia develop. Thromboembolism is less but bacterial endocarditis is more common than in mitral stenosis	Symptoms usually develop with exertion. Syncope, angina, dysrhythmias and dyspnoea develop. Prognosis is abysmal once symptoms develop	Often take years to develop. Symptoms of left heart failure, pounding palpitations, angina and dyspnoea develop Dysrhythmias are far less common than in aortic stenosis

Apex beat	Thrusting, displaced, hyperdynamic	Sustained and obvious, heaving, undisplaced, palpable systolic thrill in aortic area	Thrusting, displaced, diffuse, palpable systolic thrill	Tapping, undisplaced, parasternal heave if right side of heart involved
Heart sounds	Essentially normal S1 and S2	Soft S2 due to immobility of the aortic valve. Reversed splitting of S2. Systolic ejection click	Soft S1 due to incomplete apposition of the valve cusps. S3 present due to rush of blood back into dilated left ventricle in early diastole	Loud S1 if mitral valve not completely stenosed. Opening snap just after S2
Murmur	High-pitched, early diastolic, best heard at left sternal edge using diaphragm with patient sitting forward and holding breath in end-expiration	Ejection systolic, diamond-shaped, rough, loudest in aortic area, radiating widely over praecordium and into carotids	Pan-systolic, blowing, radiating across entire praecordium and into axilla	Low-pitched, rumbling, mid-diastolic, best heard with bell at apex with patient leaning to left side. Pre-systolic accentuation will only occur if patient is not in atrial fibrillation
Additional signs	Austin–Flint mid diastolic murmur at right sternal edge indicates passage of regurgitant jet of blood from aorta into left ventricle, hitting the mitral valve leaflets. Pulse is bounding and collapsing. Also look for Quincke's, deMusset's, Duroziez's and pistol shot femorals signs. Wide pulse pressure	Small volume, slow-rising pulse. Narrow pulse pressure		Graham–Steell early diastolic murmur in pulmonary area indicates passage of regurgitant jet from pulmonary artery into right ventricle, hitting tricuspid valve leaflets
CXR	Big left ventricle. Possible dilatation of the ascending aorta	Normal heart size. Prominent dilated aortic root. Calcified aortic valve	Big left atrium and ventricle→ cardiomegaly. Calcified mitral valve	Small heart. Big left atrium. Pulmonary oedema. Calcified mitral valve

Continued on p. 228

	Mitral stenosis	Mitral regurgitation	Aortic stenosis	Aortic regurgitation
ECG	Bifid P-wave (*P mitrale*). Tall P if pulmonary hypertension present (*P pulmonale*). Right ventricular hypertrophy — right axis deviation, tall R in V1	*P mitrale*. Left ventricular hypertrophy — deep S V1–3, tall R V4–6. Atrial fibrillation	Left ventricular hypertrophy. Left ventricular strain — ST and T ↓ in leads V_{3-6}. Usually sinus rhythm. Ventricular dysrhythmias	Left ventricular strain and hypertrophy. Dysrhythmias. May be atrial fibrillation if mitral annulus has been enlarged sufficient to cause regurgitation
Echo	Anterior and posterior leafets of mitral valve do not separate, instead they move forward together. Diastolic fluttering of tricuspid valve leaflets	Dilated left atrium and ventricle. Doppler shows regurgitant jet(s)	Thickened, calcified, immobile aortic valve. Left ventricular hypertrophy. Pressure gradient across valve on Doppler study	Vigorous cardiac contraction. Dilated left ventricle. Enlarged aortic root. Diastolic fluttering of mitral leaflets. Doppler shows regurgitant jet
Cardiac catheterization	Higher diastolic pressure in left atrium than left ventricle	Prominent left atrial pressure wave. Contrast into left ventricle regurgitates into left atrium	Pressure drop from left ventricle to aorta. If this exceeds 50mmHg, surgery reqired	Contrast into aorta regurgitates into left ventricle
Treatment	Prompt treatment of lower respiratory tract infections. Antibiotic prophylaxis of endocarditis. Diuretics for dyspnoea. Digoxin and anticoagulation for atrial fibrillation. Surgery if patient develops pulmonary hypertension	Prophylaxis of endocarditis is vital. Any evidence of cardiac enlargement warrants consideration of surgery	Warn against over-exertion. Treat angina. Prophylaxis of endocarditis. If severe pressure drop, requires valve replacement on bypass. Valvotomy little use	Prophylaxis of endocarditis is vital. Nearly always requires surgery. Perform before symptoms occur, otherwise results poor

OSCE station 3

Q. What are the causes of a mass in the right iliac fossa?
A.
- Carcinoma of the caecum
- Crohn's disease (usually an underweight, frequently young patient with scars from previous resections)
- Appendix mass or abscess
- Lymphoma
- Ileocaecal TB
- Ovarian tumour (NB ovarian tumours often rise out of the pelvis centrally)
- Transplanted kidney
- (Amoebiasis)
- (Schistosomiasis)
- (Carcinoid tumour)

Q. What would be your next investigation for this right iliac fossa mass?
A.
- Plain abdominal radiograph, looking for . . .
  - Obstruction (air/ fluid levels)
  - Calcification (tuberculosis)
  - Bowel wall oedema thickening (CD)
- Chest radiograph
  - TB
  - Metastatic disease
- Abdominal ultrasound scan
- Abdominal CT scan
- Small bowel meal and follow through for Crohn's disease
- Diagnostic laparoscopy

Q. What are the causes of a mass in the left iliac fossa?
A.
- Colonic carcinoma
- Diverticular mass
- Transplanted kidney
- Ovarian tumour
- Faeces

Q. What are the causes of an epigastric mass?
A.
- Hepatomegaly (see OSCE 4, p. 230)
- Gastric malignancy
- Pancreatic
  - Pseudocyst
  - Malignancy
- Lymphoma

Q. What are the causes of an enlarged kidney?
A.
- Renal carcinoma
- Hydronephrosis
- Hypertrophy of a solitary kidney
- Adult polycystic kidney disease
  - May have had a previous nephrectomy (for a painful non-functioning kidney) so that only one kidney is palpable
  - Cysts develop from all segments of the nephron during adolescence. Patients present with renal pain, treatment resistant hypertension, haematuria and stone symptoms
  - Renal failure occurs later in life (10% of chronic renal failure)
  - Various associations exist [see EMQ Answers 19 (2), p. 142]

Q. What are the symptoms and signs of uraemia?
A.
Clinical features of uraemia . . .
- Symptoms
  - Nausea, vomiting
  - Diarrhoea
  - Fatigue
  - Breathlessness:
    Anaemia
    Pleural effusion
    Pericardial effusion
    Impaired ventricular function
  - Weakness
  - Itching
- Signs
  - Pallor (anaemia)
  - Scratch marks (pruritus)
  - Bruising
  - Pericarditis (pericardia rub or effusion)
  - Hypertension
  - Oedema
  - Confusion
  - Muscle weakness
  - Fistula (for dialysis)

OSCE station 4

Q. What are the causes of hepatomegaly (without splenomegaly)?

A.

- *Malignancy*
  - **Secondary tumours** mainly
  - Primary hepatocellular carcinoma
  - Lymphoma
  - Leukaemias:
    CML
    CLL
    Myelofibrosis
- **Cirrhosis**
  - NB Late alcoholic cirrhosis causes a small fibrotic liver
- **Blood**
  - *Cardiac failure*
  - Tricuspid regurgitation (pulsatile liver)
  - Budd Chiari syndrome (hepatic vein thrombosis)
  - NB Hepatic engorgement can give abnormal LFTs (obstructive picture)
- **Bile**
  - Primary biliary cirrhosis
  - Common bile duct obstruction:
    Stones
    Strictures
    Tumours
    Lymph nodes
- **Infections**
  - *Viral hepatitis* A, B (D), C
  - Leptospirosis
  - Infectious mononucleosis
  - Others:
    TB, syphilis, brucellosis
    Tropical, e.g. malaria, kala-azar
- **Infiltrations**
  - Amyloid
  - Sarcoid
  - Wilson's disease
  - Haemachromatosis
  - Glycogen storage diseases

Q. What are the causes of splenomegaly?

A.

- **Blood**
  - Portal hypertension (late cirrhosis with a small liver)
- **Busy spleen**
  - Infections:

Hepatitis A, B (D), C
Leptospirosis (Weil's disease)
Infectious mononucleosis
Others:
  TB, syphilis, brucellosis
  Tropical infections, e.g. malaria, kala-azar
- Haematological malignancy:
  CML* and CLL*
  Polycythemia vera
  Myelofibrosis*
  Lymphoma
- Haemolytic anaemias (splenic filtration)
- **Others**
  - Connective tissue disease:
    SLE
    RA
  - Sarcoidosis
  - Amyloidosis

Q. What are the causes of hepatosplenomegaly?
A.
As above; however, haematological malignancy and infections feature more prominently.

Q. How can you differentiate an enlarged spleen from an enlarged liver?
A.
There is a mass in the left/ right hypochondrium extending down towards the pelvis. It moves with respiration. It is resonant to percussion (over lying air filled bowel). The upper border can be palpated (unlike a spleen or liver which have their upper pole under the ribs). You can ballot the mass bimanually assessing the size, shape and consistency. Look for abdominal scars (?nephrectomy on the opposite side). Look also for an AV dialysis fistula over the distil radius.

	Kidney	Spleen
Enlarges?	Inferiorly	To RIF
Ballotable?	Yes	No
Resonant?	Yes	No
Get above?	Yes	No

*Cause massive splenomegaly (as likely to be found in an examination)

OSCE station 5

A 48-year-old female sits in front of you in your OSCE. You are asked to take a thyroid-based history from her.

Q. What questions would you ask her?
A.

Has your weight changed recently?
'Oh yes, I've lost over a stone in the last 3 months alone.'

Have you been trying to lose weight?
'No.'

Has your appetite changed?
'It has. I eat like a horse and yet I continue to lose all this weight. In fact, I'm getting a bit concerned, as this is what happened to my mother shortly before she was diagnosed with cancer.'

Have you noticed any change in your behaviour?
'Not really, but my husband says that I've changed of late; that I'm crabby and irritable all the time. I just thought it was "the change", you know. He also says that I'm unable to sit still and I suppose he's right about that really. I just like to keep active.'

Have you noticed any weakness of your muscles?
'Not as such, though in saying that, I have noticed that of late I've found it a bit of a trial climbing up the stairs, especially if I'm carrying the washing.'

Have you noticed any trembling of your fingers or hands?
'It's strange you should say that, because just the other day I was writing a letter and I noticed that I couldn't stop my hand trembling. Now I'm beginning to notice it more and more, even when I'm holding a cup of tea.'

Have you had any palpitations?
'All the time. But that's nothing new, I've had them for years. I've got an irregular heart beat, you know.'

Are you as a rule a 'hot' or a 'cold' person?
'I'm always red hot. And sweat? I could sweat for England, even when everyone else in the room is perfectly happy with the temperature.'

Have you noticed any change in your bowel habit over the last year or so?
'Well I am a bit "looser" than I used to be in that department.'

Have you noticed any change in your appearance?
'Well my son says that my eyes are "goggly", but I don't really see any change.'

Have you noticed any changes in your vision?
'I do occasionally suffer a bit of double vision, mainly when I'm tired.'

Have you noticed any changes in your periods?
'Yes, they're becoming much more infrequent. Very hit-and-miss. But I suppose I'm at that time of life, aren't I?'

You are asked to perform a thorough examination of the person's thyroid status.

From the end of the bed you note a **thin**-looking woman who is very jittery and **fidgets** incessantly with her hands. You ask her to hold her hands out straight in front of her and close her eyes. You place a sheet of paper on top of her hands to accentuate the **very fine tremor** that is present. Her hands are **warm** and her palms are **flushed**. There is neither clubbing, swollen fingers nor periosteal bone formation. You palpate her pulse, and note a rate of 98/min, **irregularly irregular**. Blood pressure is **161/91**. JVP is not raised. In her face you note exophthalmos, and to confirm this you stand behind the patient, looking down from on top of their forehead to check that there is genuine protrusion if the eyeballs. You check for lid lag and there is none present. There is no clear loss of acuity, ophthalmoplegia or conjunctival oedema, and no goitre in the neck. The apex beat is normally located, but it is **hyperdynamic**. Heart sounds are normal and the chest is clear. There is no peripheral oedema, although there is evidence of a rash on both shins. Comprehensive neurological examination reveals questionable wasting of the limb girdle musculature, and **decreased power** in both pectoral and pelvic muscles (MRC grade 4).

Q. What is the cause of this woman's clinical situation?
A.

This woman is hyperthyroid and is displaying nearly all of the characteristic signs and symptoms. Like all types of thyroid disease, hyperthyroidism is more common in females, patients with autoimmune disease and those with a family history of thyroid disease.

Q. What are the common causes of hyperthyroidism?
A.

The commonest cause of hyperthyroidism, and the only one associated with thyroid eye disease, is **Graves' disease**. It is due to autoantibodies directed at the **TSH re-**

ceptor. It typically causes a **fluctuating** clinical picture, with alternating relapse and remission.

Other causes of hyperthyroidism include . . .
- **Toxic multinodular goitre**: difficult to treat, traditional antithyroid drugs rarely successful
- **Single toxic adenoma (Plummer's disease)**: similarly difficult to treat
- **Iatrogenic hyperthyroidism** (excessive levothyroxine replacement)
- **Drug-induced hyperthyroidism** (e.g. due to lithium, amiodarone)
- **Transient thyroiditis** (e.g. de Quervain's viral-mediated transient thyroiditis, post-partum thyroiditis)
- **Thyrotoxicosis factitia** (patient takes thyroxine, but attempts to conceal this)

Q. What investigations would you perform to confirm your diagnosis?

A.

In all cases of primary hyperthyroidism, **TSH will be suppressed**, and this is the initial investigation of choice. When this is combined with a **raised serum T_3 or T_4**, then the diagnosis of hyperthyroidism is made. **TSH-receptor autoantibodies** will be present in cases of Grave's disease, but these are not commonly measured. Surprisingly, the microsomal and thyroglobulin autoantibodies associated with hypothyroidism are also often found in Grave's disease.

In very rare situations, a pituitary tumour will be the cause of hyperthyroidsim, and TSH will be raised. The differing laboratory findings in thyroid diseases are summarized in the table below . . .

Thyroid state	*Thyroxine (T_4)*	*Triiodothyronine (T_3)*	*TSH (pituitary)*	*TRH (hypothalamus)*
Hyperthyroidism				
Graves' disease	Raised	Raised	Decreased	Decreased
Toxic multinodular goitre	Raised	Raised	Decreased	Decreased
Pituitary tumour	Raised	Raised	Raised	Decreased
Hypothyroidism				
Primary	Decreased	Decreased	Increased	Increased
Secondary	Decreased	Decreased	Decreased	Increased
Tertiary	Decreased	Decreased	Decreased	Decreased

Q. What are the treatment options available?

A.

Treatment of hyperthyroidism is complex, and depends on the underlying cause and the clinician's choice. In general, however, it can be split into three options . . .

1. **Radioiodine**: a safe treatment option that usually leads to euthyroidism in **3–6 months. I^{-131}** is given and it accumulates in the thyroid, destroying the gland. The patient should be rendered euthyroid before treatment is given, with anti-thyroid medicaitons

2. **Antithyroid drugs**, e.g. carbimazole, propylthiouracil, methimazole: if these are going to work, they will usually restore a euthyroid state in **4–12 weeks**. They are less likely to lead to permanent remission than either of the other main treatment options, and long-term therapy may be necessary. Side effects can be severe, and include hepatotoxicity, vasculitis and agranulocytosis

3. **Surgery**: the least favoured treatment option of non-neoplastic causes of hyperthyroidism because of the morbidity, expense and free availability of alternative effective treatments. The procedure of choice is a sub-total thyroidectomy, and this should only be performed in patients rendered euthyroid with antithyroid drugs. The drugs should be stopped 2 weeks before surgery and **potassium iodide** given to reduce the vascularity of the gland

Whatever treatment option is chosen **β-blockers** are a useful adjunct to treatment because they block the sympathetic side effects that are so distressing in hyperthyroidism. Propranolol also has the ability to **block peripheral conversion of T_4 to T_3**.

Q. What is thyroid storm?

A.

This is also known as thyrotoxic crisis, and is a condition

with a **20–50% mortality**, despite optimal management. It occurs as an exaggerated manifestation of hyperthyroidism, and is precipitated by **major stressors**, such as infection, trauma, major surgery, diabetic ketoacidosis, MI, CVA, PE and withdrawal of thyroid medications. It presents with an **overactivated sympathetic nervous system** (palpitations, tachycardia, tachyarrhythmia, cardiac failure, anxiety, agitation), and typically a **very high fever**. Jaundice is a late and ominous sign.

Diagnosis should be made clinically, as thyroid function tests often fail to be grossly deranged. Treatment is . . .

- ALS stabilization of airway, breathing and circulation
- Commencement of an **intravenous fluid infusion**
- **β-blocker infusion** to block adrenergic effects
- **Cooling blankets**
- **Paracetamol**
- **Propylthiouracil** to block production of new T_4
- **Iodine** to block release of pre-formed T_4

Do not give the iodine until the propylthiouracil has had chance to work (90 min) otherwise there is a risk of making the thyroid storm worse. Treat any precipitating factors that may be present.

OSCE station 6

You arrive at an OSCE station and are asked to **examine a patient's breasts** (this will almost always be on a dummy; hence, you would be expected to both *show* what you *would* do and *describe* what you *would* do because the limitations of the model mean that you cannot physically demonstrate what you would like the patient to do).

- **Introduce** yourself to the patient, stating full name and grade
- **Explain** what it is that you propose to do, and that there will be a nurse chaperone present at all times
- Gain **consent**
- Give the patient time to get undressed in private if she is not already de-robed
- Ensure that you have a **female nurse chaperone**
- Once undressed, uncover the patient from lower ribs upward
- Begin with **inspection**: inspect in a number of ways . . .
  - With the patient sitting comfortably at rest with her arms **by her sides**
  - With the patient's hands in the air **above her head**
  - With the patient's hands **on her hips**; ask the patient

to push in on her hips to tense the pectoralis musculature
  - With the patient **leaning forward slightly**
- On inspection you are looking for a number of things . . .
  - Obvious lumps or masses
  - Scars (previous neoplastic, augmentative or reductive surgery)
  - Sinuses
  - Bruising (old fine needle aspiration site)
  - Inflammatory changes in skin (*peau d'orange*)
  - Colour of skin (if darkened, may suggest previous radiotherapy)
  - Irregular skin thickening
  - Retraction
  - Dimpling
  - Asymmetry
  - Nipple changes [e.g. indrawing, eczema (Paget's disease), differing directions, inversion]
  - Lactation
  - Fungation or ulceration
- Move on to **palpation** of the breast tissue itself. The best position to have the patient in is **supine, with the hand behind the head**.
- There are a number of ways to palpate the mass of the breast; which one you use does not matter **as long as you cover the whole of the breast tissue**. Expect the palpation of a single breast to take **3 minutes**. Either . . .
  - Split the breast into four quadrants and palpate each quadrant in turn using small circular movements with the pads of the fingers, about the size of a 50 pence piece; *or* . . .
  - Start just anterior to the axilla and circle around the periphery of the breast in an ever-decreasing circle; *or* . . .
  - Start just anterior to the axilla and palpate circularly up and down the breast tissue moving from lateral to medial
- If you find any abnormality you must describe its . . .
  - **Site** on the breast (and on which breast): often giving a time in the *'o'clock'* form helps; also site within the breast (superficial or deep)
  - **Size** in cm
  - **Shape** (circular, ovoid, elongated)
  - **Surface** (regular or irregular)
  - **Consistency** (soft or hard)
  - **Tender** or non-tender
  - Overlying **skin** (tethered or mobile)
  - Underlying **fascia** (tethered or mobile)

- **Temperature** (any evidence of inflammation)
- **Transillumability** (can you shine a light through it or not)
- Once you have completely described it, move on to palpate the rest of the breast tissue from where you left off; just because you have found one abnormality does not mean there are not more to find (there usually are in the OSCE)!
- Describe each abnormality in the same way
- Once you reach the **nipple**, you must bi-manually palpate it by placing two fingers either side and gently rocking the nipple, with the specific purpose of palpating any masses behind the nipple, and also of expressing any abnormal secretions or galactorrhoea from the nipple itself
- Move on the **axilla** (it is best to sit the patient up again to do so) . . .
  - Begin with **inspection**, looking for signs of masses, infection (*hidradenitis suppuritiva*), rashes or unusual skin pigmentation (*acanthosis nigricans*)
  - Palpate any breast tissue you suspect to be deep in the axilla (do not forget that the **axillary tail of Spence** can reach far into the axilla in some women)
  - Then palpate for **lymph nodes**. Support the arm of the patient with your non-examining hand, and, starting as high in the axilla as you can, palpate the medial and lateral axillary walls, attempting to trap any nodes against the chest wall or medial humerus respectively as you do so. Warn the patient that this part of the examination may be the least comfortable
- Describe any abnormalities found in the same way as for a breast lump
- Complete your palpation by feeling for any enlarged **supraclavicular lymph nodes** *from behind*
- *Immediately* cover the patient up, thank them and turn to the examiner to present your findings

Be aware that you may get asked to examine a patient who has had a **previous mastectomy**. Do not panic! Begin by inspecting the mastectomy scar and axilla, looking for signs of masses or nodularity. Note especially the colour of the skin (radiation) and the presence of lymphoedema (impaired lymph drainage post-surgery). Move on to palpation: palpate *gently* along the scar (it is often exquisitely tender), and then move on to the rest of the chest wall in a similar way as if the breast was still present. Take special care in palpating the axilla, looking for lymphadenopathy.

The way to differentiate between the most common three breast masses is shown in the table below . . .

	Breast cyst	Fibroadenoma (breast mouse)	Carcinoma
Age of patient	Early middle age, aged 35–50 years; uncommon post-menopause except in women on HRT	Young, aged 15–30; rare after age 50 years	Older, aged 35–100+; usually patient is >50 years
Shape of lesion	Spherical	Spherical, discoid or lobular	Irregular
Consistency of lesion	Soft	Firm	Hard
Surface of lesion	Delineated from surrounds	Delineated from surrounds	NOT delineated from surrounds
Tender or not	Usually	Rarely	Rarely
Tethering	Moderately mobile	Very mobile	Commonly tethered to skin or fascia
Number of lesions at one time	Commonly multiple	Can be multiple, but usually single	Usually single

Continued

	Breast cyst	Fibroadenoma (breast mouse)	Carcinoma
Additional signs	Can be inflamed and hot. May transilluminate if skin overlying is thin		Retraction can be present

OSCE station 7

A 77-year-old obese man presents with a 12-h history of **increasing shortness of breath**, on a background of chronic ankle oedema and regular attacks of classical angina. There is no history of MI. You are asked to examine the patient . . .

From the end of the bed you note an **obese** patient who is **tachypnoeic** (RR 26 b.p.m.) with evidence of **peripheral cyanosis** and **oedema** to the mid-thigh. You note that around the bed there is a pink GTN spray, cigarettes and a huge clear plastic bag of medications. He has a **capillary refill time of 2–3 s**, cold peripheries, tar-stained fingers and koilonychia. Heart rate is **143, irregularly irregular**. Blood pressure is **93/65**. JVP is up to the level of the ears. There is moderate pallor of the conjunctivae, central cyanosis, xanthelasma, arcus sennilis and a deep groove is noticed that runs across the extent of the earlobe. The apex beat is impalpable. On auscultation of the heart you note a **soft first heart sound, reversed splitting of the second heart sound**, a **third heart sound** and a **pan-systolic murmur** loudest at the apex of the heart but audible over the entire praecordium. The lung fields demonstrate **bilateral fine inspiratory crepitations** extending from both bases to the mid-zones. You find that the oedema noted from the end of the bed is indeed **pitting**, and whilst sitting the patient forward to auscultate the lung bases, you also noted a degree of **sacral oedema**. On palpation of the abdomen you note a **4-cm expansile pulsatile mass** in the supraumbilical region that is non-tender, and a 1–2cm palpable liver edge. Dorsalis pedis and posterior tibial pulses are impalpable bilaterally due mainly to oedema. Popliteal pulses are present, and equal. The feet are cool, but pink, and are not painful to palpation.

Q. What would be the three most valuable initial investigations to undertake in this patient?
A.
1. ECG: demonstrates **irregularly irregular** rhythm, rate 156, with left axis deviation, bifid P-waves, pathological Q-waves in leads II, III and aVF, and mild ST segment depression in leads I, aVL, V5–V6. In other words, the ECG shows atrial fibrillation, P mitrale (?mitral stenosis), probable old inferior infarct (?silent) and ischaemia in lateral leads
2. CXR: shows cardiomegaly (cardio:thoracic ratio >50%), peri-bronchial cuffing, upper lobe venous diversion, 'bat's wing' peri-hilar oedema, Kerley-B lines, and bilateral pleural effusions. In other words, the patient has all the chest radiograph signs of cardiogenic pulmonary oedema
3. FBC: demonstrates haemoglobin of 9.9, white cell count of 15, MCV of 75 and platelets of 215. In other words, the patient has a microcytic anaemia (likely to be an anaemia of chronic disease), a raised white cell count suggesting infection somewhere, and a normal platelet count

Q. What would your initial management consist of?
A.
  A *Airway*: ensure protected airway safe
  B *Breathing*: high flow oxygen, check respiratory rate and oxygen saturations, auscultate chest
  C *Circulation*: check heart rate and blood pressure, auscultate the heart
  D (in this case) *Diuretics!* Usually in the form of IV frusemide
    Also stands in this case for *digoxin*, because the patient is in fast atrial fibrillation, compounding the acute-on-chronic heart failure. Remember, give digoxin in chronic AF to rate control where cardioversion is unlikely to be successful, and give amiodarone in acute AF to chemically cardiovert where this is likely to be successful.

Following these initial manoeuvres, one must monitor all vital signs carefully. **Urine output should be monitored**, usually by the introduction of a Foley catheter. If the patient is significantly dyspnoeic, the administration of **intravenous diamorphine** in titrated amounts will alleviate the subjective distress. **Nitrate venodilation** in the form of sublingual spray or tablet, or indeed an intravenous GTN infusion, will alleviate some of the stress placed on the heart by decreasing preload, though this should only be used when the systolic BP is over 100 mmHg. Repeated doses of diuretic can be given, as dictated by the blood pressure response (Swan–Ganz catheter insertion may help guide therapy). If all of the above manoeuvres fail to improve the patient's situation, then consideration should be given to introduction of **inotropic agents**. This is usually done on the coronary care unit, or intensive care. In situations of acidosis, consideration of non-invasive positive pressure ventilation (NIPPV) can be made.

Q. What are the most common causes of heart failure?
A.
Although the heart usually fails as a whole, it is theoretically possible to split up cardiac failure into predominantly left- and right-sided entities (see table below). When right- and left-sided cardiac failure co-exist, the term 'congestive cardiac failure' is used. It is also possible to split cardiac failure into 'predominantly systolic failure', 'predominantly diastolic failure', 'acute failure' and 'high-output failure' (see MCQ [1], p. 49).

Causes of left-sided cardiac failure	Causes of right-sided cardiac failure
Chronic myocardial damage secondary to ischaemic heart disease	Left-sided cardiac failure
Systemic hypertension	
Aortic valve disease	Chronic lung disease
Mitral valve disease	Tricuspid valve disease
	Pulmonary valve disease

OSCE station 8

Q. Take a history from this patient with dyspepsia. What features in the history and examination of a patient with dyspepsia would give you cause for concern?
A.
Ask about . . .
• **Age >50 years**
• **New symptoms** or recurrent

• Pain features
  • Onset
  • Duration
  • Location
  • Radiation
  • Aggravating and relieving factors
  • Effect of food:
    DU improved by food (patients may gain weight)
    GU relieved by food
• Appetite and **weight loss**
• **Swallowing**
  • **Dysphagia (especially for solids)**
  • Reflux
  • Waterbrash (an unpleasant acidic fluid in the mouth; associated with GORD)
• **Premature satiety**
• **Vomiting**
• **Symptoms of anaemia**
  • Breathlessness
  • Tiredness
  • Dizzyness
• Alteration in bowel habit
  • **Melaena**
• Previous treatment
  • Use of antacids plus other over the counter medicines, e.g. H_2 antagonists
  • Previous *H. pylori* eradication
  • Surgery
• Risk factors
  • Previous endoscopies and other investigations
  • Previous treatment including *H. pylori* eradication therapy
  • **Family history of upper GI malignancy**
  • **Smoking history**
  • **Alcohol history**
  • NSAID usage (even prophylactic low dose aspirin)
  • Warfarin therapy
  • Previous endoscopy/ *H. pylori* eradication therapy

(**Emboldened features are concerning**)

Q. Do all patients who present with dyspeptic symptoms require an initial endoscopy?
A.
No. As dyspepsia is a common problem and the likelihood of finding malignancy in the young is low, **only patients who have alarm symptoms or who are newly presenting over the age of 50 years** require prompt endoscopy.

Q. What is the approach to the initial management of dyspepsia?

A.

- Following a history and examination, unless there are 'alarm symptoms' or the patient is over 50 years of age; patients can be given appropriate life-style advice (smoking, alcohol and weight loss) and a trial of antacids can be given
- Those that fail to resolve are tested for their *H. pylori* status, and given eradication therapy if positive
- Those patients who fail to improve need go onto endoscopy

See diagram summarizing the process below:

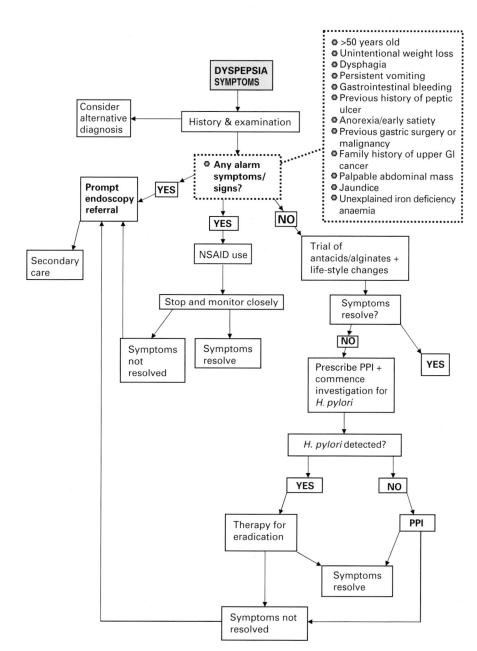

Q. *What is the role of H. pylori in dyspepsia?*
A.

- *Helicobacter pylori* is found in 50% of the population. Person-to-person spread is suggested on epidemiological grounds. It is more common in the lower socio-economic classes
- Found in **90% of patients with DU**. However, only 15% of patients who are infected get a DU. Chronic inflammation occurs especially in the laminia propria layer of the antrum of the stomach. The exact mechanism of the resultant increase in acid production is unclear
- Eradication of *H. pylori* will lead to resolution of symptoms and their non recurrence for the majority of patients (only 5% relapse compared to 60% relapse rate in those not treated)
- **Found in 70% of patients with GU**
- **Strongly associated with gastric cancer**. Chronic infection with *H. pylori* leads to a chronic superficial gastritis, which in some patients progresses to intestinal metaplasia (columnar epithelium). This change is premalignant

Q. *How is H. pylori detected?*
A.

- **Breath testing**: *H. pylori* produce a urease enzyme that cleaves ammonia and CO_2 from urea. If given ^{14}C-labelled urea orally, $^{14}CO_2$ can be measured in the breath. A sensitive and specific, non-invasive test
- **Direct urease testing** of gastric biopsies at endoscopy. The gastric biopsy is placed on a gel containing urea and a pH indicator which changes colour if ammonia is produced indicating *H. pylori* infection
- **Serology**: non-invasive but remains positive for long periods after eradication therapy, making the effectiveness of eradication difficult to asses by this method

Q. *Should all patients found to have H. pylori be given eradication therapy?*
A.

- Yes. Even those found to be positive at endoscopy who are have otherwise normal examinations (so called non-ulcer dyspepsia)
- This is because the association of *H. pylori* with chronic inflammation, DU and gastric malignancy is so strong

Q. *What is Zollinger–Ellison syndrome?*
A.

A rare (1 in 1 000 000 of the population) **gastrin-secreting tumour**, usually of pancreatic origin (other sites include the stomach and duodenum). It may occur (30%) as part of the multiple endocrine neoplastic (MEN type I) syndrome, in which cases tumours are more likely to be malignant (normally 50%). The resultant hyper-gastrinaemia causes **multiple duodenal and gastric ulcers**, which are resistant to usual measures and proton pump inhibitors (PPIs). Diagnose by finding high fasting gastrin levels and CT scanning for the tumour location (however, many are less than 1 cm). Treatment is with very high doses of PPIs and surgery.

OSCE station 9

Q. *Take a history from this patient with asthma.*
A.

Key areas to cover include . . .

- **Family history of asthma or other atopic illness** (supportive for the diagnosis of asthma)
- **History of episodic . . .**
  - Wheeze
  - Shortness of breath
  - Cough
  - Chest tightness
  - Nocturnal symptoms
- **Symptom pattern in asthma**
  - Variable
  - Worse at night
  - Intermittent
  - Provoked by various triggers:
    Cold air
    Post-exertion
    Emotion
    Pets (cats and dogs)
    Dusts
    Drugs (NSAIDS and β-blockers)
- **Smoking history** (quantity, duration and attempts to quit)
- **Occupation** (especially dust, pollen and animal exposure)
- **Markers of severity**
  - Admissions to hospital (?ITU)
  - Visits to the A&E department

- Attends hospital outpatients (most asthmatics are managed in primary care)
- Recent use of steroids
- Days off work
- Limitation of activity
- Home nebulizer
- **Asthma medications**
  - Metered dose inhalers/ breath actuated inhalers
  - Nebulizers
  - Dose and frequency of use (especially β_2 agonists indicating possible need to increase prophylactics)
  - Spacer devices
  - Recent changes (?progression up the standard treatment algorithm)
  - **Inhaler technique:** have they been shown how to use them? Ask the patient to show you
  - Use of oral steroids recently (indicating exacerbations)
- **How is the asthma monitored and followed up?**
  - GP or consultant follow up?
  - Does the patient measure peak flow at home and keep a peak flow diary

Q. What is asthma?
A.
Asthma is reversible narrowing of the small airways. The narrowing gives rise to symptoms of dyspnoea, cough and wheeze. Predisposition to asthma occurs in atopy, which is an inherited (autosomal dominant with incomplete penetrance) tendency to produce excessive amounts of IgE in response to non-specific stimuli (cold air, dust, exercise, house dust mite). The other atopic illnesses are eczema, hayfever and urticaria. Often, immediate family members of an asthmatic patient frequently either have asthma or other atopic illnesses to a variable degree. Asthma can arise for the first time at any age.

The airway narrowing in asthma has three components . . .

1. **Smooth muscle spasm** and hypertrophy in the small airways. Hyperreactivity of airway smooth muscle in asthma is a characteristic feature
2. **Oedema due to inflammatory infiltrate** (mast cells, eosinophils and lymphocytes) in the walls of the small airways
3. **Mucus secretion** into the lumen of the small airways

Asthma affects 15% of the population and the incidence is increasing. This in part may be due to increased recog-nition by doctors. It is more common in western societies and one popular theory for this is that failure to be exposed to 'dirt' in infancy results in a failure of immune system conditioning (tolerance), and subsequent overproduction of IgE in response to a variety of immune stimuli.

Q. How is the diagnosis of asthma made?
A.
- Asthma can present in a variety of ways. However, cardinal symptoms include **cough, wheeze, chest tightness and shortness of breath**. Any of these should prompt the clinician to think of the possibility of asthma
- A **20% or greater variability in the peak flow rate** (of at least 60 L/min difference) on at least 3 days during a week of monitoring makes the diagnosis of asthma very likely
- The introduction of bronchodilator treatment (e.g. a 2-week course of prednisolone at 30 mg per day, or nebulized salbutamol 5 mg) should bring about an improvement of the peak flow rates and an improvement in reported symptoms

Q. What are the pitfalls in the diagnosis of asthma?
A.
- Patients **unfamiliar with peak flow measurement technique** often have spuriously lower peak flow rates when they first perform the test. Practice alone then brings about improvement, misleading the unwary clinician. Allowing the patient to record the peak flows for a week before introducing treatment can help avoid this
- **Compliance** with oral steroids; many patients are afraid of steroid side effects, so reassurance that short courses do not lead to long-term side effects is required
- **Poor inhaler technique**, if used for a diagnostic trial
- Patients with **intermittent symptoms** may have a normal peak flow measurement between episodes
- Many patients *with asthma* will have **peak flow variability <20%**
- **Using too low a dose of therapy for too short a trial period**
- The **diagnosis is not asthma**. Asthma must be differentiated from . . .
  - COPD
  - Cardiac failure

- Restrictive (fibrotic) lung disease
- Fixed local airway obstruction e.g. tumour, lymph nodes
- Bronchiectasis
- PEs
- Aspiration
- Anxiety/ hyperventilation

Q. Take a peak flow measurement from this patient.
A.
The test is in two parts . . .
1. The explanation, demonstration and measurement of the PEFR
- Assume the patient has no experience
- Explain the procedure and why it is helpful
- Demonstrate the technique to the patient first. Hold the peak flow meter by the sides so as not to impede the marker. Place your lips **around** the tube
- Ask the patient to perform the peak flow to maximum effort three times
- Give encouragement
- It is legitimate to comment if you feel the patient has not given maximum effort or if the technique was poor (unlikely in an examination as the patient is probably well practiced)
- Take the highest of the three values as the recorded peak expiratory flow rate
2. The comparison of the result with age, sex and height predicted normal values
- A normogram should be available to plot the peak flow against. The value is corrected for the patient's age and height

Q. What do you think of this result?
A.
- Remember that **severe asthma** is indicated by a peak flow value <50% of the *expected or best ever* and the **life-threatening asthma** by a peak flow <33%
- You would therefore like to know the patients best recent peak flow rate
- Isolated peak flow rates are less useful than observing a trend over a 2-week period of measurement
- The result must always be taken in the context of the clinical picture (i.e. reported symptoms and findings on examination); if the result is low, ask the patient if they know their best ever peak flow rate is within the last year. It is likely (if the patient appears well and not distressed) that the patient will have COPD and there-

fore will record chronically low values, with occasional further dips during exacerbations
- Remember also to make an assessment of the validity of the result (particularly if the value is low) in terms of the technique and amount of effort the patient performed the test with (frequently poor in clinical practise)

Q. What is the value of teaching the patient to measure and record their own peak flow rate at home?
A.
- Patients who keep a peak flow diary will develop good peak flow technique giving representative values
- It allows the patient to monitor their own asthma and seek medical help when the values dip
- It provides a record for the clinician as to the interval history since last seen
- Involves the patient in the management of the condition, and helps the patient to assume responsibility for it

Q. What is the stepped care management of asthma?
A.
The stepped care program for asthma is a set of guidelines produced by the **British Thoracic Society** for progressively increasing the intensity of treatment in asthma according to the severity of the disease. Patients are moved up the scale of treatment until their symptoms are controlled. (Some physicians argue, however, that new asthmatics should be given aggressive treatment initially to provide immediate control. Then this can be gradually scaled back.) Nevertheless, the guidelines provide a valuable scheme for routine asthma management.

Summary of British Thoracic Society adult asthma management guidance 2004
- **Step 1. Mild intermittent asthma**
  - Inhaled short-acting β_2 agonist used as required
- **Step 2. Regular preventer therapy**
  - Add inhaled steroid, e.g. beclomethazone 200–800 mcg/day
- **Step 3. Add on therapy**
  - Add inhaled long-acting β_2 agonist (LABA)
  - If still inadequate control, increase inhaled steroid to 800 mcg/day
  - If no response:
    Stop LABA
    Increase inhaled steroid to 800 mcg/day

Consider leukotriene receptor antagonist or SR theophylline
- **Step 4. Persistent poor control**
  - Increase inhaled steroids to 2000 mcg/day
  - Addition of fourth drug if necessary:
    Leukotriene receptor antagonists
    SR theophylline
    β_2 agonist tablet
- **Step 5. Continuous or frequent use of oral steroids**
  - Use lowest effective dose
  - Consider specialist referral

Regular review and stepping down of treatment should be considered after three months. A 25–50 % reduction in drug dosage is recommended at each step down.
[See EMQ 24 (4), p. 158 For the management of life-threatening asthma.]

OSCE station 10

You arrive at one of your OSCE skills stations and are asked to cannulate a peripheral vein on a mannequin . . .
- **Introduce** yourself
- **Explain** what you are about to do and why it is necessary: i.e. *'I am going to put a drip in your arm, which is a small tube through which we can give you fluids and medications. It involves a needle, though the needle is removed immediately after the drip is in place'*.
- Gain consent: *'Are you happy for me to go ahead?'*
- Get your **equipment** ready. For this procedure you will need . . .
  - An alcohol swab (e.g. a Steret ®)
  - A tourniquet
  - A selection of cannulae of differing sizes
  - A cannula dressing
  - Some gauze and tape (e.g. Micropore ®) in case you fail
  - 10 mL normal saline or water for injections
  - 10-mL syringe
- Place the tourniquet high in the arm, e.g. over the midpoint of the upper arm, and tighten it to a reasonable degree of tension
- Select a vein by sight and by palpation; acceptable sites in upper limb are dorsum of hand or antecubital fossa
- **Clean** the area of skin over the vein with the alcohol swab
- Take the cannula, remove the covering over the needle and tube
- With your non-dominant hand, exert tension on the skin distally so that it does not move when the cannula is inserted
- Insert the cannula at a shallow angle (20–30°) directly over the vein
- Continue to insert the cannula slowly but unerringly until you see flashback in the barrel of the cannula
- At this point, stop pushing on the cannula, slightly withdraw the needle so that its tip is no longer protruding from the end of the tubing (0.5 cm should do), then advance the entire length of tubing into the vein, with the needle *in-situ* to give the tubing a degree of rigidity
- Undo the tourniquet
- Remove the cap from the base of the needle of the cannula and hold it in your dominant hand
- With your non-dominant hand, exert pressure with thumb or forefinger over the end of the cannula in the soft tissues of the patient
- Withdraw the needle with your dominant hand, maintaining pressure on the end of the cannula with your non-dominant hand
- **Safely discard your sharp**: the only way to do this is to put it in a yellow sharps bin, not on the bed or in the kidney dish in which you have your equipment
- Cap the end of the cannula
- Secure the cannula in place with the adhesive dressing
- Draw up your flush, checking what it is and the **expiry date** on it (only normal saline or water for injections should be used for this)
- Flush the cannula with sufficient fluid to clear the length of tubing of blood
- Cap the cannula
- Tidy any spills
- **Thank** the patient
- Dispose of all your rubbish

It is important to be aware that on removal of the needle, you may wish to **take samples** from the cannula for various blood tests. Once the cannula has been flushed, it should not be used for taking blood samples. Rather than connect the cap to the end of the cannula, you may be asked to connect a bag of fluid to it. If you are, you should follow the following procedure . . .
- Look at the intravenous infusion prescription **carefully**: be sure of the fluid you are about to give. Is there any **additive** written up to go into the bag?
- Take the correct bag of fluid, in the **correct volume**: double check the type and volume of fluid required

- Inspect the **expiry date** and whether or not the fluid is clear (are there any **'floaters'**?)
- Feel the temperature of the bag of fluid: ensure it is not abnormally warm or cool
- Connect the bag to a **giving set**: aseptically, remove the tear-off seal from the fluid bag's port and the sheath from the sharp end of the giving set, and insert the sharp introducing device of the giving set through the port on the bag of fluid
- Be careful not to pierce the bag with the sharp end of the giving set
- Remove the cap from the other end of the giving set
- Ensure the flow limiting device (usually a wheel) is open
- Squeeze fluid into both chambers of the giving set so that they are half full each
- Over the sink, run all the air out of the giving set tubes to avoid air embolus in the patient
- Stubborn bubbles in the giving set can be encouraged upward by flicking the tube with the flow limiting device closed
- Re-check the prescription
- Connect the giving set to the cannula in the patient and commence infusion at the desired rate
- Tape down the tubes of the giving set to avoid the cannula being pulled out of the patient by the weight of the tubes

This procedure is essentially identical when **giving blood** with the exceptions of . . .
- A giving set with a **filter** should be used when giving blood
- A **warming device** may be necessary if the blood is straight out of the fridge
- Blood and blood products which have the potential of causing fatal transfusion reactions should be **triple checked**: the patient, their date of birth and blood group should be cross-checked against the label on the blood/blood-product, and this should be cross-checked against the separate form that is always issued with blood/blood products —**if in doubt as to compatability, don't give it!**

OSCE station 11

A 44-year old female presents to her GP with a 4-day history of **blurring of the vision in her left eye**, 'like looking through frosted glass'. She wears contact lenses and was initially concerned that it was a problem caused by these, but following 3 days without wearing them, the problem has persisted. She tells you that the vision **deteriorated even further following her aerobics class** last night, and the final straw was when she developed a mild but definite **aching within the eyeball** itself during the course of today. She goes on to tell you that a similar problem has occurred **twice over the last 6 months**, but has never before lasted so long, and she has never previously experienced this 'aching' sensation. When prompted she divulges occasional, intermittent numbness of the right side of her face, but that this has been 'nothing to worry about'. Otherwise, she is fit and well, visiting the gym three times per week.

On examination, the patient looks fit and well. Examination of the CVS, RS and GI system are unremarkable. You summarize your neurological examination as below . . .

GCS 15 (e4v5m6)
AMTS 10/10
Normal gait
Romberg's –ve
Speech normal

CNS

I	Not tested
II	Acuity: 6/6 R eye, 6/12 L eye
	Fields: grossly normal L+R
	Fundoscopy: **?swollen optic disc L eye compared to R**; otherwise NAD
	Pupils: equal and reactive to light and accommodation
	No inattention
III, IV, VI	Normal pupillary movements
V	Normal facial sensation
	Normal movement of muscles of mastication
VII	Normal facial movement
VIII	Grossly normal
IX	Grossly normal
X	Grossly normal
XI	Grossly normal
XII	Grossly normal

PNS

	Left arm	*Left leg*	*Right arm*	*Right leg*
Tone	Normal	Normal	Normal	Normal
Power	5	5	5	5
Reflexes	Intact	Intact	Intact	Intact
Babinski		Down-going		Down-going
Co-ordination	Normal	Normal	Normal	Normal
Sensation	Intact	Intact	Intact	Intact

Q. What is the likely diagnosis? What is the differential diagnosis?

A.

The most likely diagnosis given the age, sex and symptoms of this patient is one of **multiple sclerosis**, an autoimmune-mediated demyelinating disease of the CNS. The symptoms that she is describing acutely are those of **optic neuritis** — visual blurring and ocular pain. The vague sensory symptoms are also a clue towards MS. Such sensory symptoms are often forgotten or ignored by patient and physician, and the date of onset of MS is mistakenly taken to be the first occurrence of more spectacular symptoms such as visual loss or weakness, whereas it correctly should be the first time that the sensory symptoms occurred.

Multiple sclerosis can mimic just about any chronic disease of the CNS, and as a consequence, the differential diagnosis is wide (and complex!). The main differentials are . . .

- Adult-onset leukodystrophies
- Spinocerebellar degenerations (including Friedrich's ataxia)
- Neurosyphilis
- Wilson's disease
- Antiphospholipid syndrome
- Lyme disease
- Behçet's syndrome
- Subacute combined degeneration of the cord
- Brain tumour
- Arteritides

Q. What investigations are available to confirm/refute the most likely diagnosis?

A.

The diagnosis of MS is established in the main by **careful interpretation of clinical signs and symptoms**, including evidence of multiple levels of involvement of the CNS. This can be reinforced by a variety of non-diagnostic tests.

MRI scan of the brain and spinal cord shows abnormalities in >95% of patients with definite clinical MS. **Plaques of demyelination** are clearly seen, but these lesions are barely visible on CT scan of the same regions.

Sampling of cerebrospinal fluid will show the presence of **IgG oligoclonal bands** in 80% of patients with MS, indicating the presence of immunoglobulin to an as yet unknown antigen. The CSF may also show a lymphocytic or polymorphonuclear pleocytosis, especially during exacerbations of the condition. Note that **oligoclonal bands are not specific for MS**, and may be seen in any condition where there is demyelination, e.g. neurosyphilis, encephalitis, meningitis, cerebral lupus, etc.

Measurement of **visual evoked responses** (VERs) shows a **delay** compared to normal in 75%. **Auditory evoked responses** may also be measured, and these are delayed in 60% of patients.

Q. What is the treatment?

A.

Treatment can be split into supportive and therapeutic . . .

- **Supportive**
  - Treat all infections expeditiously
  - Complete bed rest during exacerbations
  - Intensive physiotherapy to combat the otherwise severe spasticity that develops
  - Benzodiazepines, dantrolene and tizanidine are effective in reducing spasticity
- **Therapeutic**
  - **Corticosteroids**: evidence that high doses may arrest progression and alleviate symptoms in acute exacerbation; not thought to alter long term prognosis

- **Immunosuppression**: thought to reduce the frequency of relapses; drugs used include azathioprine, methotrexate and cyclosporine; much debate remains as to the true beneficial effects
- **β-interferon**: reduces exacerbations by 30% over 2 years; also thought to slow progression of plaque formation and hence improve the prognosis. This therapy is expensive and cost–benefit balance has slowed its generalized introduction over the last few years; however, its use is now on the up, mainly in relapsing–remitting MS and in secondary progressive MS (see below)

Q. How may MS be classified?

A

Numerous clinical classifications have been postulated in MS. The one most widely accepted has eight different classifications . . .

1. *Relapsing-remitting MS:* the classical form. Often begins in late teens or 20s with a severe attack, followed by recovery. Further attacks occur at **unpredictable intervals**, affecting **unpredictable parts of the CNS**, with a steady baseline between attacks. Tends to transform into the secondary progressive form by the late 30s (see below)

2. *Primary progressive MS:* runs a steady deteriorating course without superimposed relapses. Rate of progression is variable, but in its worst form this pattern can terminate in death within a few years. Typically later age of onset

3. *Secondary progressive MS:* follows relapsing-remitting MS and takes the form of the primary progressive type

4. *Relapsing progressive MS:* patient has primary progressive form of MS, with superimposed relapses without significant recovery

5. *Benign MS:* MS where the patient is able to be gainfully employed or provide care for family for at least 10 years after the onset of the first symptoms. These patients have a normal lifespan with only occasional mild symptoms

6. *Spinal MS:* presents with symptoms and signs predominantly of spinal cord involvement from the outset and continues in the same fashion

7. *Neuromyelitis optica:* MS presenting with acute transverse myelitis followed by optic neuritis

8. *Marburg-variant MS:* rare and malignant form with a fulminating course. Leads to rapid deterioration and death

OSCE station 12

Q. Report on this chest radiograph.

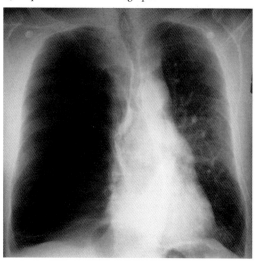

A.

Pneumothorax of the right side with complete lung volume collapse. There is evidence of mediastinal shift suggesting it is a *tension pneumothorax*

This case for obvious reasons will be dealt with theoretically, usually as an emergency question or chest film interpretation. Be prepared to describe the presentation and physical signs of acute pneumothorax or acute tension pneumothorax. Tension pneumothorax is a medical emergency because the 'valve' type leak can produce a rapid progression of increasing respiratory distress. Remember that chest pain is often the first symptom of a pneumothorax (particularly in small spontaneous pneumothoraces), followed by breathlessness.

Q. What are the possible examination findings in an acute tension pneumothorax?

A.

The patient would be (extremely) **distressed**, centrally **cyanosed** with **raised respiratory rate**. There would be **tachycardia and hypotension**. The **JVP would be elevated** (raised intrathoracic pressure in tension pneumothorax) and the **trachea would be deviated** (tension) away from the side of the pneumothorax. **Chest expansion is reduced** on the affected side and there is **hyperresonance** (in reality a difficult sign to elicit) on the affected side. **Breath sounds are reduced** on the side of the lesion.

Q. What is the approach to managing a pneumothorax?
A.
As chest drain insertion is such a potentially hazardous and unpleasant procedure, the approach to the management of pneumothoraces is to minimize their use to all but the most essential cases. Following oxygen therapy, the management of pneumothoraces can be divided as follows . . .

1. *Primary (spontaneous) pneumothorax*
- These patients have **no underlying pulmonary pathology**. They are **associated with smoking** and the rupture of small sub-pleural blebs is thought to be responsible. Commonly they occur in tall, thin young men. They should be **encouraged to stop smoking.**
- **Patients who require observation only**
  - Patient criteria:
  Young (<50 years of age)
  Small (air rim <2 cm) spontaneous pneumothorax
  Asymptomatic (or relatively asymptomatic) with no evidence of respiratory compromise
  - These patients can be **discharged** (with smoking cessation advice) from Casualty with an appointment for follow up in 1 week for repeat chest radiograph.
- **Patients who require aspiration**
  - These patients have either:
  Larger (**air rim >2 cm**) spontaneous pneumothorax, *or*
  Breathlessness
  - These patients require a **trial of simple aspiration**. If this is successful the patient can be discharged
  - If aspiration fails, repeat aspiration can be considered followed by discharge if this is successful
  - If repeat aspiration fails, an intercostal chest drain is inserted followed by admission. If this is successful the drain can be removed after 24 h (without clamping) and the patient discharged
  - If the intercostals drain fails, the patient should be referred to a chest physician for consideration of suction to the drain followed by referral to a cardiothoracic surgeon after 5 days
2. *Secondary pneumothorax*
- These patients have pneumothoraces **secondary to underlying lung disease,** e.g. COPD, pulmonary fibrosis, bronchiectasis

- These patients cannot be just observed
- **Aspiration as an initial measure**
  - Patient profile:
  Asymptomatic
  Young (<50 years of age)
  Small (air rim < 2 cm) pneumothoraces
  - Following successful aspiration, patients are admitted for observation for 24 h. If aspiration fails an intercostal drain is inserted.
- **Intercostal drain insertion initially**
  - Patient profile:
  Symptomatic
  Over 50 years of age
  Larger (air rim > 2 cm) pneumothoraces
  - If this is successful, the drain is removed after 24 h and the patient can be considered for discharge
  - If the drain fails to resolve the pneumothorax, the patient should be referred to a cardiothoracic surgeon

Q. Describe how you would perform an aspiration of a suspected pneumothorax.
A.
- Explain procedure to patient and obtain consent
- Sterile technique is employed
- Lignocaine is infiltrated into **2nd anterior intercostal space in the mid clavicular line** staying immediately superior to the third rib, so avoiding neurovascular bundle
- Slowly insert 16g venflon with 20-ml syringe with gentle aspiration until air is drawn back (not blood!). Leave the plastic tube of the venflon *in situ*, withdraw the needle and syringe and immediately replace with a 50-ml syringe connected to a three-way tap (turned such that the pleural space is not connected to the atmosphere)
- Proceed to aspirate air until the patient experiences any discomfort or starts to cough (suggesting successful reinflation), or if 2.5 L removed (suggesting continued air leak)
- Remove the venflon and immediately cover with airtight dressing. Then repeat the CXR

Q. *You are asked to see a 26-year-old male patient known to have advanced cystic fibrosis who has become acutely short of breath. You find an extremely distressed patient with central cyanosis, tachycardia and hypotension. His neck veins are distended and the trachea is deviated to the left. The chest is hyperresonant with reduced breath sounds on the right. Describe your immediate management?*

A.

- You would (if not already told by the examiner) **suspect a tension pneumothorax** as the diagnosis
- **Needle release:** you would immediately insert (do not wait for a chest X-ray) 16g venflon with an attached syringe containing saline. The plunger is then removed and the air bubbles up through the saline, which acts as a makeshift seal. The patient should improve rapidly
- The patient would be placed on **100% O$_2$** (unless COPD)
- Then you would request an **urgent portable CXR** and prepare to **insert a chest drain**

Q. *What are the indications for insertion of an intercostal chest drain?*

A.

- Pneumothorax
  - Tension pneumothorax (after needle release)
  - Recurrent pneumothorax following simple aspiration
  - Pneumothorax in a ventilated patient
  - Secondary pneumothorax where the patient is symptomatic or aged over 50 years
- Malignant pleural effusion
- Empyema
- Traumatic haemopneumothorax
- Postoperative after cardiac or thoracic surgery

Q. *Describe the procedure for insertion of an intercostal chest drain.*

A.

- Explain the procedure to the patient and obtain consent
- Ensure the CXR is to hand and correctly orientated
- Re-examine the patient
- Get the tubing and water seal container ready and ensure it all fits together properly
- Adopt no-touch sterile technique. Infiltrate the skin and subcutaneous tissue down to the pleura in the **5th**

intercostal space in mid-axillary line with 10–20 mL of 1% lignocaine

- Once skin is anaesthetized, make a 3-cm incision along the line of the intercostal space avoiding the neurovascular bundle. Have the chest drain ready with the trochar removed and discarded. Use a technique of blunt dissection down to the pleura using scissors and gloved finger
- A small hiss of air usually indicates that the pleural space has been entered. Insert the chest drain into the pleural space. A pair of large curved forceps may be used initially to help feed the tube into the chest. Feed the tube manually up towards the apex of the lung for 10–15 cm
- Immediately connect to sealed drainage system which should start producing bubbles; the water in the drainage system 'swings' with the respiratory cycle
- Use a 'purse string' suture and occlusive dressing to secure the drain. Repeat the chest X-ray to check the position of the drain

OSCE station 13

Q. *Examine this patient's abdomen for ascites.*

A.

- Introduce yourself and ask to examine the patient
  - Stand at the end of the bed and look for abdominal distension, also look from the side
  - Look quickly for other signs of chronic liver dysfunction (see OSCE 44, p. 303)
- **Examine for shifting dullness** by percussing laterally from the umbilicus to the flank (towards yourself) until the percussion note becomes stony dull. Without removing the percussing finger from the abdomen ask the patient to roll onto his opposite side (away from you). Then percuss again, the note now becoming resonant. Continue by percussing away from yourself, back to the midline with the patient still lying on his side until the note becomes dull again. Note that normally at least 1.5 to 2.0 litres of fluid must be present for there to be shifting dullness
- **Examine for a fluid thrill** by asking the examiner to help you by placing the ulnar border of his hand and distil forearm in the midline of the patient's abdomen. Demonstrate this to the examiner first. Tell the patient what you are going to do. Give a brisk flick

to the side of the patient's abdomen whilst feeling for a transmitted 'thrill' with the palm of your other hand placed on the opposite side of the abdomen. The examiners hand prevents skin transmission of the impulse

Q. What is the differential diagnosis of generalized abdominal distension?
A.

Fat, foetus, flatus, faeces and fluid.

Q. What are the causes of ascites?
A.

The common causes are **malignancy, chronic liver disease and congestive cardiac failure**.

The full list is similar to that for pleural effusions . . .
- **Exudates (protein content >30 g/L)**
  - Malignancy:
  Bowel
  Ovarian
  Liver
  Pancreas
  - Infection:
  Spontaneous bacterial peritonitis in ascites
  TB
  Surgical intra-abdominal sepsis
  - Inflammation:
  Acute pancreatitis
  Connective tissue diseases: RA, SLE
- **Transudates (protein content <30 g/L)**
  - Via portal hypertension:
  Congestive cardiac failure
  Chronic liver disease (although this is not the complete reason)
  Budd Chiari syndrome
  Constrictive pericarditis
  - Via hypoprotinaemia:
  Nephrotic syndrome
  Malnutrition
  - Via SIADH:
  Hypothyroidism

Q. What is the mechanism causing ascites in chronic liver disease?
A.

The cause of ascites in liver disease is multifactorial . . .
- **Hypoalbuminaemia** reduces plasma oncotic pressure

- **Secondary hyperaldosteronism due to reduced renal blood flow** and reduced metabolism of aldosterone leads to salt and water retention
- **Portal hypertension**
- **Nitric oxide** (failure of liver metabolism) results in vasodilatation, further secondary hyperaldosteronism and is implicated in the pathogenesis of hepatorenal syndrome

Q. How would you manage ascites in a patient with chronic liver disease?
A.
- **Restrict oral sodium** intake (40 mmol/day)
- **Bed rest**
- **Spironolactone** (an aldosterone antagonist) **and frusemide** used in combination to create a diuresis. Note that diuretics should be used to produce a gradual diuresis with a weight loss of about 0.7 kg/day. Renal function should be monitored for rising creatinine. Stop if >180 mmol/L or if hypokalaemia develops
- **Monitor daily weight, U and Es and urine output**: aim for 500 g loss in weight per day to avoid hypovolaemia, hyponatraemia, uraemia and hepatorenal syndrome. Note that diuretics can precipitate hepatic encephalopathy and hepatorenal syndrome
- **Perform a diagnostic tap of the ascetic fluid** to check features of infection. Note that a neutrophil count >250/mm^3 can be used as sufficient evidence to assume infection, prior microscopy and culture
- **Drain the ascites** (paracentesis; see below) to . . .
  - Relieve patient discomfort
  - Allow eating
  - Prevent respiratory compromise
  - Remove 5 L only

Q. What is transjugular intrahepatic portosytemic shunting (TIPS)?
A.

TIPS is a method of relieving portal hypertension. A guide wire is passed into the jugular vein and down the IVC and into the portal vein. A metal catheter is then pushed into the hepatic tissue until a connection is made into a portal vein. The resultant channel then drains blood from the portal system directly into the IVC. It is used for . . .
- Ascites refractory to diuretics
- Re-bleeding from oesophageal varices after sclerotherapy has failed

Q. Describe how you would perform paracentesis.

Q. Perform paracentesis on this model.

A.

Paracentesis is performed using a 'Trocath' peritoneal dialysis catheter, which has numerous side perforations down its length. The catheter is introduced under aseptic conditions in the midline ≈3 cm below the umbilicus following infiltration with local anaesthetic and a 5-mm skin incision. The catheter is inserted using its trocar *in situ* but with one gloved had holding it firmly 5cm from the tip to prevent trauma once the tip has passed through the layers of the abdominal wall. The catheter is then fed into the pelvic area over the trocar, which is simultaneously removed. The catheter is fixed to the skin by taping down the metal plate that slides over the catheter and lies next to the skin. It is then connected to the drainage tube.

Note that draining the ascitic fluid can precipitate hypovolaemia due to rapid reaccumulation from the circulation; therefore, co-administration of a plasma expander (e.g. dextran, human albumin solution) is used to help prevent this. The procedure should be avoided if the patient has renal impairment or very advanced liver failure.

Q. What tests would you perform on the ascitic fluid?

A.

- Neutophil count (?bacterial infection)
- Amylase (?pancreatitis)
- Protein content (?exudates or transudates)
- Gram stain, microscopy and culture (?bacterial infection)
- Cytology (?malignancy)

Q. What are the risks of ascites?

A.

- **Spontaneous bacterial peritonitis**: a very serious complication thought to be due to haematogenous spread of organism. The incidence is in the order of 10% per year amongst cirrhotic patients with ascites, but rare amongst people with non-cirrhotic ascites. There is 50% mortality. Often expected features of pain and high temperature may be absent, so suspect in those patients where there is a clinical deterioration. Diagnose on a raised neutrophil count (>250/mm^3) on paracentesis. Suspect TB if cells predominantly lymphocytes. Take cultures (inoculate into blood culture

bottles) and start IV antibiotics immediately (e.g. cefotaxime)
- **Impairment of respiration** due to splinting of the diaphragm

OSCE station 14

A 76-year-old man presents to A&E having **suddenly collapsed** at the golf club upon rising from a seated position following eating his evening meal. On falling, he banged his head on the dining table. When questioned by the doctor, the patient admits to noticing that **his heart 'thumped'** in his chest, 'as if it missed a beat', although he does state that he has noticed this phenomenon before, and it has not been associated with subsequent collapse. There was a doctor present in the club-house, who told the ambulance crew that following the collapse, the patient was **very pale**, and in the immediate post-collapse period, **his arms 'jerked a little'** and it was **very difficult to feel any pulse** at all at the radial or carotid artery. In his past medical history, the patient has a **recent diagnosis of heart murmur** made by the GP, and nil else. He takes no regular medications. You are asked to examine the patient . . .

On examination from the end of the bed, you note a **pale but otherwise well-looking** patient, GCS currently 15. He has a **2-cm laceration** on the right forehead above the eye, which is not bleeding. His heart rate is **59, regular.** His pulse is of **normal character and volume.** His blood pressure is **105/61.** There is no postural drop. There is no conjunctival pallor. JVP is normal. Auscultation of the heart reveals a grade 2–3 **ejection systolic murmur**, loudest in the second right intercostal space, but audible over most of the praecordium. Auscultation over the carotids is unremarkable. His lung fields are clear. The abdomen is soft and non-tender. There is no evidence of peripheral oedema. He has no focal neurological signs. His ECG is entirely normal, showing sinus rhythm, rate 61.

Q. On the basis of the history and examination, what is the most likely cause of the collapse?

A.

It is most likely that this patient has had a syncopal episode brought on by a combination of **bradyarrhythmia** and **post-prandial splanchnic diversion of cerebral blood supply.** The evidence for this is in the subjective sensation of palpitation just before collapse, the recent diagnosis of heart murmur, the post-prandial timing of the collapse, the demeanour around the time of collapse, his thready, difficult-to-feel pulse at the time, and the relatively quick recovery.

Syncope is defined as '*loss of consciousness and postural tone due to transient global cerebral hypoperfusion*'. There are myriad causes of syncope, summarized in the table on p. 250, along with a number of syndromes that classically masquerade as syncope. The cause of the patient's collapse is **unlikely to be related to his heart murmur**, because he has the murmur of aortic *sclerosis*, and none of the signs of aortic *stenosis* (slow rising pulse, narrow pulse pressure, murmur that transmits to the carotids, cardiac failure), so this is a red herring. Another red herring is the jerking of the patient's arms around the time of the collapse. **Jerking is *not* always related to epilepsy**, and it is not uncommon for the hypoxia present during a syncopal episode to lead to a small degree of jerking of the limbs. This is to be distinguished from true grand mal epilleptiform collapse, where there will commonly be rhythmic and violent jerking of limbs and trunk, tongue biting, loss of continence and a drowsy post-ictal phase. Distinguishing between causes of syncope is not easy and requires assimilation of numerous investigations before a definitive cause can be assigned.

Q. What three investigations would you perform on the patient during his stay in Casualty?
A.
1. **ECG**: vitally important in all cases of collapse where the cause is unknown, especially in this patient who has complained of palpitations and is still mildly bradycardic. ECG alone provides the diagnosis in 5% of cases of syncope, and it may guide further investigation by revealing structural/ functional/ biochemical abnormalities. These further investigations may include echocardiography, Holter monitoring, tilt-table testing, angiography and blood biochemistry tests
2. **Lying and standing BP**: given the history of the patient, a lying and standing blood pressure check is vital to discover whether orthostatic syncope played a role in his collapse. **Medications** are the commonest cause of a significant (>15 mmHg) drop in systolic or diastolic BP when going from a lying to a standing BP, and a thorough review of medications is indicated in all patients presenting with a significant discrepancy in lying and standing BPs
3. **Skull X-ray**: do not let elucidating the causes of a syncopal episode distract you from treating the consequences. Typically, patients collapsing due to cardiogenic syncope do so **without aura or warning** and commonly injure themselves with varying severity. In this patient a skull radiograph will suffice to rule out a fracture, though if he had a fluctuating GCS, confusion, severe headache or focal neurological signs, a CT scan of his head would be indicated

Q. Does this patient require admission to hospital, given that he has entirely recovered from his symptoms?
A.
The decision on whether to admit patients who have undergone a suspected syncopal episode can be difficult, especially if the patient themselves have recovered, and are keen to go home. As a rule, *strong indicators* of need for admission are . . .
- Patients with heart disease or likely cardiogenic cause of collapse (i.e. patients with history of coronary artery disease, cardiac failure, or abnormal ECG findings)
- Patients with chest pain accompanying the collapse
- Patients who have had a stroke or focal neurological signs/symptoms in association with the collapse

More *moderate indicators* of the need for admission include . . .
- A collapse during exertion
- Advanced age (>70 years)
- A sudden collapse with associated injury
- Moderate postural drop in BP
- Increasing frequency of collapses
- Poor social support

OSCEs

Problem	Mechanism	Precipitating factors	Predisposing factors	Prodromal manifestations	Postural associations	Recovery
Vasodepressor syncope – the 'simple faint' or 'neurocardiogenic syncope'	Sudden peripheral vasodilation, especially in skeletal muscles without a compensatory rise in BP. BP falls	Strong emotions, e.g. fear, pain	Tiredness; hunger; hot humid environments	Restlessness, weakness, pallor, nausea, salivation, sweating, yawning	Usually occurs when standing, though can occur whilst sitting	Prompt once lying down. Pallor, weakness, nausea and slight confusion can persist for a time
Postural hypotension, or 'orthostatic syncope'	*Inadequate vasoconstrictor reflexes* causing venous pooling, decreased cardiac output and hypotension	Standing up	Peripheral neuropathies; disorders of the autonomic nervous system; antihypertensives; vasodilators; prolonged bed rest	Usually none	Patient stands from sitting or lying; becomes light-headed	Prompt once lying down
	Hypovolaemia causing inability to maintain cardiac output and BP, especially in the erect posture	Standing after haemorrhage or dehydration	GI bleeding; trauma; potent diuretics; vomiting; diarrhoea; polyuria	Lightheadedness; fast palpitations upon rising to stand	Patient stands from sitting or lying; becomes light-headed	Improves once lying flat, but may not resolve if the hypovolaemia remains uncorrected

Cardiac syncope						
Arrhythmias (Stokes–Adams disease)	Decreased cardiac output due to tachy- or bradyarrhythmias	A sudden change in rhythm	Organic heart disease; old age	None; loss of consciousness occurs suddenly	Can occur in any position	Prompt return to normal unless hypoxic brain damage has occurred (rare)
Aortic stenosis and hypertrophic cardiomyopathy	Vascular resistance falls with exertion but cardiac output cannot rise	Exertion	Cardiac disease	None; particularly sudden onset	During or immediately after exertion	Prompt once exercise has ceased
Myocardial infarction	Sudden arrhythmia or decreased cardiac output	Variable	Coronary heart disease	None	Any position	Variable
Massive pulmonary embolism	Sudden hypoxia or decreased cardiac output	Variable	DVT	None	Any position	Variable
Cough syncope	Increased intrathoracic pressure causing decreased venous return to the heart	Severe paroxysm of coughing	COPD	Cough	Any position	Prompt once coughing has ceased

Continued

Problem	Mechanism	Precipitating factors	Predisposing factors	Prodromal manifestations	Postural associations	Recovery
Micturition syncope	Unclear	Emptying bladder, usually after getting out of bed to pass urine	Male sex; nocturia; old age; prostatism	None	Standing	Prompt
Disorders resembling syncope . . .						
Hypocapnia	Hyperventilation and hypocapnia lead to cerebral vessel constriction	Stressful situations	Predisposition to anxiety attacks and hyperventilation	Dyspnoea; palpitation; chest discomfort; numbness and tingling	Any position	Only once hyperventilation stops or patient breathes into bag
Hypoglycaemia	Not enough glucose to maintain cerebral metabolism	Fasting	Insulin therapy	Sweating; tremor; palpitations; hunger; headache; confusion; abnormal behaviour; coma	Any position	Variable, depending on severity of hypoglycaemia and speed of treatment
Fictitious faint	Patient feigns faint to avoid stressful situation	Stressful situation	Hysterical personality; psychiatric history	Variable	Any position; rare to see injuries	May be prolonged and variable

OSCE station 15

A 74-year-old right-handed female presents to Casualty following an episode of **collapse** at home. Her husband states that she was making breakfast when she 'came over queer'. She sat down and progressively, over the course of a few minutes, developed **pins and needles** down her right arm and leg, and subsequently developed **severe weakness** of the right arm and leg which has now progressed to the extent that she is unable to move either right arm or right leg. She has also developed **slurring** of her speech, and when given a cup of tea by the nurse at triage, was **unable to swallow** it without choking. The patient denies headache, dizziness or loss of consciousness. There is no history of head trauma. You are asked to perform a full neurological examination on the patient . . .

On examination, you note from the end of the bed that the patient is leaning to the right, and is not moving either right arm or leg. You also note some drooping of the right corner of the mouth. You summarize your neurological findings as below . . .

GCS 15 (e4v5m6), significant slurring of speech

CNS

I	Grossly normal
II	Acuity: 6/6 L+R eyes
	Fields: grossly normal L+R
	Fundoscopy: normal L+R, no papilloedema
	Pupils: equal and reactive to light and accommodation
	Right-sided inattention
III, IV, VI	Normal pupillary movements
V	Normal facial sensation
	Normal movement of muscles of mastication
VII	**Flatness of nasolabial fold on right; weakness of right side of mouth** (orbicularis oris); no other noticeable weakness of facial movement — can wrinkle forehead, raise eyebrows and close eyes tightly bilaterally
VIII	Grossly normal
IX	Grossly normal
X	Chokes upon swallowing water
XI	Grossly normal
XII	Grossly normal

PNS

	Left arm	Left leg	Right arm	Right leg
Tone	Normal	Normal	Hypotonic	Hypotonic
Power	5	5	0	0
Reflexes	Intact	Intact	Absent	Absent
Babinski		Down-going		Up-going
Co-ordination	Normal	Normal	Affected by weakness	Affected by weakness
Sensation	Intact	Intact	Globally decreased	Globally decreased

Gait is not assessable due to right leg weakness. AMTS is not assessable due to difficulty with speech, although there is no evidence of confusion. Initial assessment of speech reveals that the patient has slowed, slurred speech that is appropriate, but is reduced in amount. The patient appears frustrated by her lack of ability to speak.
Examination of CVS, RS and GI systems are unremarkable.

Q. What has happened to this patient? Where is the likely lesion?

A.

This patient has had a stroke. Given the hemiplegia, it is likely that an infarction has occurred in the middle cerebral artery supplying the internal capsule of the brain on the left side (giving contralateral signs). The fact that the infarction has affected speech in this right-handed woman further suggests that the problem is in the left side of the brain (the dominant hemisphere in a right-handed person). The stroke appears quite extensive, given that it is also affecting the facial nerve in an upper motor neurone lesion pattern (contralateral side, lower face only).

Q. What are the differences between an upper motor neurone lesion and a lower motor neurone lesion?
A.
The term 'upper motor neurone (UMN) lesion' refers to any lesion affecting proximal systems of motor control, beginning at either motor cortex of the cerebral hemi-spheres, through the internal capsule, through the decus-sation of the corticospinal tracts in the medulla of the brainstem, down to where the corticospinal tracts termi-nate, either in the motor nuclei of cranial nerves, or the anterior horn cells of the spinal cord. UMN lesions are also known as 'pyramidal' lesions.

The term 'lower motor neurone (LMN) lesion' refers to any lesion affecting peripheral systems of motor con-trol, from the cranial nerve nucleus or anterior horn cell proximally, through the peripheral nerve, to the motor end-plate.

The symptoms caused by these distinct patterns of motor nerve lesion are summarized in the table below . . .

UMN lesion	*LMN lesion*
Drift: outstretched arms drift downward and medially on affected side; forearm tends to pronate and fingers flex	**Fasciculation**: caused by visible contractions of individual motor units; electrical sampling shows fibrillation potentials
Weakness: acute lesions (e.g. internal capsule stroke) cause sudden dense hemiparesis; progressive lesions (e.g. neoplasms) cause progressive hemiparesis affecting extensors before flexors in arms, and flexors before extensors in legs; lesions above medulla cause contralateral weakness, those below medulla cause ipsilateral weakness	**Weakness**: in LMN lesions, the weakness is of *all* muscle groups in the affected region, i.e. weakness of flexors = weakness of extensors
Loss of skilled movement: fine finger and toe control diminishes	**Muscle contractures**
Increase in tone — spasticity: initially following acute UMN lesion, the patient's limbs will be flaccid, but increased tone follows within a few days owing to loss of inhibitory effects of corticospinal pathway; hypertonia preferentially affects stronger muscles; resistance to movement typically fluctuates — 'clasp knife' rigidity (suddenly gives way); clonus will accompany the increased rigidity	**Decrease in tone — flaccidity**
Hyperreflexia: patient with acute UMN lesion is initially arreflexic, but within a few days becomes hyperreflexic, with extensor plantar reflexes in the affected leg	**Arreflexia**
No muscle wasting	**Muscle wasting**: becomes clinically apparent within 3 weeks of lesion
Normal electrical excitability of muscles	**Trophic changes in skin and nails**

Remember that everything goes down in a LMN lesion — power down, tone down, reflexes down, muscle bulk down and plantars down.

Common causes of UMN lesions can usually be split into one of two patterns . . .

- **Hemiparesis** (weakness of the arm and leg of one side of the body): usually caused by a lesion **within the brain**, e.g. haemorrhage, infarction, tumour, trauma, plaque
- **Paraparesis** (weakness of both lower limbs): usually caused by a **spinal cord lesion**, e.g. plaque, tumour, trauma, compression

Common causes of LMN lesions can be divided based on where the lesion is on the nerve . . .

- **Cranial nerve nuclei**: Bell's palsy, MND, poliomyelitis
- **The anterior horn**: cervical and lumbar disc protrusion
- **Peripheral or cranial nerve itself**: nerve trauma, nerve entrapment, mononeuritis multiplex

Q. What are the common clinical patterns of stroke, based on cerebral blood supply?
A.
The blood supply to the brain is via the **common carotid and the vertebrobasilar arteries**. These come together at the base of the brain to form the circle of Willis, comprising the **anterior, middle and posterior cerebral arteries** (with anterior and posterior communicating arteries). A simplistic way to think of cerebral blood supply is that the anterior cerebral artery supplies blood to the antero-superior part of the brain; the posterior cerebral artery supplies blood to the postero-inferior part of the brain; and all the important bit in between is supplied by the middle cerebral artery (including the speech areas; the middle cerebral also supplies a branch to the macular cortex of the occipital lobe, vital for normal visual functioning).

Strokes may be classified based on this blood supply . . .
- **Anterior circulation (carotid territory) stroke**: this is split further into . . .
  - *Middle cerebral artery syndrome*: total occlusion (also known as a **TACI** — total anterior circulation infarct) leads to contralateral hemiplegia, hemianaesthesia, homonomous hemianopia, deviation of head and eyes towards side of lesion. If affecting left side of brain, more likely to cause global dysphasia. If affect-

ing right side of brain, more likely to lead to unilateral neglect of contralateral side. However, branch occlusions are more common than total ones (also known as **PACI** — partial anterior circulation infarct), and these lead to incomplete syndromes, e.g. branch occlusion of upper middle cerebral artery leads to expressive (Broca's) dysphasia, whereas branch occlusion of the lower middle cerebral artery leads to receptive (Wernicke's) dysphasia
  - *Anterior cerebral artery syndrome*: total occlusion leads to contralateral paralysis of the leg (leaving the arm spared), gegenhalten rigidity (patient opposes all attempts at movement of their limb), perseveration (constant repetition of a meaningless or inappropriate word or phrase), contralateral grasping reflex and urinary incontinence
- **Posterior circulation stroke** (also known as **POCI** — posterior circulation infarct), which leads to . . .
  - *Posterior cerebral artery syndrome*: ataxia, vertigo, diplopia, visual field defect (hemianopia or quadrantanopia), mild contralateral hemiparesis and hemianaesthesia, dyslexia, memory loss
- **Lacunar infarction** (also known as **LACI**): infarcts in small penetrating vessels — the lacunar arteries — leading to a number of bizarre pure or mixed motor or sensory syndromes; often a consequence of hypertension

---

OSCE station 16

Q. Take arterial blood gases from this patient (dummy).
A.
A frequent OSCE station. The candidate is asked to demonstrate (on a dummy) the technique for arterial blood gas sampling either from the radial artery or from the femoral artery, or comment on blood gas analysis data.
- Explain the procedure to the patient and obtain informed consent (dummy): it is a painful procedure
- Palpate the radial artery where it is superficial to the distal radius at the wrist. Use two fingers lightly so as not to occlude the vessel and carefully plot out the direction of the vessel
- Note that different blood gas syringe packs (a larger needle for the femoral stab) exist
- The syringe contains heparin to prevent coagulation of the sample. This must be expelled after pushing the plunger up and down to coat the syringe

- Warn the patient of the impending 'sharp scratch' and introduce the needle **slowly** with bevel facing the direction of flow (towards the heart), either perpendicular or slightly angled (bevel tilted up) to the skin
- The flash back of blood should spontaneously fill the gas syringe without the need for aspiration. Remove the sample having some cotton wool to press firmly on the puncture site as soon as the needle is removed
- Advice is given to the patient to press firmly for a short time, or engage an assistant if the patient is not able to do this
- The needle of the syringe should be made safe by insertion in the rubber bung provided or else removed and the syringe capped
- The sample must be analysed immediately or else put in ice for urgent transfer to the lab

You should be familiar with various patterns of acid–base disturbance. (See EMQ 9, p. 96)

OSCE station 17

A 71-year-old female is presented to you in your OSCE. You are asked to examine her.

From the end of the bed you note a pale, mildly obese woman with **dry, straw-like hair** and rather masculine features. It is a sunny May afternoon and she is wearing an overcoat and a bobble hat. When you introduce yourself to her she **speaks slowly**, in a gruff low voice. Her pulse rate is 62 and regular. There is no tremor of her hands, though they are cold. Her BP is 149/89. Her central pulse is of normal character and volume. Her JVP is not elevated. There is mild pallor of her palmar creases and conjunctivae. There is no central cyanosis, though her tongue is large. Her apex beat is normally located and is of normal character. Her heart sounds are normal with no added sounds or murmurs. Her chest shows a few mild bi-basal crepitations on auscultation; otherwise there is good air entry throughout. Her abdomen is soft and non-tender. There is mild pitting ankle oedema. On comprehensive neurological examination, you note only that the patient appears **weak (power 4/5) in both upper and lower limb girdle muscles** (flexion at the hip, abduction at the shoulder) and has **reflexes that remain contracted longer than normal** following stimulation. She demonstrates mild ataxia and dysmetria on both the finger-nose and dysdiadochokinesis tests.

Q. This woman has an endocrine disorder. What is it most likely to be?
A.
This woman has the classical features of hypothyroidism. Hypo- is commoner than hyperthyroidism, affecting **5–8% of randomly screened populations**, and like all types of thyroid disease, is commoner in women, the elderly, those patients with autoimmune disorders and those patients with a family history of thyroid disease.

Q. If you had been asked to take a thyroid-based history on this patient, what questions would have been relevant?
A.
- *How are your energy levels?*
- *Has you weight changed over the last 6 months/ year?*
- *How is your appetite?*
- *Do you tend to feel hot or feel cold as a rule?*
- *How is your memory?*
- *Have you noticed any change in your appearance/ voice?*
- *How is your mood/ libido?*
- *Have you noticed any changes in your skin/ hair?*
- *Have you noticed any change in your periods?*
- *Have you noticed any change in your bowel habit?*

Q. Name three causes of primary hypothyroidism.
A.
The causes of hypothyroidism can be split into primary (**thyroid gland dysfunction**), secondary (**pituitary dysfunction leading to TSH deficiency**) and tertiary [**thyroid-releasing hormone (TRH) deficiency**] . . .

Primary causes of hypothyroidism
- **Hashimoto's and other forms of autoimmune thyroiditis:** the **most common** cause of hypothyroidism, occurring due to the presence of **microsomal autoantibodies,** leading to chronic lymphocytic infiltration of the gland, and subsequent fibrosis. Patients with Hashimoto's may have a goitre, and often have an initial phase of disease where they are hyperthyroid — known as **Hashi-toxicity.** Along with antimicrosomal autoantibodies, these patients typically have **antithyroglobulin autoantibodies**
- **Previous treatment for hyperthyroidism**
- **Subacute thyroiditis**
- **Iodine deficiency or excess:** especially seen in mountainous areas, leading to endemic goiter
- **Medications,** e.g. lithium, amiodarone
- **Genetic dyshormonegenesis;** when this is associated with sensorineural deafness, it is known as Pendred's syndrome

Secondary causes of hypothyroidism

- **Post-partum pituitary necrosis (Sheehan's syndrome)**: heavy post-partum bleeding leads to infarction of the pituitary
- **Space occupying pituitary neoplasm**
- **Infiltrating disease (e.g. TB)**

Tertiary causes of hypothyroidism

- **Hypothalamic granuloma (e.g. TB)**
- **Hypothalamic neoplasia**
- **Hypothalamic radiation**

Q. What investigations would you use to diagnose the patient?

A.

Serum thyroid stimulating hormone (**TSH**) is the most sensitive marker of thyroid dysfunction, and hence is used as the mainstay of diagnosis. Primary hypothyroidism can be diagnosed if the **level of TSH is high in the presence of low thyroxine (T$_4$)**. TSH may be low or normal in hypothalamic and pituitary disease, and a finding of a low T$_4$ in this situation suggests secondary hypothyroidism (see table, p. 232).

The finding of thyroid specific (e.g. microsomal or TSH-receptor) autoantibodies would help to confirm the diagnosis of autoimmune hypothyroidism. Other supportive findings would include **hyponatraemia**, **macrocytic anaemia**, elevated creatine kinase MM isoform (CK) and increased liver transaminase levels.

Q. What is the treatment?

A.

The treatment of hypothyroidism is by **oral replacement of levothyroxine** for the rest of the patient's natural life. Initial dose should be low: *start low, go slow*. The progress of treatment should be assessed at 4–6 weeks by measurement of TSH, the aim being to **restore it to as near normal levels as possible**. Dosage should initially be attenuated in patients who are elderly or have cardiac disease due to the risk of cardiac ischaemia. Full resolution of symptoms even when the patient is on optimal treatment can take up to 6 months. Always bear in mind the possibility of concurrent autoimmune conditions as a cause of persisting symptoms despite optimal treatment.

Q. What is myxoedema coma?

A.

This is a life-threatening complication of hypothyroidism with profound lethargy, **bradycardia** and **coma** accompanied by **hypothermia** (<35°C). A very important clue can be extremely slow-relaxing reflexes, progressing to **arreflexia**. It arises due to a variety of **physiological stressors**, such as infection, trauma, surgery, prolonged exposure to cold temperatures or sedative/ narcotic drugs. Mortality approaches **50%**, even if it is recognized and treated early. Treatment is with the ABCs, with mechanical ventilation if indicated (GCS < 8), **re-warming** (warmed IVIs, Bair-Huggers®) and intensive care unit monitoring. Drug treatment should incorporate **intravenous thyroxine**, glucocorticoids and intravenous hydration.

OSCE station 18

Q. Examine this patient's respiratory system.

The patient who may be **thin** and **dyspnoeic** has a respiratory rate of 24 b.p.m. There is (maybe) a square area of **telangiectasia over the sternum** (following radiotherapy). The sputum pot contains clear/ purulent/ blood-stained sputum. There is an oxygen mask/ nebulizer/ walking aid/ nutrient drink supplement beside the bed. There is **clubbing** of the fingers. There are **palpable lymph nodes** in the cervical area. There is facial flushing and **dilated veins over the anterior chest wall** (possible SVC obstruction). There is **stony dullness** at the left base (pleural effusion). There is a **fixed monophonic wheeze** (suggesting localized bronchial partial obstruction due to tumour).

The likely diagnosis is a carcinoma of the bronchus.

Q. Comment on this chest radiograph.

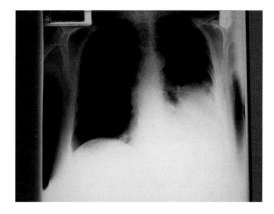

A.

There is a unilateral pleural effusion on the left side (most likely to be an exudate). A 5-cm round opacity can be seen above the effusion (partially obscured by the effusion). The likely diagnosis is carcinoma of the bronchus.

Other chest radiograph appearances of carcinoma of the bronchus include . . .
- Unilateral pleural effusion; no mass lesion seen
- Solitary 'coin' lesion
- Lobar collapse distil to an obstruction
- Hilar lymphadenopathy

Q. What complications of bronchogenic carcinoma do you know?

A.
- **Horner's syndrome**
  - Unilateral **ptosis, enopthalmos** (recessed eye)**, miosis** (small pupil) and **anhydrosis** (loss of sweating) over the orbital area
  - Due to an **apical lung tumour that has invaded the T1 sympathetic ganglion**
  - Remember that the pathway of the sympathetic innervation to the eye originates in the mid-brain and descends the cord to T1 and T2 where efferent fibres enter the sympathetic trunk and ascend to the stellate ganglion. Post-synaptic fibres ascend around the internal carotid artery and ophthalmic fibres pass along the ophthalmic division of the trigeminal nerve. Thus, any damage (e.g. tumour, trauma, demyelination, vascular event) that causes disruption to the sympathetic supply along its path may cause Horner's syndrome
  - **Differential diagnosis of ptosis . . .**
    Horner's syndrome (unilateral)
    CIII nerve palsy (eye down and out)
    Facial myopathy (bilateral):
       Myasthenia gravis
       Dystrophia myotonica
    Congenital:
       Congenital ptosis
       Congenital Horner's syndrome (the most common cause). Associated with heterochromia (different coloured irises)
    Structural, e.g. tissue laxity with age, lid pathology
- **Pancoast's syndrome**
  - Due to an apical tumour
  - Invasion of the lower trunks of the brachial plexus (C8 and T1)

- Intractable pain down the inner arm (all unexplained shoulder pain needs a chest X-ray)
- Wasting of the intrinsic small muscles of the hand occurs (T1)
- **Superior vena cava obstruction**
  - Dilated veins in the neck with collaterals over the anterior chest wall
  - Facial redness and oedema may occur
  - Morning headaches may occur
- **Hoarse voice**
  - Recurrent laryngeal nerve involvement (remember this loops down and through the aortic arch before passing back up to the larynx)
  - A chronic hoarse voice in a smoker always requires investigation
- **Invasion of mediastinum structures**
  - Oesophagus (dysphagia)
  - Aortic arch (massive haematemesis)
  - Phrenic nerve (hiccough, weak respiratory effort, elevated hemi-diaphragm on chest X-ray)
  - Pericardium (effusions, pericardial tamponade)
  - Throracic spine (cord compression and UMN signs in the legs)

Q. What are the various cell types of bronchogenic carcinoma?

A.
- **Small cell** carcinoma (APUD or oat cell)
  - 25% of cases
  - Early metastases occur
  - Ectopic hormones production may occur (ACTH, ADH, PTH)
  - There is no response to radiotherapy but chemotherapy improves survival minimally
- **Squamous cell** carcinoma
  - 35% of cases
  - Late metastasis
  - Cavitates
  - Radiosensitive
- **Large cell** carcinoma
  - 25% of cases
  - Early metastasis occur
- **Adenocarcinoma**
  - 20% of cases
  - Often in the lung periphery
  - *Not* related to smoking
- **Alveolar** cell carcinoma
  - 1% of cases
  - Often in the lung periphery

- Large volumes of mucus occur
- Associated with asbestos exposure

Q. How does carcinoma of the bronchus typically present?

A.

- Pneumonia (recurrent or non-responsive to treatment)
- Chronic cough
- Haemoptysis
- Chest pain or shoulder pain
- Weight loss

Q. What are the available treatments for carcinoma of the bronchus?

A.

- Only 20% are amenable to **surgery**, which offers the best chance of a cure (25% 5-year survival in selected cases)
- **Radiotherapy** can be used in palliation for bone pain and SVC obstruction
- Small cell tumours have a very poor prognosis (weeks) but are the only ones which have any response to chemotherapy (months)

Q. What features of bronchogenic carcinoma contraindicate surgery?

A.

Only 20% are amenable to surgery. Surgery is not possible if . . .

- The patient is too weak or debilitated
- The FEV1 is less than 1.5 L (respiratory reserve too small)
- Small cell tumours (have usually spread at time of diagnosis)
- Factors causing operative technical difficulty
  - Tumours close to the carina (within 2 cm of start of either main bronchus)
  - Phrenic or recurrent laryngeal nerve involvement
  - Pericardial involvement

Q. What is the relationship between smoking and carcinoma of the bronchus?

A.

There is a linear relationship between number of cigarettes smoked, duration of smoking and disease incidence except for adenocarcinomas (not related to smoking). Following stopping, risk declines over ten years to the base line again.

OSCE station 19

Q. Take a history and examine this patient who has experienced chronic diarrhoea and weight loss.

A.

The patient, who is **thin and pale**, may have a history of **bulky and loose stools** for weeks or months. There will be a history or evidence of significant **weight loss**. There is **apthous ulceration** in the mouth. The patient may be **breathless** (?anaemia), have **proximal muscle weakness** (?osteomalacea due to vitamin D malabsorption) and have **oedema** (hypoprotinaemia). The abdomen will be thin, non-tender, with no masses (?unless complicated by small bowel lymphoma). The history and examination findings suggest **malabsorption**, the most common cause in western countries being coeliac disease. **The diagnosis is coeliac disease.**

Q. What is the aetiology of coeliac disease?

A.

Allergy to gluten, especially the α-gliadin component, resulting in inflammation (largely T mediated) and sub-total villous atrophy of the jejunal mucosa. Gluten is contained in wheat, barley and rye cereals. Withdrawal of gluten from the diet reverses the pathological and clinical abnormalities.

Q. How and when does coeliac disease present?

A.

At any age but especially childhood and later life (1 in 1000 prevalence in the UK). The onset may be acute with diarrhoea, weight loss and abdominal pain or sub-clinical, with weight loss, lethargy and anaemia (especially the elderly).

Q. What are the associations of coeliac disease?

A.

- **Other associated autoimmune illness,** e.g. type I diabetes, hypothyroidism, Addison's disease, pernicious anaemia and fibrosing alveolitis
- **Other GI disease:** inflammatory bowel disease, small bowel lymphoma, splenic atrophy (Howell–Jolly bodies)
- **Skin diseases:** dermatitis herpetiformis
- **HLA types; B8 and DRW3** in 90%
- **Northern climates** (especially Ireland; it is suggested that the reliance on potatoes for carbohydrate fails to expose the immune system to gluten at a certain critical

point if life for the development of immunological tolerance)

Q. How is the diagnosis of coeliac disease made?

A.

- **Endomysial autoantibodies**: a good screening test for first-line investigation
- **Jejunal biopsy** and the finding of subtotal villous atrophy
- **Clinical improvement after withdrawal of gluten from the diet**

Q. What type of anaemia occurs in coeliac disease?

A.

- **Folate deficiency and iron deficiency**: giving a mixed blood picture of a macrocytosis and a microcytosis (dimorphic blood picture). Howell–Jolly bodies (nuclear remnants in the RBCs) are also seen due to splenic atrophy which may occur
- Vitamin B12 deficiency **is rare**: vitamin B12 absorption relies on functioning gastric mucosa to produce intrinsic factor to bind and transport the molecule, and the terminal ileum to absorb it. Coeliac disease involves the jejunum which is in between these critical areas

Q. Ask this patient who has had (chronic) diarrhoea some questions?

A.

Ask about . . .

- Duration of the illness
- Travel
- Contacts with cases of diarrhoea
- Weight loss
- Drugs
- Vomiting
- Blood in the stool
- Bulky loose motions (?steatorrhoea)
- Abdominal pain
- Fluid intake/ passing urine

Q. What is the differential diagnosis?

See EMQ 13 (5), p. 117.

OSCE station 20

You are asked to examine a patient without taking any history from them in your OSCE . . .

On examination from the end of the bed you note a slim, middle-aged female patient, who looks weak and miserable. You note several areas of vitiligo over her forearms and shins. She has a heart rate of 71, regular and a blood pressure of 130/82. There is a **postural drop** in blood pressure to 98/60 on standing. The patient has a normal JVP. On looking in her mouth, you see no evidence of central cyanosis, but there is **brown pigmentation of the gum line**. Her trachea is central. Her apex beat is undisplaced, her heart sounds are normal and her chest is clear. Her abdomen is **slightly tender** all over, and there is an apparent decrease in total body hair. An old hysterectomy scar appears brown. Neurological examination is entirely unremarkable.

Routine blood tests reveal . . .

Na$^+$	130 mmol/L
K$^+$	5.0 mmol/L
Ur	8.3 mmol/L
Cr	98 μmol/L
Haemoglobin	10.2 g/dL
WCC	6.1 x 10^9/L
MCV	90 fL
Platelets	290 × 10^9/L

Q. The examiner says to you that this patient has an endocrine condition. What is it likely to be?

A.

This patient has the typical nondescript signs of Addison's disease, a condition that gives classically vague, creeping signs and symptomatology. When something is wrong, but the clinical situation is vague, always have Addison's disease in the back of your mind. It has in the past been described as *'the unforgiving master of nonspecificity and disguise'*. Although the features are nonspecific and difficult to recognize, Addison's can be fatal if unrecognized and untreated, so it is vitally important to include it in the differential diagnosis where appropriate. The blood picture typically shows mild **hyponatraemia, normokalaemia, hyperuricaemia and a normocytic anaemia**.

Q. What questions would you ask to take a disease-focused history in this patient?

A.

The history in Addison's should encompass the following . . .

- Fatigue
- Weakness

- Depression (gloomy thoughts, disturbance of sleep, early waking, etc.)
- Weight loss
- Anorexia
- Dizziness on standing
- Abdominal pain
- Nausea
- Vomiting
- Diarrhoea
- Hyperpigmentation (especially of old scars)
- Vitiligo
- Symptoms of other autoimmune disease, including thyroid disturbance, pernicious anaemia, etc.

It is a very difficult history to take as there are no 'meaty' symptoms to get your teeth into.

Q. What is the pathogenesis of the condition?
A.
Addison's is **primary adrenocortical insufficiency due to destruction of the entire adrenal cortex**. This leads to deficiency of all adrenocortical hormones: glucocorticoid, mineralocorticoid and sex steroid production are all reduced. **Tuberculosis** is the leading cause worldwide, but in the UK the most common cause is **autoimmune** destruction of the adrenal cortex. This shows a marked **female preponderance** and is associated with the presence of other autoimmune diseases. Other, more rare causes of adrenocortical insufficiency include . . .
- Surgical removal
- Haemorrhage/infarction (occurs in meningococcal septicaemia—waterhouse–friderichsen)
- Infiltration (by malignancy or amyloid in amyloidosis)
- Adrenal leukodystrophy (Schilder's disease): the commonest cause of Addison's disease in males

Secondary adrenocortical insufficiency can be caused by disturbance in the hypothalamic-pituitary axis, but this is rare and leads only to a lack of glucocorticoid and sex steroid (mineralocorticoid production remaining intact due to stimulation by angiotensin II).

Q. What is the cause of the hyperpigmentation in this disease?
A.
In Addison's disease, lack of cortisol leads to positive feedback on the hypothalamus and pituitary, causing high levels of corticotrophin releasing factor (CRF) and adrenocorticotrophic hormone (ACTH) in the blood. It is the **persistently high levels of ACTH** that lead to the buccal hyperpigmentation and pigmentation of palmar creases, flexor regions and scars due to an effect on melanocytes within the skin.

Q. How is the diagnosis made?
A.
Once Addison's disease is suspected, investigation should be carried out expeditiously. The gold standard in diagnosing Addison's is the **ACTH-stimulation test** (Synacthen test; a synthetic ACTH analogue). There is both a short and a long version of the Synacthen test. The *short* Synacthen test is most commonly employed to demonstrate Addison's. Essentially, an intramuscular or intravenous injection of Synacthen is given at time 0, and blood cortisol levels are taken at times 0 and +30 min. A normal patient would be expected to show either a total cortisol greater then 600 nmol/L at +30 min, or a rise of greater than 330 nmol/L from 0 to +30 min. Patients with Addison's disease show an **absent or a diminished cortisol response**.

The value of random serum cortisol measurements is much debated. A high early morning cortisol (>550 nmol/L) almost rules Addison's out, and similarly a very low early morning cortisol is very suggestive of Addison's.

Other clues to the diagnosis include a hyponatraemia combined with a normo- or hyperkalaemia, a raised urea, hypoglycaemia, hypercalcaemia, mild normocytic anaemia, lymphocytosis, eosinophilia, and the presence of adrenal autoantibodies.

Remember also that Addison's disease is one of the medical causes of acute abdominal pain, along with inferior MI, diabetic ketoacidosis, basal pneumonia, sickle cell anaemia, gastroenteritis, thyroid storm, malaria and lead poisoning. These causes can be remembered with the following mnemonic: **S**urgeons **L**ove **B**eing **G**od, **T**hough **M**edics **D**isagree **A**bout **I**t!

- **S** Sickle cell crises
- **L** Lead poisoning
- **B** Basal pneumonia
- **G** Gastroenteritis
- **T** Thyroid storm
- **M** Malaria
- **D** Diabetic ketoacidosis
- **A** Addisonian crisis
- **I** Inferior MI

Q. What is the treatment?

A.

The treatment of Addison's disease is with . . .

- **Glucocorticoid replacement**: use the smallest dose needed to relieve symptoms, e.g. hydrocortisone 20 mg p.o. a.m., 10 mg p.o. p.m. Alter the dose based on clinical symptoms
- **Mineralocorticoid replacement**: e.g. fludrocortisone 100 µg q.d.s.
- Encourage salt and water intake
- Monitor potassium levels
- Increase glucocorticoid dose in times of stress, e.g. infection, surgery, fever. May need to double or triple the normally taken dose
- Advise wearing of **Medic-Alert®** bracelet

Acute hypoadrenalism can be fatal, and it is vital to recognize this early. It occurs due to deficiencies of salt, steroid and glucose, and presents with dehydration, hypotension, shock, acute abdominal pain, hypoglycaemia, fever and gross electrolyte disturbances. The treatment is ALS-based management of airway, breathing and circulation, with early, large-bore intravenous access. Give a **rapid infusion of 2–3 L of normal saline over 1 h**. Give a bolus injection of **100 mg hydrocortisone** and repeat every 6 h. Identify and treat the trigger. Dextrose should also be infused if the patient is hypoglycaemic. Consider invasive monitoring of filling with a central venous catheter. Many litres of intravenous fluid may be required if the patient is severely dehydrated. Mineralocorticoid replacement is not necessary acutely.

OSCE station 21

Although traditionally an uncommon OSCE station, with the advent of more sophisticated and more robust models, a station where the candidate is asked to perform a lumbar puncture (LP) is on the increase. You must know the theory and practice of how to perform this initially difficult practical procedure, even though it is relatively unlikely that you will have had chance to perform a significant number of these procedures as an undergraduate.

- **Introduce** yourself to the patient
- **Explain** what you are about to do — 'We need a sample of the fluid surrounding your spinal cord to help us manage your illness the best that we can. This involves us taking a sample of this from your back. You should only feel a little pushing since we will be using local anaesthetic on the skin. You may experience some discomfort during the procedure when we are taking the sample itself, and you may have a headache afterwards. There is a theoretical risk also of bleeding and infection'.
- Obtain **consent**
- Ensure that you have all the **equipment** you need . . .
  - Nursing assistance
  - Antiseptic solution (e.g. Betadine ®)
  - Local anaesthetic, with syringe and needle
  - Sterile gloves
  - Sterile surgical towels
  - Sterile gown
  - Spinal needle with stylet
  - Three empty sterile plain tubes labelled 1–3
  - One empty sterile chemical pathology tube (for protein and glucose analysis)
  - One empty sterile tube for meningococcal DNA analysis (usually an EDTA tube)
  - Gauze swabs
  - Dressing
- Place the patient in the preferred **position** for performing the procedure—either curled up in the left lateral decubitus position, or sitting up on the edge of the bed, hunched over a pillow or table; with either technique, aim for maximal forward flexion of the spine, whilst keeping the spine in line
- Palpate the **posterior superior iliac spines**, imagining a transverse line connecting the two across the back: this localizes the **L4–L5** area
- Palpate the space between the L4–L5 spinous processes; consider marking this space with an indelible pen
- Clean the area, and prepare the surroundings with sterile surgical drapes
- Infiltrate with plain 1% **lignocaine**, both superficially and deep, right down to the periosteum, which is exquisitely sensitive to the probings of spinal needles
- Take the spinal needle with the stylet *in situ* and insert it in the **sagittal plane**, angling slightly upwards toward the umbilicus
- Continue to advance until a slight 'give' is felt; withdraw the stylet and await the slow issuing forth of the straw-coloured cerebrospinal fluid (CSF)
- If there is no CSF forthcoming, replace the stylet and advance slightly further, removing the stylet and checking for CSF at frequent intervals

- Once CSF does appear, take **3–5 drops** into each of the numbered plain tubes in order of their numbering. Take a similar amount of CSF into the chemical pathology and meningococcal DNA tubes
- After you finish sampling CSF, replace the stylet into the needle, and withdraw the whole appliance *en masse*
- Exert pressure on the area with the sterile gauze swabs until all bleeding has ceased. Place sterile dressing over area
- Remove all sterile towels from the patient, **clean** them up, **thank** them, and instruct them to remain laying flat on their bed for at least 1 h. Even after this, they should only mobilize if absolutely necessary for a total of 3–4 h, during which hourly neurological observations and frequent checks on BP should be performed
- Dispose of your sharps carefully

If you are having trouble accessing the interspinous space at L4–L5, it is perfectly acceptable to attempt the same procedure at the L3–L4 interspace. Don't forget that the spinal cord ends at L1–L2, so even the L2–L3 space is safe if you are really struggling.

Q. What are the indications for LP?
A.
LP can be either **diagnostic** (meningitis, subarachnoid haemorrhage, encephalitis, meningeal carcinomatosis, tertiary syphilis) or **therapeutic** (administration of intrathecal drugs, benign intracranial hypertension).

Q. What are the contraindications to LP?
A.
1. Any **source of infection** along the potential path of the spinal needle is a contraindication to LP, e.g. cellulitis of the overlying skin, epidural abscess, etc.
2. Suspected significantly **raised intracranial pressure** is also a definite contraindication to LP, e.g. the patient who is vomiting, drowsy, bradycardic, hypotensive or has papilloedema. In this circumstance, to proceed without CT scan of the head would be seen as medico-legally indefensible
3. The third and final major contraindication to LP is the presence of **coagulopathy** or **anticoagulation therapy**

Q. What are the potential complications of LP?
A.
Despite being feared by the general public, the complications of LP are relatively few . . .
- **Herniation of the cerebellar tonsils:** if the intracranial pressure is very high or if there is a posterior fossa space-occupying lesion
- **Infection:** more likely if the patient has a bacteraemia
- **Post-procedural headache:** this occurs in approximately **one-quarter** of all LPs, starting from a few minutes to two days after the procedure. It is more likely to occur in young, female patients with a previous history of similar
- **Subdural or epidural haematoma:** very rare
- **Minor backache:** very common
- **Disc herniation:** theoretically possible if the needle is pushed far and hard enough, although in practice is rarely seen
- **Implantation of epidermoid neoplasms** and **aspiration of nerve roots** is much less likely if the needle used for the procedure has a stylet

---

OSCE station 22

Q. Examine this patient's respiratory system.
A.
The patient appears **breathless** from the end of the bed. The respiratory rate is raised at . . . . The patient has evidence of finger **clubbing**, there is fluctuance of the nail bed with loss of the nail fold angle and increased longitudinal curvature of the fingernails. There is no flap of CO_2 retention. The pulse is elevated at . . . . The patient has evidence of **central cyanosis** on inspection of the buccal mucosa. The JVP is normal (or elevated; suggesting cor pulmonale). The apex beat is normally located (or displaced laterally). The chest shape is normal. Chest expansion is normal and symmetrical. Tactile vocal fremitus and percussion of the chest wall are unremarkable. There are **fine bilateral end inspiratory crackles** at both lung bases heard to the mid-thorax.

The diagnosis is fibrosing alveolitis

Q. Comment on this chest X-ray?

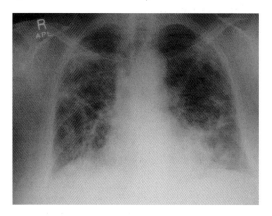

A.

The chest X-ray shows diffuse bilateral 'honey comb' reticular shadowing spreading from the bases. This suggests pulmonary fibrosis; the most likely diagnosis is fibrosing alveolitis.

Q. What is the differential diagnosis?

A.

The differential is that of lung fibrosis. The most common cause (especially in the elderly) is cryptogenic fibrosing alveolitis (CFA).

Other causes of pulmonary fibrosis

- **Pulmonary sarcoidosis** [see EMQ 16 (1), p. 123]
- **Extrinsic allergic alveolitis**
  - Various inhaler organic spores
  - Various types:
    Farmer's lung, due to *Micropolyspora faeni*
    Maltworker's lung, due to *Aspergillus clavatus*
    Humidifier fever
    Bird fancier's lung, due to feather proteins
  - Leads to recurrent inflammation and eventual fibrosis
- **Inorganic dust**
  - **Coal:**
    Simple pneumoconiosis: dust on the chest X-ray with micro-nodular shadowing; debatably little effect on lung function
    Progressive massive fibrosis: produces large upper lobe fibrotic masses and emphysematous changes. A large lung function deficit occurs, with a mixed obstructive and restrictive picture
    Caplan's syndrome: the occurrence of fibrotic

nodules in patients with coal dust exposure and rheumatoid disease
- **Silica:**
  Very fibrogenic even in small quantities with calcification of lymph node rim (egg-shell calcification)
- **Asbestos:**
  Various outcomes from asbestos exposure occur
  Any asbestos exposure is relevant no matter how brief or how long ago
  The outcomes include . . .
    Asbestosis: honeycomb fibrosis (major differential of CFA)
    Pleural plaques: frequently calcify (common spot chest X-ray) See the irregular calcification in the lower zones bilaterally in the chest film below

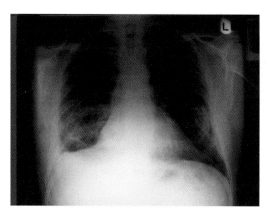

Pleural thickening: causing a restrictive deficit
Carcinoma of the bronchus: the risk with smoking is synergistic
Mesothelioma: pain and shortness of breath (see CXR, p. 178)
- **Drugs**
  - Bleomycin
  - Amiodarone
  - Antiretrovirals
  - High concentration prolonged oxygen therapy
- **Poisons**, e.g. paraquat
- **Radiation**
- **Mitral stenosis**
- **Uraemia**
- **Histiocytosis**
  - Various patterns of multisystemic Langerhan cell granulomatous lung infiltrations resulting in fibrosis (including the lung) occur
  - Of unknown aetiology

- **Connective tissue disease**
  - Systemic sclerosis
  - SLE
  - RA
  - Ankylosing spondylitis:
    Apical fibrosis—remember the **7 As** of ankylosing
    spondylitis (see EMQ 18, p. 131)

Q. What are the typical findings on spirometery?
A.
- The typical defect is **'restrictive'**. Although the FEV1 is
  reduced, the reduction in FVC (lung volume) is pro-
  portionately greater. Therefore, the ratio FEV1/FVC
  rises by >80%. This is unlike in 'obstructive' defects
  (such as asthma and emphysema) where the FEV1 is
  proportionately more affected than the FVC and so the
  FEV1/FVC is reduced <80%
- Any defect that reduces lung volume may produce this
  restrictive pattern . . .
  - Mesothelioma
  - Chest wall injury
  - Large pleural effusion

*Q. What are the associations of cryptogenic fibrosing
alveolitis?*
A.
Several other autoimmune illnesses . . .
- Rheumatoid arthritis
- Ulcerative colitis
- SLE
- Chronic active hepatitis

Q. What other investigations would you request?
The way to approach any question on the investigation of
any disease is in essentially two parts . . .
1. You would order tests to confirm the diagnosis and
exclude other conditions in the differential diagnosis,
and . . .
2. You would want to assess the progression and functional effect of the disease in question. Very often both
stages are performed by single investigations
A.
- Chest X-ray
- Spirometry
- High resolution CT scan of the chest: invaluable in
  visualizing the fine architecture of the fibrosis or
  otherwise
- Autoantibodies
  - ANF positive in 30%

- Rheumatoid factor positive in 50%
- Broncho-alveolar lavage
  - Typically neutrophils in CFA
  - ?Asbestos bodies
  - ?Lymphocytes in extrinsic allergic alveolitis
  - ?TB

Q. What is the prognosis?
A.
Various patterns of disease are recognized in fibrosing
alveolitis dependent upon the detail of the chest CT scan.
Overall, unfortunately, the prognosis is poor, with 5-year
survival at 50%.

OSCE station 23

You arrive at an OSCE station and are asked to examine a
man's testicles . . .
- Introduce yourself to the patient, stating your full
  name and grade. The patient in question will often be a
  dummy with special examination testicles attached—
  although this is a strange situation, you should be no
  less courteous or professional
- Explain what you propose to do and why this is neces-
  sary. Explain that there will be a male chaperone pres-
  ent at all times throughout the examination
- Gain consent
- Allow the patient private time to get undressed if he has
  not already done so
- Return with a male chaperone
- Lay the patient supine and uncover: ideally you need to
  see from the lower ribs down to the knees
- Put on a pair of examination gloves
- Begin by inspecting the scrotum for . . .
  - Scars
  - Asymmetry
  - Colour (blueness may suggest underlying
    varicocoele)
  - Obvious underlying masses
  - Rashes
  - Epidermoid cysts
  - Carcinoma of the skin
  - Pustules
  - Ulcers
- Ensure that you lift the scrotum up gently so that you
  can see the posterior surface fully
- Next, move on to the palpation of the scrotal contents:
  take each testis and palpate between two fingers and

thumb around its entire circumference. Palpate similarly the epididymis and any associated intrascrotal soft tissue, including the spermatic cord with its vas deferens from epididymis to superficial inguinal ring. For any abnormality describe . . .

- **Site** on the testicle or within the scrotum
- Whether **confined to the scrotum or not**
- **Size** in cm
- **Shape** (circular, ovoid, elongated?)
- **Surface** (regular or irregular?)
- **Consistency** (soft or hard, worm-like?)
- **Tender** or non-tender
- Overlying **skin** (tethered or mobile, thickened, ulcerated?)

- **Temperature** (any evidence of inflammation?)
- **Transillumability** (can you shine a light through the mass or not?)
- Examine each side of the scrotum in turn, taking approximately 2 min per side
- Palpate the inguinal region bilaterally for the presence of lymphadenopathy and herniae
- *Immediately* cover the patient up, thank them and write your findings in the notes, asking the chaperone to sign in addition. Wash your hands (before using your pen)
- Present your findings to the examiner

The examination findings for the majority of common scrotal lumps is shown in the table below . . .

Pathology	Confined to scrotum?	Testicle separate to epididymis?	Trans-illuminates?	Tender?	Additional findings . . .
Hernia	No	Yes	No	Only if strangulates	Can be reducible; cough impulse
Infantile hydrocoele	No	No	Yes	No	No cough impulse
Epididymitis	Yes	No	No	Yes	Overlying scrotum reddened, vas deferens tender; co-existent UTI or prostatitis confirms diagnosis
Orchitis	Yes	No	No	Yes	Overlying scrotum reddened; seen in mumps and other viral infections; unilateral
Testicular cancer	Yes	Yes	No	No	Testis affected feels heavier
Epididymal cyst	Yes	Yes	Yes	No	Often multiple, may be bilateral
Adult hydrocoele	Yes	No	Yes	No	Also known as non-communicating
Torsion of the testicle	Yes	No	No	Yes	Peak incidence in second decade of life; surgical emergency; fix both sides as long as testis is not infarcted (if it is → orchidectomy)

Continued

Pathology	Confined to scrotum?	Testicle separate to epididymis?	Trans-illuminates?	Tender?	Additional findings . . .
Torsion of the hydatid of Morgagni	Yes	No	Yes — blue	Yes, often less severe than testicular torsion	The torted hydatid at the upper pole of the testis may be palpable or be visible through the scrotal wall on transillumination as a 'blue dot' on the scrotum; of no consequence, except that it presents the same way as a testis torsion; bilateral removal not indicated
Varicocoele	No	No	No	No	Said to feel like a bag of worms; commoner on left; cough impulse; can disappear on laying flat
Syphilitic gumma	Yes	No	No	No	Irregular, non-tender lump
Idiopathic scrotal oedema	Yes	Yes	No	Slight	Occurs in boys <10 years of age, presenting with scrotal redness and oedema; testis feels normal

OSCE station 24

A 56-year-old **lifelong smoker** presents to A&E complaining of **sudden onset** 30 minutes ago of **crushing, central chest pain**, with associated dyspnoea and nausea, but no palpitations. The pain is still present despite the ambulance crew administering the patient with 3 mg of buccal suscard and 300 mg of aspirin, and according to the patient it is now **getting worse than ever** and is **beginning to radiate down her left arm** and into the **temporomandibular joint of her jaw**. You are asked to examine the patient . . .

On examination from the end of the bed, you observe that the patient is **sweaty and tachypnoeic**, rate 30 b.p.m. and shallow. BMI is 19. You find there is a **sinus tachycardia**, rate **126** at the radial pulse, and the brachial pulse is of **normal character and volume**. The fingers are heavily tar-stained. The blood pressure is **180/110**, and the patient states that she has 'always had blood pressure'. The JVP is within normal limits. Heart sounds 1 and 2 are present, but there is **a further heart sound just prior to S1**. There are no murmurs, and the lung fields are clear. All peripheral pulses are intact, but dorsalis pedis and posterior tibial pulses are faint. There is no oedema. There is nil else to find on examination.

The ECG taken on this patient shows one small square of definite ST-segment elevation in leads V1–V4, T-wave inversion in the same leads, but no other abnormality.

Q. What is the significance of this patient's heart sounds?
A.
The patient in the above question has normal heart sounds 1 (due to closure of mitral and tricuspid valves) and 2 (due to closure of aortic and pulmonary valves), but she also has a ***fourth*** heart sound, known as *atrial sound* or *atrial gallop*. This sound classically occurs just before S1, and is **dull and low in pitch**, being heard best with the bell. It can occasionally be heard in an apparently normal person, especially in the elderly or athletes. However, much more commonly it is due to **increased ventricular wall stiffness during atrial contraction** (remember that patients in atrial fibrillation *cannot* have a

fourth heart sound, because they have no coordinated atrial contraction).

Causes of a left-sided S4 include . . .
- Hypertension
- Coronary artery disease
- Aortic stenosis
- Cardiomyopathy

This is best heard at the apex with the bell in the left lateral position, and it is said to have the cadence of *'Tennessee'*.

The much less common right-sided S4 is usually caused by . . .
- Pulmonary hypertension
- Pulmonary stenosis

This is best heard along the lower left sternal border or below the xiphisternum.

When S4 coexists with a third heart sound, the four sounds together are described as a **'summation gallop'** or a 'quadruple rhythm'.

Q. Should this patient be thrombolysed on the above findings?
A.
No. The indications for thrombolysis are clear and concise, and should be followed to the letter to avoid potentially life-threatening complications of this otherwise potentially life-saving intervention. First, the patient must have **cardiac-sounding chest pain**. If the patient has no chest pain, it is against protocol to thrombolyse, regardless of what the ECG looks like. Secondly, as long as the patient has cardiac-sounding chest pain, then they **must have one of only two ECG changes** before thrombolysis can be considered . . .
  either . . .
1. **ST-segment elevation** greater than **2** small squares in two consecutive anterior chest leads (V1–V6) or greater than **1** small square in two consecutive limb leads (I, II, III, aVR, aVL, aVF) . . .
  or . . .
2. **New-onset left bundle branch block**

The patient in the question clearly has cardiac-sounding chest pain, but the ECG changes are currently insufficient to thrombolyse. Don't forget to check for contraindications to thrombolysis, because a single absolute

contraindication will rule out thrombolysis as a therapeutic option.

Absolute contraindications to thrombolysis
- Previous haemorrhagic stroke at any time
- Other strokes or cerebrovascular events within 1 year of proposed thrombolysis
- Known intracranial neoplasm
- Active internal bleeding, not including menses
- Suspected aortic dissection

Relative contraindications to thrombolysis
- Severe or uncontrolled hypertension on presentation (BP > 180/110)
- Current use of anticoagulant therapy in therapeutic doses (INR > 2–3)
- Known bleeding diathesis
- Recent (within 2–4 weeks) trauma
- Prolonged (>10 min) CPR
- Recent major surgery (within 3 weeks)
- Non-compressible vascular punctures
- Pregnancy
- Active peptic ulcer
- Age >75 years
- History of proliferative retinopathy
- (For streptokinase) exposure within 5 days to 2 years in the past

Q. What should your initial management be, given that thrombolysis has temporarily been ruled out?
A.
As with any medical emergency, always answer this question 'A,B,C . . .'. Ensure the patient has a patent airway and no potential C-spine injury. Give **oxygen**, initially high-flow, but being aware that this patient has a higher than average chance of type II respiratory failure, so acquire an arterial blood gas reading at the first appropriate opportunity to ensure that she is not retaining CO_2. Monitor SpO_2. Gain intravenous access. Take routine blood tests. Consider intravenous infusion. Place patient on a cardiac monitor. Obtain a full and definitive 12-lead ECG. Regularly measure non-invasive blood pressure (NIBP). Consider arterial line for beat-to-beat monitoring of BP.

Control cardiac pain: give buccal nitrate, sublingual GTN spray and intravenous diamorphine (+anti-emetic) if required. Opiate will also assist with uncomfortable subjective sensations of dyspnoea. If pain continues/recurs, consider intravenous infusion of nitrate.

Give antiplatelet therapy: give all patients 300 mg aspirin, even if they have already had their 75 mg dose today, and almost always regardless of peptic ulcer/gastritis history. Consider administration of clopidogrel 300 mg in patients who have ECG changes consistent with acute coronary syndrome.

Limit the size of the infarct: intravenous administration of β-blocker in the situation of acute MI is proven effective but is much underused in the UK. Remember it cannot be used in patients with bradycardia or hypotension. Early introduction of ACE inhibitors is another proven important therapeutic manoeuvre in acute MI.

NB It is important to be aware of the rise of **primary percutaneous coronary angioplasty (PCA)** as a favourable alternative for acute reperfusion in MI in centres where catheter labs and well-trained interventional cardiologists are constantly available. Importantly, in randomized controlled trials, primary PCI offers better flow rates, more sustained infarct-related artery patency and fewer haemorrhagic complications than does thrombolytic therapy.

OSCE station 25

Q. Take a history from this patient who has been experiencing some swallowing difficulties.
A.
The history in dysphagia is extremely important for diagnosing malignancies of the oesophagus and gastro-oesophageal junction. The candidate must take a detailed history of the symptoms.

Ask about . . .
- **Duration**
- **Intermittent or a constant feature**
  - Constant features suggest a malignancy or stricture
  - Intermittent problems suggest a possible neurological cause (e.g. myasthenia gravis)
- Is the problem **with swallowing** (e.g. pain, choking or obstruction) **or does food stick once swallowed?** If swallowing is problematic the problem is likely to be neurological

- Is it **progressive** (getting worse)? Highly suggestive of malignancy
- **Solids or liquids or both**
  - Ask which foods cause difficulty
  - Dysphagia for liquids rather than solids suggests a possible neurological cause (e.g. stroke causing pseudobulbar palsy)
- **Painful** swallowing
  - Infections
  - Foreign body
  - Neurological illness
  - Late feature of malignancy
- **Regurgitation**
  - Suggests a structural blockage
- History of **choking or recurrent chest infections**
  - Suggests aspiration due to either a problem (probably neurological) with the swallowing reflex
  - Aspiration of regurgitated food
  - Aspiration of refluxed gastric contents
- **Weight loss**
- **Risk factors** for strictures or malignancy
  - History of dyspeptic symptoms
  - GORD for peptic stricture
  - Excessive alcohol intake (units per week) and smoking for oesophageal carcinoma
  - Previous diagnosis of anaemia for Plummer–Vinson syndrome
- **If you suspect a neurological cause, enquire about possible associated symptoms plus risk factors**, e.g. history of stroke, atrial fibrillation, diabetes, hypertension, hyperlipidaemia, difficulty with limb function, vision, speech or balance
- **Previous investigations and interventions**
  - Endoscopy: stents, dilatation of strictures?
  - Treatment for *H. pylori*
  - Surgery

Q. What are the typical clinical features for a patient with oesophageal carcinoma?
See EMQ 12 (1), p. 102.
A.
There is difficulty in swallowing initially solids (not liquids), becoming progressive. The patient may have presented with bolus obstruction. Pain is a late feature but may occur with advanced and erosive disease; it may be constant or just with swallowing. The history is typically short (weeks or months). Weight loss occurs which

is often massive. High alcohol intake and smoking predispose.

On examination . . .
- Weight loss
- Lymphadenopathy
- Anaemia
- Jaundiced
- Hoarse voice
- Cough/choking (suggesting aspiration)
- Hepatomegaly

Q. What is the differential diagnosis for oesophageal carcinoma?

A.

Other structural lesions . . .
- **Peptic stricture** (secondary to GORD) the most likely alternative. Ask about previous reflux symptoms. Treatment with balloon dilatation, high dose PPIs
- **Plummer–Vinson syndrome**: a rare association with iron deficiency anaemia and more common in women. A post-cricoid web-like obstruction occurs. Other features of iron deficiency anaemia may be present (e.g. koilonychias, angular stomatitis, glossitis). There is a raised incidence of oesophageal carcinoma
- **Pouches**
- **Impacted foreign body**
- **Extrinsic compression** from lymph nodes, goitres and carcinoma of the bronchus
- **Systemic sclerosis** can cause fibrosis of the GIT causing strictures, impaired motility and malabsorption due to bacterial overgrowth (analogous to blind loop syndrome)
- **Infections** (think AIDS) CMV, *Candida* and HSV

Q. What is the management of patients with GORD?

A.

See EMQ 12 (2), p 102.

Q. What are some neurological causes for dysphagia?

A.
- **UMN lesions** (pseudobulbar palsy)
  - **Stroke**: the most common neurological cause of a swallowing problem. Involvement of the lower cranial nerve nuclei (C IX, X, and XII), producing a UMN *pseudobulbar* palsy. Emotional lability, a small spastic tongue and a brisk jaw jerk may occur also
  - **Motor neurone disease**: causing both a pseudobulbar and bulbar palsy
  - **Multiple sclerosis**

- **LMN lesions** (bulbar palsy)
  - **Poliomyelitis**
  - **Syringobulbia**: the enlarging 'syrinx' causes progressive and often asymmetrical damage to the motor nuclei
- Neuromuscular
  - **Achalasia**: the lower oesophageal sphincter does not relax due to a degenerative process of unknown aetiology affecting the myenteric plexus in the oesophagus. Solids and liquids both cause difficulty. Retrosternal pain a typical feature. Some weight loss may occur. A chest film may show a fluid level behind the heart (?hiatus hernia) with tapering 'rats tail' narrowing at the lower end
  - **Chagas' disease**: American trypanosomiasis. A late feature of the disease is damage to the myenteric plexus of the gastrointestinal tract resulting in dilatation. In the oesophagus this results in a disease very similar to achalasia. Dilation of other parts of the gut (constipation) can occur along with a cardiomyopathy
  - **Diffuse oesophageal spasm**: the 'corkscrew oesophagus' on barium swallow. Chest pain due the spasm can occur. Oesophageal manometry records very high pressure and non-functional oesophageal peristalsis. There is an association with oesophageal carcinoma
  - **Myasthenia gravis**: fluctuating weakness. Other muscle groups involved (facial, limbs). Worse after exercise or chewing?

Q. What is globus pharyngeus?

A.

A common functional disorder that consists of feeling a lump or obstruction in the throat, often with discomfort. The feeling may be persistent between meals, but there is no problem with swallowing. Neither regurgitation nor weight loss occur. Treatment is with reassurance.

Q. What investigations would you like to arrange for this patient who has dysphagia?

A.
- **Routine blood tests** may be helpful if the patient has been vomiting (U and Es) or bleeding (FBC). The liver function tests may reveal a low albumin (malnutrition) or a raised bilirubin and alkaline phosphatase with secondary tumour deposits
- A **chest X-ray** may show a fluid level behind the heart and oesophageal dilatation in achalasia. It may also

show an aspiration pneumonia (classically in the right lower lobe)

- **Upper gastrointestinal endoscopy**: to visualize the lesion, remove a bolus obstruction, take biopsies, dilate a benign stricture or insert a stent
- **24-h pH probe testing and manometry**: allows for definitive proof and severity of GORD as well as diagnosing dysmotility disorders. The normal pH in the lower oesophagus is 5–7; values <4 suggest significant reflux
- **CT scan of chest** may help to further evaluate a malignancy or look for extrinsic compression or erosion

OSCE station 26

Q. Examine this patient's chest.

A.

On inspection the **respiratory rate is increased**. There are signs of accessory muscle usage and flaring of the alar nasae from the end of the bed. There is (or may be) **central cyanosis**. There is (or may be) lymphadenopathy in the cervical area. The JVP is (or may be) elevated. The trachea may be shifted away from the side of the lesion. **Expansion may be reduced** on the affected side. **On percussion there is a stony dull area** at the (right or left base). There is **reduced air entry on the affected side** with crepitations and (possibly) an area of bronchial breathing (lung compression) above this.

The patient has evidence of a pleural effusion.

Q. What is the differential diagnosis?

A.

- Consolidation due to pneumonia
- Collapse distil to an obstruction (tumour/lymph nodes/ foreign body)

Q. What investigation(s) would you perform next?

A.

- **Routine blood tests**
  - **FBC**: possible raised WCC in infection, anaemia of chronic disease in malignancy
  - **U and Es**: possible low sodium and potassium if the patient is taking diuretics; also possible low sodium due to SIADH leading to effusion
  - **Liver function tests**: for possible hypoalbuminaemia or underlying liver disease with raised transaminases

- **Urine dip test for protein**
- **Chest radiograph**
  - Loss of the normally sharp costophrenic angle as an early sign of fluid collection. The effusion grows with an ascending meniscus towards the chest wall
  - Check to see whether the effusion **is unilateral (?exudates) or bilateral (?transudate)**
  - If bilateral, look for other **features of cardiac failure**; upper lobe venous diversion, cardiomegaly, 'bat's wing' shadowing of pulmonary oedema
  - Look closely for an **associated mass (coin) lesion** in bronchogenic carcinoma, either sitting on top or within the effusion
  - Look for other evidence of a cause:
    Hilar lymphadenopathy (TB, malignancy, lymphoma)
    Bony metastases
    Mastectomy
- **Pleural fluid aspiration** for . . .
  - **Biochemical analysis** of aspirate for protein estimation (?exudates or transudates), glucose, and amylase
  - **Cytology** (malignancy) and cell count (polymorphs in bacterial infection, lymphocytes in TB)
  - **Immunology** for antinuclear antibody, rheumatoid factor and complement levels
  - **Microbiology** for microscopy and culture including for acid–alcohol fast bacilli (TB)
- **Pleural biopsy** if the diagnosis is still in doubt after the above investigations
- **CT scan** of chest for further evaluation of a mass lesion or intrinsic chest pathology

Q. How you would drain the effusion?

A.

- Explain the procedure to the patient and obtain informed consent
- Get a chest X-ray to confirm the effusion and give its size
- Sit the patient forward holding knees; enlist assistant to help you and comfort patient. Percuss back of chest and locate the area of maximum stony dullness in mid scapula line. Have X-ray available to check this
- Clean the area with iodine solution: adopt 'no touch' sterile technique
- Infiltrate down to the pleura in the intercostal space immediately superior to lower rib (in order to avoid the neurovascular bundle) with 5–10 mL of 1% lignocaine

- Advance a green cannula with a 10-mL syringe along the line of infiltrated tissue, again staying close to the superior surface of the lower rib. Gently aspirate as you advance until you draw back fluid into the syringe
- Remove inner needle and attached 10-mL syringe from the cannula and immediately connect 50-mL syringe with a 3-way tap (ensuring the tap is closed to the drainage port, i.e. not connecting the pleural space to the atmosphere) to the remaining *in situ* plastic tube.
- Remove 50 mL of fluid at a time and turn 3-way tap to empty into a jug. Take early specimens in clear universal containers for laboratory analysis (see notes above). Continue until no further fluid can be aspirated
- Remove the cannula and immediately cover with air-tight dressing, e.g 'Tegaderm' or 'Opsite'. Re-examine the patient and repeat chest X-ray

Q. What are the possible underlying causes of this pleural effusion?

A.

The causes of fluid accumulations in the pleural and peritoneal space can be remembered as **HOT LIPS** . . .

   H Hydrostatic pressure increased (CCF or portal hypertension)

   O Oncotic pressure reduced (any cause of hypo-albuminaemia)

   T Tumours (primary or secondary) or Trauma (haemoperitoneum, haemopneumothorax)

   L Leaks (oesophagus, intestinal perforation)

   I Inflammation (connective tissue disorders) or Infarction (pulmonary embolism)

   P Pancreatitis (pleural effusions or ascites)

   S Sepsis (pneumonia, abscess)

The causes of pleural effusions are divided by the protein content into exudates (>30 g/L, high cell count) or transudates (<30 g/L, low cell count)

Exudates
- **Infection**
  - Pneumonia
  - TB
- **Infarction**
  - Pulmonary embolism
- **Malignancy**
  - Primary or secondary

- **Others**
  - Connective tissue disease:
    RA
    SLE
  - Acute pancreatitis (raised amylase in pleural aspirates)
  - Rare causes:
    Familial Mediterranean fever
    Dressler's syndrome
    Yellow nail syndrome
    Meig's syndrome (ovarian tumour and right-sided effusion)

Transudates
- **Hypoprotinaemia**
  - Low protein manufacture:
    Chronic liver disease
  - Protein loss:
    Nephrotic syndrome
    Gastrointestinal loss
    Malnutrition/malabsorption
- **Raised pulmonary venous pressure**
  - Cardiac failure
- **Others**
  - Hypothyroidism (via SIADH)

Q. How would you manage a patient with a pleural effusion?

A.
- The cause of the pleural effusion must be investigated as above and the underlying problem treated depending on the cause
- For symptomatic effusions causing breathlessness, drainage by insertion of an intercostal drain or needle aspiration should be performed
- Recurrent problematic pleural effusions may be treated with surgical pleurodesis

---

OSCE station 27

You are presented with a patient with **tremor**. You are asked to examine him . . .

On examination you are presented with a patient who appears to be in their 60s. From the end of the bed you note that there is a tremor present of the right arm whilst the patient is at rest. It is a **fine tremor**, with a frequency that you estimate as being **5 Hz**. You note especially that there is **repeated apposition of forefinger and thumb**. Interestingly, it seems that when the patient moves the right arm to itch the face and shake your hand, the tremor seems to **lessen in intensity**. You note that the patient **looks miserable**, and that their **expression changes little** even during what would normally be engaging conversation. You also think that **speech appears slow and monotonous**.

On examination, the extremities are warm, heart rate is 90, blood pressure is 131/89, and heart sounds are normal. The chest is clear with good air entry throughout. Abdomen is soft and non-tender. GCS is 15 (e4v5m6). AMTS is **6/10** (fails on time of day, short-term memory recall, name of monarch and counting backwards). There is no focal abnormality of the cranial nerves. Examination of the PNS is summarized below . . .

	Left arm	*Left leg*	*Right arm*	*Right leg*
Tone	Increased; rigidity uniform through range of movement	Normal	Increased; rigidity uniform through range of movement	Normal
Power	5	5	5	5
Reflexes	Brisk	Brisk	Brisk	Brisk
Babinski		Downgoing		Downgoing
Co-ordination	Normal	Normal	Normal	Normal
Sensation	Intact	Intact	Intact	Intact

You ask the patient to stand. He takes **longer than you might expect** to begin the process of rising from his position on the examination couch, and the whole process takes longer than normal. Romberg's test is negative. You ask the patient to walk. You note that he takes **small, shuffling steps that seem to get quicker** as he walks in a straight line, and his balance appears unsteady to the extent that you are concerned he may fall. Turning to walk back towards you takes an excessively long length of time.

Q. What are the four cardinal features of Parkinsonism?
A.
The cardinal features of Parkinsonism may be recalled with the aid of the mneomonic **'TRAP'** . . .

 T   **tremor**, which is a **resting tremor** with a frequency between 4 and 7 Hz; it is usually **lessened with movement** and **exacerbated by high emotion**; repeated apposition of finger and thumb is classical in Parkinsonism, and is referred to as **'pill-rolling'**

 R   **rigidity**, which is present throughout the range of movement at a particular joint, i.e. the **lead-pipe** form of rigidity; often **begins unilaterally in the upper limbs**, before affecting neck and trunk, eventually spreading to involve the lower limbs; simultaneous movement of the contralateral limb can distract the patient sufficiently to allow full assessment of the tone in a given limb; when the increased **tone is combined with tremor**, the lead-pipe rigidity is broken up, giving the phenomenon of **cogwheeling**

 A   **akinesia**, which is poverty or slowing of movement (**bradykinesia**); there is **difficulty initiating movements** or altering a movement which is being performed; fine finger movements are especially affected, e.g. playing the piano and writing; akinesia of the facial muscles gives the characteristic **dour look** of Parkinsonism, and akinesia affecting the extraocular muscles gives rise to the characteristic **staring gaze** with **decreased frequency of spontaneous blinking**

 P   **postural changes** lead to a bowing of the head, stooping of the trunk and a shuffling gait with **poor**

arm swing; balance is impaired and the gait remains narrow—a recipe for frequent falls; patients with Parkinsonism fall characteristically 'stiffly' with their arms by their sides, often producing spectacular head injuries

Other features seen in Parkinson's disease include: **monotony of speech** developing into **tremulous slurring dysarthria**; dribbling; dysphagia; late decline in cognition; constipation; weight loss; greasy skin; excessive sweating; and urinary difficulties.

Although not known for their florid imaginations, neurologists deemed Parkinsonism the disease in which they would let their vocabulary run free. As in all examination situations, producing the correct buzz-words at the right time can set the examiner purring, so fit in as many of the following as possible . . .
- **Pill-rolling** tremor
- **Lead-pipe** rigidity
- **Cogwheeling**
- **Mask-like** facies
- **Serpentine** stare
- **Festinating** gait
- **Simian** stance
- **Tree-like** falls

Q. Other than idiopathic Parkinson's disease, what are the other causes of Parkinsonism?
A.
Parkinsonism simply refers to the collection of symptoms outlined above, all of which are caused by a **decrease in the activity of the neurotransmitter dopamine in the pars compacta of the substantia nigra of the basal ganglia**. Although idiopathic Parkinson's disease is the most common cause, this collection of symptoms may also be caused by . . .
- **Post-encephalitic Parkinsonism**: first described following epidemic of encephalitis lethargica (viral encephalitis)
- **Arteriosclerotic Parkinsonism**: follows infarction and damage to substantia nigra, nigrostriatal pathways or the basal ganglia, disrupting dopaminergic systems in the brain
- **Drug-induced Parkinsonism**: metoclopramide, phenothiazine, butyrophenones and thioxanthines may all produce Parkinsonian effects. Usually, but not always, reversible. Anticholinergic drugs can be used to alleviate some of the effects of the causative agents
- **Toxic Parkinsonism**: excessive exposure to manganese, carbon monoxide, cyanide, methanol or man-made toxic designer drugs like MTPT can produce Parkinsonian effects
- **Post-traumatic Parkinsonism**: recovery from severe closed head injury has been witnessed in some individuals to lead to a Parkinsonian syndrome

Q. What are the other causes of a resting tremor? What other types of tremor exist?
A.
Tremor is described as '*a sinusoidal regular oscillation of a part of the body*'.

Resting (or static) tremors are **most prominent at rest**. They usually **disappear with spontaneous movement** and **worsen with increased stress and emotion**. Other than Parkinson's disease, causes of resting tremor include **anxiety**, **β-adrenoceptor agonists** (e.g. salbutamol), **alcohol intoxication**, **alcohol withdrawal**, **thyrotoxicosis**, and **benign familial resting tremor** (also known as benign essential tremor, inherited as an autosomal dominant trait).

Intention tremors are **absent at rest** and only become manifest when the affected limb becomes active. If trying to point at a target, the limb affected by intention tremor demonstrates **increased intensity of coarse tremor the closer to the target it gets**. Causes include **disorders of the cerebellum**, e.g. MS. Titubation (a nodding tremor of the head), dysdiadochokinesis and nystagmus may all also be present.

Flapping tremors are coarse to-and-fro movements of the hands at the wrist in response to being asked to hold the arms out to the front and fully extend the hands at the wrist. After a variable interlude, flapping will begin in patients with **advanced liver disease** and in patients with **retention of CO_2**

Some authors identify a further category: *postural tremors*. These are described as fine, rapid tremors that only become manifest when the affected part is made to maintain a posture, e.g. holding the hands out straight. Frequency is in the region of 8–12 Hz. Causes include the previously mentioned hyperthyroidism, anxiety, fatigue and benign essential tremor. It does not worsen on movement.

Depending on the cause, tremor may be **treated with low-dose β-blocker** (e.g. propranolol). Alcohol can also reduce tremor, but in some patients it can make the involuntary movements worse.

OSCE station 28

Dermatology OSCE spot diagnoses

Nails
Q. *Examine this patient's fingernails.*
A.
Possible diagnoses include . . .
- **Clubbing**: early increase in nail bed fluctuance followed by progressive loss of the nail fold angle. Discuss the usual causes. The causative mechanism remains unknown
- **Splinter haemorrhages**: single or multiple nail vascular lesions. Associated with active bacterial endocarditis (immune complex vasculitis) and other causes of vasculitis, but often traumatic in origin
- **Leukonychia**: nail pallor in hypoalbuminaemia
- **Beau's lines**: transverse linear grooves following episodes of systemic illness (e.g. pneumonia) or trauma. May occur with atopic eczema
- **Kolionychia**: spoon-shaped nails in iron deficiency, haemochromatosis and thyrotoxicosis
- **Onycholysis**: separation of the distil nail from the nail bed. Occurs in psoriasis, thyrotoxicosis (known as Plummer's nails), hypothyroidism, systemic sclerosis and fungal nail infections
- **Yellow nail syndrome**: thickened, curved (laterally) and yellow nails. Associated with a lymphatic system deficiency, resulting in peripheral oedema and various pulmonary problems, e.g. pleural effusions, bronchiectasis and malignancy
- **Nail-patellar syndrome**: small (atrophic) fingernails associated with absent or rudimentary patellae. An autosomal dominant condition
- **Linear pigmentation**: streaks of pigmentation running longitudinally with nail growth. Seen in subungual malignant melanoma, naevi and Addison's disease

- **Darier's disease**: triangular defects in the nail tips with longitudinal lines running back to the nail bed from their apices. An autosomal dominant skin condition with associated greasy, brown papular skin eruption and palmar pits. There is occasionally mental subnormality and infertility
- **Terry's nails**: transverse brown discoloration seen in liver and cardiac failure, but also may be normal in the elderly
- **Pits**: small pits as if from a pencil indentation. Seen in psoriasis, alopecia areata and lichen planus
- **Onychogryphosis**: thickened and opaque nails often due to chronic fungal infection of the nail lamella
- **Nail fold dilated capillaries**: may be seen in dermatomyositis, RA and systemic sclerosis
- **Nicotine staining**
- **Paronychia**
- **Biting** (splitting and horizontal ridges), trauma and artefact

Psoriasis
Typical silvery well demarcated scaling lesions. Largely on the extensor surfaces and scalp areas. Look for nail pitting, subungual hyperkeratosis and onycholysis. Seven per cent of cases have an associated seronegative arthropathy [five types of arthropathy are found; see EMQ 23 (4), p. 155] . . .

Q. *What types of psoriasis do you know?*
A.
- **Plaque psoriasis**
- **Guttate psoriasis**: small frequent lesions. Follows streptococcal throat infections, often in younger patients
- **Pustular psoriasis**: often localized on the palms and soles, occasionally generalized
- **Erythrodermic psoriasis**: a potentially serious variant that may follow the use of topical steroids or tar treatment

Q. *What is the Köebner's phenomenon?*
A.

The Köebner (also known as the isomorphic) phenomenon is the development of a skin lesion at the site of trauma, e.g. scratching or surgery. It occurs with psoriasis, lichen planus, molluscum contagiosum and vitiligo.

Q. What factors may exacerbate or trigger psoriasis?

A.

- Drugs, e.g. β-blockers, lithium, ACE inhibitors, antimalarials, NSAIDs, alcohol
- Infections, e.g. streptococcal (guttate psoriasis), HIV
- Psychological, e.g. stress, anxiety or depression
- Trauma to the skin, e.g. UV light, burns

Eczema

Itchy, scaly, erythema on a background of dry skin. A flexural pattern is usual after infancy. Ask about a personal or family history of atopic conditions (eczema, asthma, hay fever) and urticaria.

Q. What does the term atopy mean?

A.

Atopy is an inherited predisposition (autosomal dominant with incomplete penetrance) leading to the production of abnormally large amounts of IgE in response to non-specific stimuli (e.g. cold, trauma, stress, certain foods, house dust mite). It is associated variably with one or more of the clinical conditions asthma, eczema, hay fever and urticaria.

Q. What is the management of eczema?

A.

- Emollients: form the basis of treatment. Frequent and regular use
- Prevent and/or treat secondary infection (most commonly due to *Staphylococcus aureus*, *Candida*, or HSV), using, e.g., antiseptics, topical fucidin, occasional courses of oral flucloxacillin/aciclovir
- Steroid creams (minimum effective potency for short periods) for inflamed areas
- Avoidance of triggers where possible, e.g. woollen clothes, house dust mite
- For difficult eczema: phototherapy (UVB, PUVA) or systemic immunosuppressant drugs (cyclosporin or azathioprine)

Lichen planus

Discrete, shiny, flat-topped, violaceus (light purple) lesions. Usually on the volar aspect of the wrists. Look in the mouth for the lace-like white lesions of Wickham's striae on the buccal mucosa. Look for associate nail dystrophy (onycholysis, longtitudinal grooves or occasional complete absence/malformation). The lesions are intensely itchy.

Q. Do you know any causes of lichen planus type eruptions?

A.

Various drugs and chemicals can result in so-called 'Lichenoid eruptions', e.g. gold, non-steroidals, β-blockers and penicillamine.

Malignant melanoma

Irregularly pigmented (occasionally amelanotic) lesions of the skin and occasionally nail. Often on the lower limb. Say you would like to examine the local lymph node groups and liver.

Q. What is the prognosis in malignant melanoma?

The prognosis is related to the depth of penetration of the tumour (known as the Breslow thickness) . . .

<1.5 mm	gives a 90% 5-year survival
1.5–3.5 mm	gives a 75% 5-year survival
>3.5 mm	gives a 50% 5-year survival

Q. What types of melanoma do you know?

A.

- **Superficial spreading**
- **Nodular**: the most aggressive form because of the tumour thickness
- **Lentigo maligna melanoma**: slow growing macule for several years until a nodular phase occurs. Frequently in elderly people
- **Acral lentiginous melanoma**: commonly occurs on the palms and soles. Again slowly growing until a nodular phase occurs
- **Amelanotic**: contain very little or no melanin
- **Subungual**: involving the nail

Q. What features of a pigmented naevus might cause you to suspect malignancy?

A.

- A Asymmetry
- B Border irregularity, bleeding
- C Colour irregularity (variable pigmentation)
- D Diameter >5 mm
- E Elevation irregularity

Erythema nodosum

Dusky red raised painful nodules usually on the shin, which heal with bruising. They are tender to palpation and are due to a panniculitis (inflammation of subcutaneous fat).

Q. What are the possible causes of erythema nodosum?

A.

- **Infections**
  - Bacterial: *Streptococcus*, TB, leprosy, yersinia, chlamydial psittacosis
  - Fungal: histoplasmosis, coccidiomycosis, blastomycosis
- **Drugs:** penicillin, sulphonamides, oral contraceptives
- **Sarcoidosis**
- **Inflammatory bowel disease**
- **Pregnancy**
- **Cryptogenic**

Erythema multiforme

Target lesions occurring in any possible location. Occasionally starting with a central blister. A more severe form can occur affecting the mucus membranes (mouth, conjunctiva, genitals) known as **Stevens–Johnson syndrome**.

Q. What are the possible causes of this eruption?

A.

- Infection
  - Herpes virus infection (most frequently)
  - Mycoplasma infection
  - Streptococcal infection
- Drugs: sulphonamides, carbamazepine
- Connective tissue disease: SLE, polyarteritis nodosa, Wegener's granlomatosis
- Malignancy, lymphoma
- Cryptogenic

Pyoderma gangrenosum

A bluish or pustular nodule breaks down to form an ulcer with a very irregular and undermined border. Most commonly seen on the shins.

Q. What are the possible causes of this condition?

A.

- Inflammatory bowel disease
- Rheumatological: RA, ankylosing spondylitis
- Malignancy: myeloma, leukaemia, lymphoma
- Liver disease: primary biliary cirrhosis, chronic active hepatitis, sclerosing cholangitis
- Idiopathic

Systemic sclerosis

A rare connective tissue disorder characterized by fibrosis of the skin and internal organs. Various patterns occur . . .

- When the brunt of the disease falls upon the skin it is termed **scleroderma**
- When the disease has extensive internal involvement the acronym **CREST** (Calcinosis cutis, Raynaud's, oEsophageal, Sclerodactyl, Telangiectasia)
- When the disease is confined to the skin it is recognized in plaques (**morphea**) or a linear distribution (**en coup de sabre**)

In clinical examinations, however, systemic sclerosis is common and two types of question tend to occur . . .

1. A **spot diagnosis**: e.g. the typical scleroderma faces, Raynaud's phenomenon or digital gangrene and or calcification, or an X-ray showing soft tissue calcification
2. As a **long case or EMQ** drawing upon one or more of the multisystemic features, e.g. renal, pulmonary, gastrointestinal

The features of system sclerosis may include . . .

- **Cutaneous:** initially oedema and swelling followed by sclerodactyly, Raynaud's, calcinosis, contractures, digital gangrene, pigmentation and hair loss. The typical faces have radial lines around the mouth and a tight, beak-shaped nose, with telangiectasia
- **Musculoskeletal:** arthritis, myositis
- **Pulmonary:** fibrosis, pulmonary hypertension
- **Renal:** accelerated hypertension due to renovascular disease and intense activation of the Renin Angiotensin Aldosterone axis. The most common cause of death in systemic sclerosis
- **Gastrointestinal:** fibrosis throughout the GIT leads to oesophageal reflux and strictures. Malabsorption may occur due to bacterial overgrowth (blind loop syndrome) developing within a static small intestinal lumen

Investigations include looking for the specific autoantibodies;

- Anti-centromere positive in 70% of cases
- Anti-Scl-70 positive in 30% of cases

Management can be divided into the following areas . . .

- **Symptomatic:** PPIs for reflux disease, physiotherapy for contractures, nifedipine and hand warmers for Raynaud's
- **Management of renal hypertension:** ACE inhibitors
- **Management of pulmonary hypertension:** diuretics,

anticoagulation and oxygen. Recently IV prostacycline has been used with some success
- **Control of fibroblastic activity** with immunosuppression; steroids are of no value

Blistering eruptions

- **Pemphigus vulgaris**: an autoimmune condition with IgG deposition in the epidermis, leading to **thin-walled blisters which rupture early** leaving a raw blister base which leaks fluid. Shear stress applied to the skin slides off the epidermis. (Nikolsky's sign). The blisters may be widespread and involve the mouth (?Bechet's or Herpes simplex). There is an association with thymoma and myasthenia gravis. It is rare but serious (remember pemphig**us** is serio**us,** the skin split is **su**perficial). Treatment is with steroids and immunosuppressives
- **Pemphigoid**: an autoimmune condition with IgG deposition in the dermo-epidermal junction. The resultant separation of the skin layers leads to thick-walled blisters which do not rupture as easily as pemphigus. Nikolsky's sign is negative and mouth lesions are less common
- **Dermatitis hepetiformis**: an intensely itchy, blistering rash on a background of red raised macules. Often over the elbows, knees and buttocks. It is associated with coeliac disease (often subclinical gluten sensitivity). IgA deposition at the basement membrane occurs. Treatment with dapsone can be very effective (monitor for methaemaglobinaemia) and a gluten-free diet
- **Linear IgA disease**: similar to pemphigoid. Occurs in children and adults. Bullae occur on large plaques
- **Erythema multiforme**
- **Epidermolysis bullosa conginita**: many forms occur. Children are affected. Defects in the proteins securing the epidermis to the dermis may occur in the most severe forms. When severe, contractures, scarring and defects of the hair and teeth, and GIT may occur
- **Epidermolysis bullosa acquisita**: like pemphigoid (IgG deposition at the basement membrane) blisters occur following trauma. It occurs in adults and is associated with malignancy and inflammatory bowel disease

Increased pigmentation

- **Addison's disease** (via ACTH): pigmentation over pressure areas and sites of trauma (elbows, buccal mucosa and scars)

- **Other ACTH driven**, e.g. pituitary and ectopic production from tumours
- **Racial**
- **Post-inflammatory** hyperpigmentation, e.g. acne vulgaris
- **UV light** exposure
- **Drugs**: Amiodarone (photosensitivity), oral contraceptives
- **Liver and renal failure**
- **Pellagra**: niacin deficiency—**d**iarrhoea, **d**ermatitis and **d**ementia (sun-exposed areas; Casal's necklace around the neck)

Pruritus

- **Dermatoses**: especially dermatitis herpetiformis, atopic eczema, pemphigus, lichen planus, urticaria and itch–scratch–itch
- **Parasitic**: scabies, body lice, GI worms
- **Liver disease**
- **Renal disease**
- **Haematological**: lymphoma, primary polycythemia, iron deficiency
- **Malignancy**: GIT, bronchus, breast
- **Endocrine**: hyper- or hypothyroidism
- **Drug sensitivities**
- **Neurological**: some cases of peripheral neuropathy

Alopecia

- **Male pattern baldness** (including female with a positive family history, often Mediterranean descent)
- **Alopecia areata**: autoimmune hair loss. If extensive the entire scalp hair may be lost (**alopecia totalis),** or all body hair lost (**alopecia universalis**). Exclamation mark hairs occur (narrower at base than tip)
- **Telogen effluvium**: shedding of hair following a physiological stress, e.g. surgery or pneumonia (like beau's lines)
- **Scaring dermatoses**: fungal or bacterial infection, lichen planus, SLE
- **Hair pulling** (trichotillomania) or traction due to combing or tying back
- **Iron deficiency**
- **Endocrine**: hyper- or hypothyroidism, hypopituitarism
- **Chemotherapy**
- **Malnutrition**

Cutaneous manifestations of malignancy

- **Jaundice**

- **Clubbing**
- **Pyoderma gangrenosum** (see above)
- **Tylosis:** hyperkeratosis of the feet with painful fissures; associated with oesophageal malignancy
- **Thrombophlebitis migrans:** pancreatic carcinoma
- **Acanthosis nigricans:** GIT (also diabetes, acromegaly, hypothyroidism)
- **Dermatomyositis** (when in adults)
- **Generalized pruritus**
- **Erythema gyratum repens:** bronchogenic carcinoma
- **Necrolytic migratory erythema:** glucaconoma
- **Herpes zoster:** lymphoma

Vitiligo

The importance of vitiligo lies in the cosmetic distress it can cause for patients (especially if facial or in dark-skinned individuals) and its well known association with autoimmune illness, e.g. thyroid disease, Addison's disease, pernicious anaemia, autoimmune hypoparathyroidism, type I diabetes. Vitiligo is prone to the Köebner phenomenon. There is no effective treatment (cure) although topical steroids and phototherapy can be used. Skin-colour matched camouflage creams are used for facial lesions

HIV infection

Note that in addition to the list below, a macular–papular eruption may occur during the acute seroconversion phase of HIV very like infectious mononucleosis along with generalized lymphadenopathy.

- Malignancy
  - **Kaposi's sarcoma** (30% of AIDS sufferers, 15% at the time of presentation with HIV): a tumour of vascular endothelium that produces dark nodules or plaques, especially on the lower legs. It may also involve the GIT, lymph nodes and pulmonary tract
  - **Lymphoma**
  - **Hair oral leucoplakia:** Epstein–Barr virus implicated, very specific for HIV infection
- Infections
  - *Candida*: especially oral and oesophageal (early in HIV)
  - **Pityrosporum ovale** (seborrhoeic dermatitis and pityriasis versicolor)
  - *Staphylococcus aureus* (impetigo; may be bullous)
  - **Herpes zoster**
  - **Herpes simplex**
  - **Human papilloma virus** (common warts)
- **Molluscum contagiosum**
- **Cytomegalovirus**
- Dermatoses
- **Seborrhoeic eczema**
- **Psoriasis**
- **Atopic eczema**

Leg ulcers

The differential diagnosis of an ulcer on the leg is wide. Most fall into the first three categories . . .

- **Venous stasis:** lower leg region, often medial malleolar area. Shallow and often large. There may be evidence of chronic venous insufficiency with dermatosclerosis (fibrotic woody skin which limits the otherwise inevitable oedema), haemosiderin pigmentation (brown discoloration), varicose eczema and evidence of old previously healed ulcers
- **Arterial insufficiency**, e.g. smoking related, diabetes, sickle cell disease or other haemolytic anaemia
- **Neuropathic:** usually on the sole of the foot over pressure areas. Most frequently due to diabetes
- **Traumatic:** e.g. simple skin trauma in the elderly that breaks down to form an ulcer due to poor healing. Also IV drug abusers who inject the feet after the arm veins have been occluded by repeated use
- **Malignancy**, e.g. basal cell carcinoma, squamous cell carcinoma, malignant melanoma
- **Infective**, e.g. cellulitis (streptococcal), syphilis (gumma)
- **Vasculitis**, e.g. RA, polyarteritis nodosa
- **Dermatological conditions**, e.g. necrobiosis lipoidica diabeticorum, pemphigus, pyoderma gangrenosum

Essential investigations include: sensory testing; a blood sugar; FBC; ESR (or equivalent); the brachial-popliteal doppler index; bacteriology swabs; and occasionally a biopsy (suspected malignancy or dermatological rarity).

Tuberous sclerosis

Frequently occurs as a spot diagnosis. An autosomal dominant condition with gene abnormalities on chromosomes 9 and 16. Hamartomas occur affecting the . . .

- Skin
  - **Adenoma sebaceum:** red nodular lesions around the nose
  - **Periungual fibromata:** growths from the nail bed
  - **Shagreen patches:** indurated skin coloured connective tissue naevus plaques on the trunk

- **Ash leaf macules**: pale patches seen using UV (Wood's) light
- CNS
  - Epilepsy
  - Cognitive impairment
- Kidneys
  - Cysts
- Eyes
  - Retinal hamartomas
- Heart muscle (may resolve)

Dermatomyositis
[See also EMQ 15 (5), p. 123]
Polymyosistis and dermatomyositis for practical purposes may be viewed as the same disease plus or minus the skin changes. An inflammatory (painful) myopathy (muscle wasting) occurs. The muscle enzyme CPK is raised and muscle biopsy will show inflammation and necrosis of myocytes. The cutaneous manifestations are much loved by examiners and include . . .
- Face
  - 'Heliotrope' rash; red/ purple flare around the eyes
- Hands
  - Gottron's papules: red thickened plaques over the knuckles with nail bed vasculitic lesions

Neurofibromatosis
A disease characterized by . . .
- **Skin manifestations**
  - Café au lait patches (also seen in Von Hippel Lindau syndrome and McCune Albright syndrome)
  - Neuromas (numerous soft fleshy lesions)
  - Freckling of the axillary and inguinal areas
- Neural tumours
  - Acoustic neuromas
  - Spinal cord/nerve root neurofibromas
  - Meningimomas
  - Gliomas
  - Plexiform neuromas
- Associated features
  - Scoliosis
  - Local giantism
  - Phaeochromocytomas
  - Obstructive cardiomyopathy
  - Renal artery stenosis
  - Haemangiomas, e.g. orbital
  - Fibrous dysplasia of bone
  - Pulmonary fibrosis

Note that a peripheral (type I; chromosome 17) and a central (type II, chromosome 22) form of the condition occur. In the peripheral form, the skin lesions dominate the clinical picture; in the central form, CNS tumours are the main feature.

Vasculitis
The patient has purpuric lesions over the legs. The lesions may be raised and tender ('painful palpable purpura'). Vasculitic illnesses may be primary vasculitides (e.g. Wegener's, polyarteritis nodosa, Takayasu's) or secondary causes (e.g. RA). [See EMQ 15 (4), p. 122.]

Q. Take a history from this patient.
A.
Ask about . . .
- **Systemic upset**; fever, weight loss, malaise, weakness (anaemia, renal failure)
- **Respiratory symptoms**, cough, wheeze, haemoptysis (Wegener's, PAN), shortness of breath (various conditions causing effusions and fibrosis)
- **Abdominal pain** (PAN, Henoch–Schonlein purpura)
- **Joint pain** (RA, Henoch–Schonlein purpura, SLE)
- **Neurological symptoms**; weakness (transverse myelitis), fits, headaches, visual changes (accelerated hypertension)
- **Cardiovascular**; chest pain, shortness of breath, orthopnoea.
- **Recent viral illness** (?Henoch–Schönlein purpura)
- **Drugs** (?drug induced lupus)

Malar rash
The differential of a malar redness includes . . .
- SLE
- Dermatomyositis
- Mitral valve disease (malar flush)
- Polycythemia
- Acne rosacea
- Alcohol abuse
- Superior vena cava obstruction
- Solar damage (telangiectasia and solar keratosis)
- UV light exposure

OSCE station 29

Q. This patient, who has problems with high alcohol consumption, has recurrent bouts of abdominal pain. Take a history and perform an examination.
A.
The pain is **episodic** possibly following alcohol excess. It

is often **very severe**, **central** abdominal and **radiates to the back**. **Nausea and vomiting** may occur. The pain is colicky and relieved by movement and by crouching forwards. There may be a history of steatorrhoea and weight loss suggesting malabsorption. In addition, there may be typical symptoms of **diabetes** (thirst, polyuria, weight loss, soft tissue infections).

The likely diagnosis is acute pancreatitis. (However, the differential includes acute peptic ulceraltion, cholecystitis, acute cholangitis, inferior MI, renal colic, and leaking abdominal aortic aneurysm.)

Examine the patient for . . .
- Features of hypovolaemic **shock** (hypotension and tachycardia)
- **Jaundice and other signs of chronic liver dysfunction**
- **Tetany** (hypocalcaemia)
- **Abdominal tenderness** and guarding
- Abdominal **mass** [pseudocyst, inflammatory mass (phlegmon), ascites]
- **Brusing** over the abdominal wall
  - **Cullen's sign**: peri-umbilical due to spread along umbilical vein
  - **Grey Turner's sign**; bruising in bilateral flanks due to lateral spread in the retroperitoneum

Q. What investigations would you like to arrange?
A.
- **Blood tests**
  - FBC
  - U and Es
  - LFTs
  - Glucose; raised
  - Calcium; hypocalcaemia due to deposition in the inflamed pancreas
  - Amylase;
    Also elevated in upper GI perforation, cholecystitis, ischaemic colitis and DKA; however, levels over 1000 u/L are diagnostic of acute pancreatitis
    NB Chronic pancreatitis may not produce such an elevated level as the gland is small and fibrotic (similar to the limited LFT rise following an insult to a cirrhotic liver)
  - Blood gases (acidosis and hypoxia)
- **Plane abdominal X-ray** ('sentinel' loop of small bowel next to the pancreas due to ileus; calcification in chronic pancreatitis; 90% of gallstones are invisible)

- **USS or CT scan of abdomen**

(See Paper 1, MCQ 23, p. 63.)

Q. What is the prognosis in acute pancreatitis?
A.
A poor prognosis is indicated by any of the following features in the first 48 h . . .

Age	>55 year
WBC	$>15 \times 10^9$/L
Albumin	<30 g/L
Glucose	>10 mmol/L
Urea	>16 mmol/L
LDH	>600 U/L
AST	>200 U/L
Calcium	<2 mmol/L
Oxygen	$PaO_2 < 8$ kPa

Q. What is the management of acute pancreatitis?
A.
- **Nil by mouth**
- **Analgesia**: opiates usually required
- **Intravenous fluid resuscitation**
- Prophylactic intravenous **antibiotics**
- Eneteral **nutrition** via naso-jejunal feeding tube
- Removal of possible obstructing gallstone by ERCP

Q. What is Courvoisier's law?
A.
Courvoisier's law states that if, in the presence of painless jaundice, the gallbladder can be palpated then cause is unlikely to be gallstones. This is because the chronic presence of gallstones in the gallbladder causes fibrosis and contraction of the gallbladder, which becomes impalpable.

Q What are the possible complications of gallstones?
A.
- Biliary colic
- Acute cholecystitis
- Jaundice
- Mucocele
- Carcinoma of the gallbladder
- Cholangitis
- Acute pancreatits
- Gallstone ileus

Q. What is the management of acute cholecystitis?
A.
- **Analgesia**, e.g. IV morpine 10 mg and metoclopramide 10 mg

- Send blood for FBC (?WCC), U and Es (?vomiting), amylase (?acute pancreatitis) and blood cultures
- **IV fluid resuscitation**
- **Antibiotics** to cover possible Gram-negative sepsis, e.g. IV Cefuroxime
- **Abdominal ultrasound** scan to confirm the diagnosis
- **ERCP and sphincterotomy** (of the ampulla) for stones blocking the common bile duct
- **Cholecstectomy** may be performed once the acute symptoms have settled and the patient has been adequately resuscitated

Q. What percentage of gallstones are visible on a plain radiograph?
A.

- **Only 10%**
- But plain abdominal films may pick up features that indirectly suggest gallstones . . .
  - Air in the biliary tree
  - Calcification of the wall of the gall bladder
  - Speckled pancreatic calcification in chronic pancreatitis
  - Obstruction due to gallstone ileus

OSCE station 30

Q. Examine this patient's gastrointestinal system.
A.
An **underweight** (often young) patient who appears **pale**. There may be **clubbing**. The patient may be having parenteral nutrition. There is **chelitis** of the lips and oral **aphthous ulceration.** There are numerous **scars on the abdomen** from previous resections. There may be **localized tenderness** indicating possible active disease. There may be a **possible mass** in the right iliac fossa (see differential p. 229). Rectal examination may reveal **fistulae near the anus, skin tags and fissures.**

The diagnosis is Crohn's disease.

Q. What are the complications of Crohn's disease/ ulcerative colitis?
See Paper 3, MCQ 24, p. 114

Q. What is short bowel syndrome?
A.
Although the small bowel has considerable functional reserve such that 40–50% can be removed without ensu-ing malabsorption, beyond this malabsorption will occur. In addition, perfuse diarrhoea will occur, especially if the ileocaecal valve is removed. Following resection there is hypertrophy of the remaining gut, which can result in some compensation of these symptoms.

Q. What are the causes of anaemia in inflammatory bowel disease?

- Anaemia of chronic disease (normochromic, normo-cytic or microcytic)
- B12 deficiency with terminal iliitis in Crohn's disease
- Iron deficiency
- Folate deficiency
- Iatrogenic: sulphasalazine (haemolytic anaemia)

Q. What are the characteristic radiographic appearances of Crohn's disease/ ulcerative colitis on a barium study?
A.

Crohn's disease
- Skip lesions
- Strictures of small intestine ('string sign of Kantor')
- Thickening of the valvulae coniventes
- Rose thorn ulcers
- Cobblestoning
- Fistulas
- Carcinoma (less common than in ulcerative colitis)

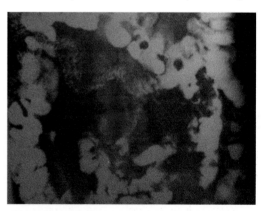

This radiograph shows Crohn's disease with stricture (centre) and cobblestoning

Ulcerative colitis
- 'Hosepiping': featureless thickened and oedematous bowel with loss of haustral pattern
- Inflammatory pseudo-polyps (islands mucosal oedema)

- 'Back wash ileitis' affecting the terminal ileum
- Megacolon (clinically; decreasing stool frequency and increasing abdominal circumference)
- Carcinoma

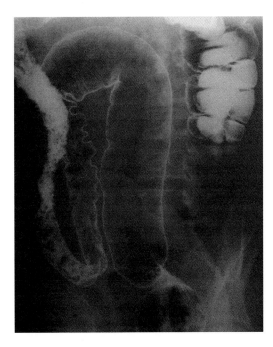

This radiograph shows ulcerative colitis with hosepiping and inflammatory pseudopolyps

Q. What is the association of smoking with inflammatory bowel disease?
A.
Smoking is more common amongst patients with CD, whereas UC tends to be more common amongst non-smokers.

Q. What are the risks of carcinoma of the large bowel?
A.
The risk of developing large bowel carcinoma in UC is related to the duration, extent and severity of the illness. All patients with active disease should have annual colonoscopy. Overall there is a **5% lifetime risk**.

In CD the risk of carcinoma is only marginally raised above that of the general population and thus regular screening is not performed.

Q. What clinical features would you look for in a severe episode of inflammatory bowel disease?
A.

- >6 stools per day
- Pyrexia > 37.5°C
- Pulse > 90/min
- Investigations
  - ESR > 30 mm/h
  - Hb < 10 g/dL
  - Albumin < 30 g/L

Q. How would you manage a patient with an acute exacerbation of inflammatory bowel disease?

- **IV access and IV fluids** for diarrhoea
- **Send blood for**
  - FBC (anaemia, neutrophilia, raised platelets)
  - U and Es (Low K^+ with diarrhoea, elevated urea with dehydration)
  - LFTs (Low albumin)
  - Glucose
  - Blood cultures
  - CRP (elevated in active disease)
- **Chest and abdominal X-ray**
  - ?Megacolon
- **Chart**
  - Weight
  - Abdominal circumference
  - Fluid balance
  - Stool frequency
  - Temperature
- **Nil by mouth/elemental diet**
- **Intravenous corticosteroids** (e.g. hydrocortisone 100 mg q.d.s.) for severe attacks; less severe episodes can be managed by oral prednisolone 60 mg daily
- Local steroids for distil bowel disease (e.g. predfoam enemas)
- Give oral **mesalazine** (5-ASA) for colonic disease (little evidence of benefit in small bowel CD)
- Give **IV antibiotics** for septicaemia and megacolon
- **Watch for megacolon** (decreasing stool frequency and increasing abdominal girth), bleeding, sepsis and perforation
- **Referral to the surgical team if . . .**
  - On admission if severe features
  - Failure to improve after a one week trial of medical therapy
  - Impending megacolon or perforation
  - Severe haemorrhage

- **NB**
  - Only UC can be cured by surgical pan-proctocolectomy; CD tends to recur
  - Agents such as azathioprine are steroid-sparing agents and have no role once steroid therapy has failed

Q. Who was Crohn?

A.

Burill Bernard Crohn was a New York surgeon who described the disease in 1932 as being a distinct disease from tuberculosis of the bowel.

Other possible inflammatory bowel disease
OSCE stations
- As a history station
- Explain the diagnosis of Crohn's disease to this patient

OSCE station 31

Q. Examine this patient's throat.

A.

- Introduce yourself and ask to examine the patient
- Use a bright torch
- Usually there is no need to use a tongue depressor which is unpleasant (especially in examinations), unless the patient really has difficulty in showing you the pharynx
- If a tongue depressor is required, press gently proximal to the highest part of the tongue so as to avoid precipitating a gag reflex. Ask the patient to say 'ah'. Check that the uvula remains central
- Inspect each area of the mouth, tongue and pharynx in turn
- Test the tongue movements for a CXII nerve palsy
- Say you would ideally check the gag reflex and observe the patients swallowing
- Palpate the tonsillar, submental, submandibular and anterior cervical lymph glands

Possible diagnoses include . . .
- **Infections**
  - Bacterial:
    Streptococcal throat infection (red, white exudate, lymphadenopathy)
    Quinsy (abscess within the tonsil)
  - Viral:
    Infectious mononucleosis (petechiae on the hard palate)

Herpes simplex type I
Coxsackie A16 (hand, foot and mouth disease)
Koplick's spots in measles (unlikely); grey lesions with an erythematous bed again on the buccal mucosa that appear early in the course of measles
- Fungal:
  Candida (diabetes, inhaled corticosteroids, HIV)
- **Malignancy**
  - Oropharyngeal carcinoma: squamous cell in smokers, look for associated lymphadenopathy
  - Kaposi's sarcoma: in HIV; dark papules; a vascular tumour
  - Leukoplakia: white atrophic patches often on the side of the tongue. Associated with alcohol and smoking. A pre-malignant condition. Note that in HIV the leukoplakia is hyperplastic giving the so-called hairy leukoplakia.
- **Wickham's striae**: lace-like white lesions on buccal (cheek) mucosa in lichen planus
- **Neurological** (likely in an exam)
  - CN XII lesion: tongue points to the side of the nerve palsy
  - CN X palatal palsy: uvula deviates away from the side of the lesion
  - CN IX palsy: absent gag reflex (do not perform the gag reflex unless specifically directed to)
  - Fasciculation and wasting of the tongue in MND (look for associated limb wasting and fasciculation)
- **Glossitis**: inflammation of the tongue. Loss of the papillae leads to a smooth appearance in vitamin B12 deficiency, folate and iron deficiency. Note geographical tongue is a normal variant where there is differential shedding of tongue papillae giving the appearance of contour lines on a map
- **Ulceration**
  - Aphthous ulceration:
    Inflammatory bowel disease
    Coeliac disease
    Behçet's disease
    Reiter's disease
    Vitamin B12, iron and folate deficiency
  - Trauma due to food or poorly fitting dentures.
  - Malignancy (risk factors include smoking and alcohol)
- **Cleft palate**
- **Lips**
  - Chelitis in Crohn's disease
  - Angular stomatitis
  - Angioedema (unlikely)

- **Dental**
  - Decay
  - Gum hyperplasia:
    Drugs, e.g. phenytoin (most likely) and cyclosporin
    Leukaemic infiltration (monoblastic leukaemia)
    Amyloidosis (and tongue)
    Pregnancy
    Scurvy (with haemorrhage into the gums)
    Familial gingival fibromatosis
    Apparent due to enlargement of the maxilla in Paget's disease and thalassaemia

---

OSCE station 32

A 32-year-old landscape gardener, who is otherwise previously fit and well, presents to his GP surgery complaining that he has been unable to go to work for the last few days due to 'having the "flu"'. On closer questioning he reveals that he has been feeling '**hot and cold**', with general malaise, **arthralgia**, cough and a generalized headache. You are asked to examine the patient . . .

On examination from the end of the bed, you observe a **very unwell looking** patient. He looks sweaty and pale. His fingernails are **clubbed**. Whilst you are checking the capillary refill time, he sharply withdraws his finger, complaining that his **fingertips have been tender** for a few days, but that 'it must be work'. His heart rate is 110, regular, of normal character and somewhat increased volume. His blood pressure is 115/69. Whilst looking for central cyanosis in the patient's mouth, you notice that there is evidence of recent dental extraction. The patient states that he had a tooth removed 'about a month back'. JVP is within normal limits. The apex beat is located normally. On cardiac auscultation, you note a **harsh pansystolic murmur**, loudest at the apex, radiating into the axilla. The chest is clear. The abdomen is generally mildly tender, and you are convinced that there is a **firm mass in the left upper quadrant** that you can neither get above, nor ballot. There is nil else to find on examination.

Urine dipstick shows ketones (+) and **blood** (++).

Q. What is the significance of the findings in this patient's hands?

A.

First of all, the patient is clubbed. This is of concern when present alongside a previously unknown heart murmur, and it should make you immediately consider a cardiac cause for the clubbing (although do not rule out the respiratory and gastrointestinal causes). Cardiovascular causes of clubbing are five in number, and should trip off the tongue without a thought in the exam situation . . .

1. **Subacute bacterial endocarditis (SBE)**
2. **Cyanotic congenital heart disease**
3. **Atrial myxoma**
4. **Brachial arteriovenous malformation**
5. **Axillary artery aneurysm**

Always recite them in the above order, because the last two are vanishingly rare, and remember that acute or fulminant bacterial endocarditis does not cause clubbing because it occurs over a much shorter time-scale than does the subacute form.

The finding of exquisitely tender fingertips should also not be overlooked in this patient. It is highly likely that he has got **Osler's nodes**, named after Sir William Osler, the Canadian physician (1849–1919). These are **tender, raised, pea-sized, purplish-red lesions** that can occur anywhere on the palms or soles, but most commonly occur on the pads of the fingers and toes. They are rare but are **pathognomonic of SBE**. They occur later than other telling signs and will disappear spontaneously and for no good reason after a few days. The pathogenesis is incompletely understood; they may result from bacterial emboli that lodge in the peripheral capillaries, or they may be an immunological reaction to the infecting organism.

Other important hand signs to look for in SBE include the even rarer **Janeway lesions**, named after the US physician Edward G. Janeway (1841–1911). These are **usually flat (but may be slightly raised), irregular and *non-tender* erythematous lesions** on the palms and the soles that disappear spontaneously. They blanch with pressure or elevation of the affected limb. They can rarely spread to form a diffuse rash over the trunk and extremities. They are thought to be due to an immunological reaction to the infecting organism, and are now rarely seen compared to a few years ago due to early detection and treatment of the underlying problem.

Splinter haemorrhages are the final hand sign related to SBE. These are small, sub-ungal splinter-like haemorrhages, that **commonly occur singularly**, but may be multiple, under the nails of either the fingers **or toes**. They probably have similar aetiology to Osler's nodes and Janeway lesions. Correct examination for splinter haemorrhages involves a **detailed close look at each of the nails**; a fleeting glance at the hands in the exam situation is insufficient for a conclusion of 'no splinter haemorrhages' to be made. They commonly occur harmlessly in patients with a manual profession, and if this patient had demonstrated multiple splinter haemorrhages, it would have been difficult to know whether this was related to disease or job.

Q. What are the most common infecting organisms likely to be in this patient?

A.

The cause of SBE in the above patient is most likely to be *Streptococcus viridans*, the cause of 50–60% of cases of native valve endocarditis. Other common causes of native valve endocarditis that warrant mention are *Staphylococcus aureus* (25–30%), **enterococci** (15%), **coagulase negative *Staphylococci*** (5–8%), **Gram-negative bacilli** (5%), **culture negative agents** (5%) and very rarely **fungi** or **polymicrobial infections**. Prosthetic valve endocarditis is more likely to be due to coagulase negative staphylococci. Endocarditis in intravenous drug users is a result of *Staph. aureus* in almost 60% of cases. Polymicrobial, fungal (usually *Candida* spp.) and pseudomonal endocarditis also occurs much more frequently in this population.

Q. Which three investigations would be most important to consider at the earliest opportunity?

A.

1. **Full blood count**: the white cell count would be raised, with a neutrophilia
2. **Blood cultures**: it is vitally important to take cultures before commencing antibiotic therapy, otherwise choosing the correct antimicrobial treatment may be difficult. For a diagnosis of endocarditis, you need to demonstrate persistent bacteraemia, defined as either . . .
   - *Two or more* culture results taken from different sites positive for the same organism, separated by at least 12 h, or . . .
   - *All of three, or the majority of four or more* blood cultures taken from a variety of sites positive for the same organism, with at least 1 h between the first and last taken culture
3. **Echocardiography**: if suspicion of SBE persists, then echo is a vital test. Transthoracic echo (TTE) is non-invasive and is highly specific if a vegetation is detected; however, it is limited by its poor sensitivity (65% in native valve SBE, 25% in prosthetic valve SBE). In contrast, transoesophageal echo (TOE) is >95% sensitive in native valve endocarditis and 90% sensitive in prosthetic valve

endocarditis. It is also vastly superior for detecting abscess formation.

In the absence of pathological proof, the diagnosis of SBE has been historically very difficult to make with certainty. Several criteria and schemes have been proposed to try to overcome this, the most widely accepted one of which currently is the *Duke criteria* (not to be confused with the Duke–Astler–Coller classification used in the staging of colorectal carcinoma). On the basis of these criteria, endocarditis can be diagnosed definitively, even in the absence of histological findings. It is validated for use in both native and prosthetic valve endocarditis. The criteria are shown below . . .

Major Duke criteria

1. Positive blood culture for infective endocarditis (has to be from at least *two* separate cultures—see above)
2. Evidence of endocardial involvement (either in the form of positive echocardiographic findings *or* new or changed regurgitant murmur)

Minor Duke criteria

1. Predisposition (e.g. predisposing heart condition, prosthetic valve or IVDU)
2. Fever ≥ 38°C
3. Vascular phenomena (e.g. major arterial emboli, septic pulmonary infarcts, conjunctival haemorrhages, Janeway lesions)
4. Immunological phenomena (e.g. glomerulonephritis, Osler's nodes, Roth spots, rheumatoid factor positivity)
5. Positive blood culture that does not meet the strict stipulations for being a major criterion (e.g. only *one* positive culture of appropriate organism)

A patient has ***definitive*** infective endocarditis if . . .
- They have both major Duke criteria, or . . .
- They have one major and three minor criteria, or . . .
- They have all five minor criteria, or . . .
- There is pathological evidence of endocarditis (demonstration and culture from vegetations, intracardiac abscesses or septic emboli)

A patient has ***possible*** infective endocarditis if . . .
- They have one major and one minor criteria, or . . .
- They have three minor criteria

OSCE station 33

Q. Examine this patient for a possible abdominal aortic aneurysm.

A.

- **Introduce** yourself and request to examine the patient
- **Expose** the abdomen adequately
- **Observe** whether patient appears comfortable or distressed (unlikely)
- Is there **nicotine staining** of the fingers?
- Look for an abnormal **prominent central abdominal pulsation** (beware that visible aortic pulsation can be a normal finding in young people)
- **Ask the patient if he has any abdominal pain** and to inform you if there is any discomfort when you examine them
- Gently place the **finger tips over the central abdomen** just above the umbilicus. Press gently and constantly until you feel an expansile (pushing and separating) mass, whist observing the patient's face for tenderness
- Gradually **palpate with your finger tips further and further apart** until the pulsations are no longer felt
- Give an **estimate of the size** of the aneurysm in centimetres
- **Listen** to the central area for a bruit (remember the actual lumen of an aneurysm may be small; also there may be associated atherosclerotic renal artery stenosis)
- Examine the **pulses below the aneurysm**
- **Examine the feet** for signs of ischaemia (pale, pulseless, cold, atrophic skin, ulceration, capillary refill), amputations, emboli (the so-called 'trash foot'; skin infarction, necrosis, punched out arterial ulcers)
- Say you would like to . . .
  - Examine the cardiovascular system in full (high prevalence of associated ischaemic heart disease)
  - Take the blood pressure
  - Dip the urine for glucose

Q. What investigations would you request if this patient were referred to out patients?

A.

In addition to routine pre-operative investigations, specific imaging would involve . . .

- **An abdominal ultrasound** would be simple and readily available; it would confirm the diagnosis and give a measurement of the size of the aneurysm

- **MRI scan** would provide detailed information pre-operatively

Q. What is the management of asymptomatic abdominal aortic aneurysms?

A.

- Aneurysms of <5 cm
  - Follow up annually
  - The risk of rupture is in the order of 1% per year
- Aneurysms of >5 cm
  - Should be repaired electively
  - The risk of death during surgery is in the order of 5%; however, the risk of spontaneous rupture is in the order of 90%

[See EMQ 19 (4), p. 143.]

OSCE station 34

A 36-year-old man brings his 66-year-old father to see you because he has noticed some behavioural changes, some difficulty with memory and fidgety hands and arms. No further history is available. You are asked to examine the patient . . .

On examination from the end of the bed you note first that the patient has an **expressionless face**. GCS is 14 (e4v4m6), patient appears confused. You also note **rapid, irregular, brief, jerky, seemingly unpredictable writhing movements of the hands and forearms**. The patient occasionally makes tic-like movements of the face, whereby he screws his face up, turns his head to one side and flicks out his tongue, like a frog trying to catch flies. His peripheries are warm, his pulse 79/min and regular, and his BP is 138/91. His heart sounds are normal, and his chest is clear with a respiratory rate of 18 b.p.m. and SpO_2 on room air of 98%. His abdomen is soft and non-tender. Throughout your examination, the strange movements of arms and face continue, and despite your best efforts to engage the patient in conversation, verbal exchange between the two of you is limited. Neurological examination is summarized below . . .

CNS

I	No gross defect
II	Acuity grossly normal (patient can read small print on newspaper with right and left eyes easily)

Visual fields normal L=R	VII Normal movements of facial muscles L=R
Fundoscopy normal L and R, no papilloedema	VIII Grossly normal hearing L=R
	IX Normal taste
Pupils equal and reactive to light and accommodation	X **On swallowing, patient chokes: ? dysphagia**
	XI Grossly normal L=R
No visual inattention	XII Patient unable to maintain protrusion of the
III/IV/VI Normal pupillary movements	tongue due to excessive twitchiness,
V Normal facial sensation L=R	although the tongue itself looks of normal
Normal power of muscles of mastication	bulk and is not wasted or fissured

PNS

	Left arm	Left leg	Right arm	Right leg
Tone	Increased (lead-pipe)	Increased	Increased	Increased
Power	5	5	5	5
Reflexes	Hyperreflexia	Hyperreflexia	Hyperreflexia	Hyperreflexia
Plantars		Equivocal		Up-going
Co-ordination	Impaired	Impaired	Impaired	Impaired
Sensation	Intact	Intact	Intact	Intact

Higher mental functioning
AMTS **4/10**

Gait
Staggering, unsteady and wide-based, with some bouncing quality due to the irregular movements which also affect the lower limb upon ambulation. There is ex-aggerated difficulty with turning. Romberg's is negative: the patient cannot balance especially well with eyes open or closed.

Speech
Speech is **slurred with difficulty in oration**. There appears to be no evidence of dysphasia.

Q. What is the most likely diagnosis, and why?
A.
The most likely diagnosis is **Huntington's disease**. The combination of lack of facial expression, choreoatheto-sis, paucity of verbal communication, dysphagia, dysarthria, so-called 'flycatcher's tongue', increased tone, hyperreflexia, abnormal plantar responses, impaired

co-ordination, cognitive impairment and ataxic gait is essentially the 'full house' of symptoms in Huntington's disease.

Q. What is the differential diagnosis?
A.
The differential diagnosis of conditions that cause chorea includes . . .
- **Drug-induced chorea** (neuroleptics, anti-Parkinsonian medications): ask about new medications
- **Metabolic chorea** (hyperthyroidism, hypoparathy-roidism, hyponatraemia, hypomagnesaemia, hypo-or hyperglycaemia): ask about new medical diagnoses
- **Cerebrovascular disease**: stroke may cause chorea, al-though this is usually limited to one side of the body
- **CNS inflammatory diseases** (SLE, sarcoidosis, Behçet's disease, MS): rare but important causes of chorea
- **Neurometabolic disorders** (Wilson's disease)
- **Neurodegenerative disease** (Alzheimer's, vascular de-

mentia, prion disease, etc.): again rarely causes chorea, but must be borne in mind
- **Post-infective chorea** (St Vitus' dance): follows either early or late after infection with rheumatic fever

Q. What is the treatment?
A.
There is **no specific treatment** for Huntington's disease, and the management is mainly supportive. Both patient *and* carers (often family) require consideration. Chorea may be decreased by **tetrabenazine** or **reserpine** (dopamine-depleting agents). Rigidity may be decreased with **baclofen**. Dysphagia may progress to necessitate the introduction of nasogastric supplementation, nasogastric feeding, and eventually formation of a percutaneous enterogastrostomy (PEG) to ensure adequate nutrition. Dysarthria may be improved with speech therapy. Little can be done to subvert the cognitive decline. Depression is a prominent symptom in Huntington's disease, and should be treated in the usual way (e.g. initial trial of a tricyclic agent or selective serotonin-reuptake inhibitor, e.g. fluoxetine).

The prognosis in Huntington's is bleak: the disease is **uniformly fatal**. The interval between diagnosis and death is approximately **15 years**, with few patients surviving beyond 20 years. Death often occurs due to aspiration pneumonia secondary to the swallowing difficulties inherent in the disease.

Q. What are the consequences for the patient's children and grandchildren?
A.
Huntington's disease is a hereditary triplet-repeat, neurodegenerative disease: it is inherited as an **autosomal dominant trait with full penetrance**, i.e. the children of an affected parent have a 50% chance of inheriting the disease. The Huntington allele is located on the short arm of chromosome 4, and consists of an extended CAG trinucleotide repeat. The phenotypic disease only occurs when the number of repeats exceeds 40. Huntington's disease is known to show the genetic phenomenon of **'anticipation'**: the number of triplet repeats may increase between generations, leading to earlier onset of the symptoms of the disease. A family history of Huntington's chorea is often deliberately or accidentally concealed: you need to look hard in your history for any early or unexplained deaths that have been put down to unsound reasons in the patients family.

A DNA test is now available that will tell the child of a patient with Huntington's whether they are in the lucky or the unlucky 50%, and will one way or the other alleviate 'the sword of Damocles' that is hanging over them. There is much controversy surrounding the value of such a test: given that there is no available treatment of the condition, why test for an illness that cannot be treated? People should only receive the test after **extensive genetic counselling**.

OSCE station 35

Q. Examine this patient's respiratory system.
A.
A **young** patient, who is **underweight** and shows evidence of **dyspnoea** from the end of the bed. The sputum pot at the bed side contains a (large) quantity of **purulent sputum** (with blood). There may be a cough productive of purulent sputum. The respiratory rate is elevated at. . . . There may be evidence of **finger clubbing**. There is no flap of CO_2 retention, the pulse is elevated at. . . . There may be **central cyanosis**. There is no lymphadenopathy. Chest examination reveals **course crepitations** throughout, with **scattered wheezing**. There may be an elevated JVP and ankle oedema if cor pulmonale has occurred.
The diagnosis is cystic fibrosis.

Q. Report on this chest radiograph.

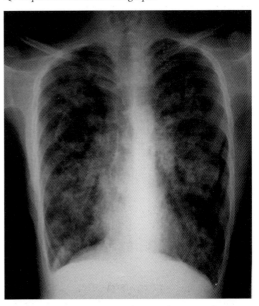

A.
The chest is **hyperinflated**. There are **multiple dilated**

airways with **thickened walls** (ring shadows) and a suggestion of **fluid levels**. In addition there are areas of **fluffy shadowing** diffusely in both mid-zones (infection). There are also areas of linear shadowing suggesting scarring. The appearances are consistent with diffuse bronchiectasis with associated inter-current infection. The most likely diagnosis in a young adult is **cystic fibrosis**. These changes are similar for bronchiectasis from any cause.

Q. What is the differential diagnosis?
A.

The differential diagnosis is that of bronchiectasis in a young patient . . .
- Childhood pneumonia including pertussis infection
- Congenital bronchiectasis
- Idiopathic bronchiectasis
- Hypogammaglobulinaemia
- Kartagener's syndrome (mucociliary clearance defect plus dextrocardia)
- Distil to an obstruction
  - Foreign body
  - Lymph nodes
  - TB

Q. What is the pathogenesis of cystic fibrosis?
A.

- An autosomal recessive condition; the frequency of the gene defect in the general population is 1 in 22
- In most cases a single gene mutation on chromosome 7 [deletion of phenylalanine in position 508 (δF508)] resulting in defective Cystic Fibrosis Transmembrane conductance Regulator (CFTR)
- This results in impaired chloride excretion into the airway lumen and an increase in sodium absorption from the lumen. Because water follows sodium the secretions are abnormally thick
- At birth the only sign is abnormally thick and viscid exocrine gland secretion:, the lungs are normal
- The brunt of the disease is on the respiratory tract. Colonization with pathogenic bacteria occurs early in childhood, leading to recurrent bouts of respiratory infection that causes progressive lung parenchymal damage
- Bronchiectasis occurs principally affecting the upper zones and an obstructive (FEV1/FCV < 80%) picture develops
- There is an inexorable progressive decline in the respiratory function, leading to pulmonary hypertension and cor pulmonale. This can be slowed but not halted by aggressive modern treatment

Q. How is the diagnosis made?
A.

- **Sweat testing**: a **sodium concentration of sweat above 60 mmol/L** is diagnostic. The test is less reliable in early childhood, becoming more reliable in adulthood. Paradoxically, the sodium concentration of sweat is raised unlike that of airway secretions, for reasons which are poorly understood
- **DNA analysis** for defective gene
- **Immunoreactive trypsin** in dried blood is decreased in patients with CF compared to normal subjects. Useful for screening but is not diagnostic
- Family history
- Early diagnosis in childhood is essential to allow active treatment (physiotherapy and antibiotics) to slow progressive impairment of lung function. Suspect in any child who . . .
  - Fails to thrive
  - Has repeated respiratory tract infections
  - Has meconium ileus
  - Has a positive family history

Q. Which bacteria colonize the respiratory tract in cystic fibrosis?
A.

Stepwise colonization occurs with age . . .
- Childhood
  - *Staphylococcus aureus*
  - *Haemophilus influenzae*
- Adolescence
  - *Pseudomonas aeruginosa*
- Adults
  - *Burkholderia cepacia*
  - *Streptococcus pneumoniae*
  - *Mycobacterium tuberculosis* (plus atypical mycobacteria)
  - *Aspergillus fumigatus*

Q. What are the complications of cystic fibrosis?
A.

- Pulmonary
  - Bronchietasis
  - Pneumothorax
  - Respiratory failure
  - Cor pulmonale

- Upper airway
  - Nasal polyps
- Hepatobiliary
  - Cirrhosis (5%)
  - Portal hypertension:
    Splenomegaly
    Oesophageal varices
  - Gallstones
- Pancreas
  - Exocrine insufficiency:
    Malabsorption
    Steatorrhoea (85%)
  - Pancreatitis
  - Diabetes (10%)
- Gastrointestinal
  - Meconium ileus in infancy
  - Meconium ileus equivalent:
    A mass of poorly digested food causing obstruction
  - Intussusception
- Subfertility
  - 95% of males due to failure of vas deferens development
  - Conception is often possible in females provided that ovulation is occurring. Secondary amenorrhoea is common

Q. How is the condition managed?
A.
- **Antibiotics**
  - Prophylactic antibiotics (nebulized tobramycin/oral flucloxacillin)
  - Antibiotics for acute exacerbations. An increasing purulence and quantity of sputum often requires admission for IV antibiotics (guided by sensitivities, e.g. cefatazidime, ciprofloxacin, gentamicin) and intensive physiotherapy
  - Nebulizers (saline for viscid secretions, tobramycin and asthma medications)
- **Physiotherapy** (during acute exacerbations and regularly at home)
- **Avoidance of colonization** with *Burkholderia cepacia* (segregation of carriers)
- **Oxygen** therapy (both for in-patient treatment and at home)
- **DNase therapy**: much of the viscid nature comes from the DNA left over from dead cells/bacteria. DNase enzyme helps to break this down and reduce the viscosity of secretions. Improvements of FEV1 of ≤20% in some patients occurs

- **Nutritional support**
  - Enzyme supplementation (powdered enzyme supplements with meals)
  - Nutritional supplements
- **Lung transplantation**

OSCE station 36

A 54-year-old man presents to his GP complaining that he has been having trouble driving due to **changes in his peripheral vision**.

On examination, you note that the patient has a very distinctive look about him, with a large nose, a prominent forehead, a protruding jaw and big hands. He has thick, greasy skin. Closer examination of his hands reveals their remarkable size. His heart rate is 95, regular. His BP is **210/110**. There is no postural drop. His JVP is slightly raised. His tongue is large, and on looking in his mouth you note a degree of **separation of his teeth**. He is very hirsute. His apex beat is mildly inferolaterally displaced. His heart sounds are normal. His lung bases reveal fine crepitations on the left and right. He has a soft, non-tender abdomen and mild peripheral oedema.

ECG is normal. Chest radiograph shows cardiomegaly, upper lobe venous diversion and small bi-basal effusions. Urine dipstick shows **glucose (+++)** and nil else.

Q. What is the likely diagnosis?
A.
The diagnosis here is **acromegaly**. The clues are in the patient's characteristic **appearance**, signs of **cardiac failure** and heavy **glycosuria**. Acromegalics tend to develop decreased glucose tolerance due to the **anti-insulin effects of growth hormone**. Patients with acromegaly usually present complaining of alteration in appearance, but the second most common complaint at presentation is of a visual field defect, usually **bi-temporal hemianopia**. Other symptoms include tightening of rings, carpal tunnel syndrome, polyuria, excessive sweating, impotence, galactorrhoea, goitre, menstrual disturbance, headaches and muscular weakness with joint pain. Any features of hypopituitarism may also be present: check for hypothyroidism, hypogonadism and postural hypotension. Acromegaly is due to a **pituitary somatotroph adenoma** in nearly all cases. Pituitary hyperplasia due to excessive hypothalamic GHRH production is rare, but can occur.

Q. What is the likely visual field defect?

A.

Patients with acromegaly develop bi-temporal hemianopia due to disruption of the fibres at the **optic chiasm** portion of the visual axis. These fibres carry information from the medial half of each retina, i.e. that portion of the retina that receives information from the lateral portion of the visual field. Patients typically complain of difficulty in driving.

Q. How would you confirm the diagnosis?

A.

The **glucose tolerance test (GTT)** is diagnostic for acromegaly. Acromegalics **fail to suppress levels of growth hormone** to less than 1 mU/L during the GTT, whereas non-acromegalic patients always would. In addition, approximately 25% of all patients with acromegaly will display a diabetic GTT. Other tests that may be useful in acromegaly include early morning growth hormone levels (expect raised levels in acromegaly, although commonly they are normal) and serum insulin-like growth factor (IGF-1) levels (made by the liver under growth hormone control and henceforth elevated in acromegalics). MRI scan of the pituitary will usually allow visualization of the adenoma.

Q. What is the treatment?

A.

The treatment of acromegaly can be either medical or surgical. What is clear is that some treatment must be forthcoming, otherwise lifespan of the patient will be attenuated, usually by death from cardiac failure, ischaemic heart disease or hypertension-related disease. Medical treatment can take the form of pharmacology or **external beam radiotherapy**. Drugs used in acromegaly are two in number . . .

1. Octreotide: a growth hormone analogue with no growth hormone effects, given subcutaneously for short-term treatment. It inhibits growth hormone production by a direct negative feedback effect on the pituitary

2. Dopamine agonists (e.g. bromocriptine, cabergoline): only used in the elderly and frail, are used to shrink tumours, but have largely been replaced by octreotide

Radiotherapy is usually only employed once other therapy has failed, or has only been partially successful, e.g. partially successful adenectomy. Used alone, the growth hormone response to radiotherapy has been shown to take up to 10 years to become manifest.

Surgery on the pituitary adenoma causing acromegaly

is usually approached **trans-sphenoidally**, although if the adenoma is large, surgery may have to proceed trans-frontally. Approximately two-thirds of patients will be placed into complete remission by surgery and will require no further therapy. The rest will need either octreotide, radiotherapy or both.

OSCE station 37

Q. Take a history from this patient who has had a long history of abdominal pain and altered bowel habit.

A.

The patient (usually **young and female**) complains of **frequent episodes** of **recurrent cramp**-like central or lower abdominal pain. There may be an associated sensation of abdominal **bloating**. The **appetite may be reduced** during an episode but there has been **no alteration in the patient's weight**. The patient may attribute the episodes to being **triggered by various types of foods**. There is **alteration of the bowel habit**. The motions may be bulky and loose or small and like 'rabbit pellets'. Defecation may partially relieve the abdominal pain for a period. There may be a history of mucus or even blood in the stool, but not melaena. The **history may date back over several years** and the episodes may occur during **periods of stress** either at home or work. There is frequently a **history of negative gastrointestinal investigations** such as barium enemas or colonoscopy.

There may be several non-GIT associated symptoms including . . .

- Painful heavy periods
- Tension headaches
- Functional bladder symptoms (frequency, a sensation in incomplete voiding)
- Fatigue symptoms
- Non-ulcer dyspeptic symptoms

On examination there is no evidence of malabsorption (weight loss, anaemia, proximal myopathy or oedema). The abdomen is not (significantly) tender and there is no organomegaly. PR examination is unremarkable.
The diagnosis is irritable bowel syndrome

Q. What is irritable bowel syndrome?

A.

It is a functional disorder of the gut where the clinical

picture consists of bouts of abdominal pain and altered bowel habit but without effect on nutrient absorption. It is common in all ages but especially young women (M:F = 3:1).

Q. How is the diagnosis made?
A.
The **diagnosis of IBS can be made clinically on the history and examination** without the requirement for further examination provided that . . .
- There are no worrying features suggesting malabsorption, inflammatory bowel disease or malignancy
- It is not a new presentation in a patient aged over 35 years

Q. What features make the diagnosis of irritable bowel syndrome likely?
A.
- A typical history
- A young patient (under 35 years of age)
- No worrying features
- A history of similar previous events
- Intermittent symptoms during the current phase ('good days and bad days')
- A clear association with stressful life events or other triggers

Q. What is the management of suspected IBS?
A.
- **Reassurance** that there is no serious pathology
- **High fibre diet** for patients where constipation or 'rabbit pellet' stools occur, *or*
- **Low fibre diet** for patients where bloating and diarrhoea predominate
- **Smooth muscle relaxants**, e.g. mebeverine or peppermint oil capsules, for cramp-like pain
- **Antidepressants** can help as a pain modulator and useful adjunct

OSCE station 38

A 60-year-old woman is brought into the resuscitation room of A&E following a **collapse in the street** whilst walking with her daughter. Immediately prior to collapse she complained of feeling **dizzy**, then developed 'a splitting headache'. Suddenly, she fell to the ground 'as if she had been shot' and became immediately unconscious. The daughter called an ambulance immediately. The ambulance crew requested resuscitation because the patient's GCS at scene was **7 (e2v1m4)**.

On examination, you note that the patient's GCS is now more like **3 (e1v1m1)**. She is currently maintaining her own airway, breathing spontaneously with SpO_2 of 99% on high flow O_2. Her chest is clear. Heart rate is 50, BP is **210/120**, heart sounds are normal, no carotid bruits. ECG shows no acute changes. Brief neurological examination of this unconscious patient reveals an entirely flaccid left side of the body, with absent deep tendon reflexes on the left. Fundoscopy reveals bilateral papilloedema. Right pupil is 6 mm and unreactive, left pupil is 3 mm and still reacting.

Q. What would be your initial management of this patient?
A.
Initial management of any acute medical problem is the same: **ABCDE** . . .
- A **Airway**: ensure **patent airway**; given patient's GCS, it is likely that even though she is currently maintaining her own airway, she will not continue to do so, and **the airway is not protected from aspiration in any patient with a GCS <8.** You must either **establish a definitive airway** (correctly sized endotracheal tube within patient's airway with cuff inflated and tube tied in place, connected to source of oxygen ± mechanical ventilator) or use **airway support techniques** (e.g. jaw thrust/chin lift, plus Guedel or nasopharyngeal airway) and call an anaesthetist to establish a definitive airway using rapid sequence induction. Ensure, if indicated, adequate cervical and/or spinal control (hard collar, sandbags, tape)
- B **Breathing**: give **high flow O_2** via tight-fitting facemask with reservoir bag attached. Check **respiratory rate**. Check **SpO_2. Auscultate chest**. This patient is tachypnoeic, RR = 30, with SpO_2 100% on high flow. Chest has crepitations at the right base, although overall air entry is good
- C **Circulation**: check **heart rate**; check **blood pressure**; check **capillary refill time** and **warmth of extremities. Auscultate the heart**. Obtain **intravenous access** and send **routine blood tests** (U+E, bicarbonate, glucose, FBC, clotting screen). HR = 50 regular, BP = 210/120, HS = normal, no added sounds or murmurs
- D **Disability**: estimate **GCS** — it is still 3. Check **BM**

E **Exposure and extremities** — patient is well covered from the elements and there is no clear abnormality of extremities on primary survey

Further management of a patient should only commence once all the above priorities have been dealt with. Only then should one be considering further tests to elucidate the cause of the clinical situation. **ECG** should be performed to rule out arrhythmia as the cause of the collapse. Discussion should be begun early with the radiologist to obtain an urgent head CT scan to elucidate any neurosurgically remediable causes of this collapse. **Frequent re-examination of the patient should be undertaken**, because various new developments, such as disappearance of pupillary reactions, will dictate the future clinical path.

In the near future, it is likely that CT- or angiographically-guided thrombolysis will become an option for ischaemic strokes, but it is not currently widely available in the UK for a variety of resource and manpower reasons.

If the cause of the stroke is likely to be a subarachnoid haemorrhage, then the calcium-channel antagonist **nimodipine** may be helpful, because it reduces the cerebral vasospasm that accompanies subarachnoid haemorrhage, thus assisting in maximal perfusion of threatened areas of brain.

Q. What is the likely diagnosis?
A.
The most likely diagnosis is a **haemorrhagic stroke**, probably due to subarachnoid haemorrhage from rupture of a congenital berry aneurysm.

Q. What are the treatment options?
A.
The patient must initially be stabilized maximally with regards ABC. If the head CT confirms the diagnosis of subarachnoid haemorrhage and the patient continues to deteriorate because the haemorrhage is acting like a fast expanding mass, then **urgent neurosurgical referral** must be undertaken (always re-examine the patient immediately before speaking to neurosurgeons to give them an up-to-date idea of the clinical situation). Their first priority, should they accept the patient, is to decompress the brain, usually by **surgical evacuation of the subarachnoid blood clot**, otherwise progression to deep unrecoverable coma and coning will ensue. Once this has been achieved, the neurosurgeons may then decide to attempt to find the location of the subarachnoid bleed

(usually an aneurysm) by **angiography**. They will then go on to either **surgically clip** or **endovascularly coil** the aneurysm to prevent further bleeding. Uninvolved aneurysms incidentally found may also be treated prophylactically.

OSCE station 39

Q. Examine this patient's respiratory system.
A.
There may be a **sputum pot** at the end of the bed (large volume of purulent material with possible evidence of haemoptysis). The patient may be **dyspnoeic, clubbed, underweight** and of **any age**. There may be **cyanosis** and features of cor pulmonale (elevated JVP, right ventricular heave, loud pulmonary component of the second heart sound, etc.). On auscultation there are **low-pitched coarse crepitations** on inspiration (secretions) which may be **localized or diffuse**. There may also be associated **wheezes**.

The diagnosis is bronchiectasis.

Q. Comment on this chest radiograph.

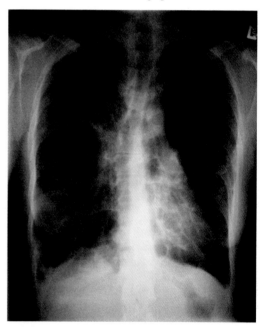

A.
This plain chest radiograph shows numerous **ring**

shadows (in this case in the proximity of the hilar areas) consisting of dilated airways with thickened walls, **tramline shadows** (as above but side on) and some **fluid levels**. The likely diagnosis is bronchiectasis. (Look also for an associated mass lesion with bronchiectasis distil to an area of airway compression).

Q. What are the causes of bronchiectasis?

A.

See cystic fibrosis, OSCE 35, p. 289

Q. What investigations would you perform to help in the diagnosis?

A.

- Chest radiograph
- High-resolution CT scan of the chest
- Sputum for culture and sensitivity
  - Common pathogens include:
    Staphylococcus aureus
    Haemophilus influenzae
    Pseudomonas aeruginosa
    Streptococcus pneumoniae
- Sweat test for cystic fibrosis
- Gammaglobulin levels
- Skin prick test for *Aspergillus* infection

Q. What is the management of bronchiectasis?

- **Physiotherapy** and postural drainage to remove thick sputum: patients are taught how to do this at home
- Regular courses of **antibiotics for exacerbations**
- **Oxygen** therapy as appropriate
- Diuretics and ACE inhibitors for cor pulmonale
- Occasionally surgical resection of localized disease

OSCE station 40

A 44-year-old female presents to her GP complaining of symptoms of generalized muscle aches, **pins-and-needles** and **weakness of her lower limbs** that she first noticed on ascending the stairs of her house 24 h previously. This weakness has subsequently progressed and she is finding it difficult ambulating around her home, and she is most concerned as to the cause. She feels as though over the last 12 h her hands have also begun to show signs of weakness. She is not complaining of loss of sensation in either arms or legs. She has no history of similar symptoms. The GP notes that she visited the surgery 3 weeks previously complaining of an upper respiratory tract infection, which was successfully treated with a course of amoxicillin.

On examination the GP notes an anxious lady. Cardiovascular, respiratory and gastrointestinal system examination is unremarkable. Her gait is normal, though she **tires easily** after walking only a few yards. Examination of her cranial nerves is unremarkable. Examination of the PNS is summarized in the table below . . .

	Right arm	*Right leg*	*Left arm*	*Left leg*
Tone	Normal	Hypotonic	Normal	Hypotonic
Power	5/5 (with effort)	4/5 — weakness as pronounced proximally as distally	5/5 (with effort)	4/5 — weakness as pronounced proximally as distally
Reflexes	Intact	Absent	Intact	Absent
Co-ordination	Normal	Unassessable due to weakness	Normal	Unassessable due to weakness
Sensation	Intact all modalities	Intact all modalities	Intact all modalities	Intact all modalities
Plantars		Down-going		Down-going

Q. What is the significance of the neurological findings?

A.

This patient has the classical clinical features of **Guillain–Barré syndrome**, an **acute symmetrical ascending polyneuropathy** that often begins with myalgia or paraesthesia of the legs, followed by weakness. The weakness often ascends to involve the pelvic girdle, abdominal, thoracic and arm muscles. Examination shows *symmetrical* **weakness with loss of tone, loss of reflexes and flaccidity. The seventh cranial nerve is frequently involved** and bilateral facial weakness is common. Other cranial nerves may be involved. Sensory loss does occur, but this is **disproportionately less than the motor involvement**. It is thought to follow 1–3 weeks after an upper respiratory or GIT infection (may be subclinical), and occurs due to **lymphocytic sensitization to a peripheral nerve antigen**, leading to **diffuse patchy segmental demyelination of peripheral nerves**.

Miller–Fisher syndrome is a rare proximal variant of Guillain–Barré syndrome in which there is ophthalmoplegia ($\rightarrow$ diplopia), ataxia and arreflexia, without significant weakness or sensory signs.

Q. What is the differential diagnosis?

A.

Differential diagnosis of the neurological symptoms includes . . .

- **Poliomyelitis**: characterized by initial pyrexia, severe myalgia and subsequent *asymmetrical* flaccid paralysis and no sensory involvement
- **Botulism**: occurs in groups from food poisoning; begins with visual symptoms (diplopia)
- **Heavy metal neuropathy**: onset of symptoms is much slower
- **Periodic paralysis**: onset of symptoms is more sudden; respiratory involvement is absent and there is an accompanying hypo- or hyperkalaemia

If the patient presents with acute neuromuscular respiratory failure, then the diagnosis of Guillain–Barré should be one of exclusion once other known causes of neuromuscular respiratory failure have been ruled out. The treatment of neuromuscular respiratory failure is the same regardless of the cause: regular measurement of forced vital capacity (FVC); if FVC falls below 1 L, then consideration of intubation and intermittent positive pressure ventilation (IPPV) should be undertaken (as a rule, only commence in reversible conditions such as Guillain–Barré).

Q. What is the prognosis? What are the complications?

A.

The prognosis of Guillain–Barré syndrome is good: approximately **85% of patients make a complete or almost complete recovery**. The acute paralysis commonly progresses for 10 days, remains unchanged for 2 weeks, and then slowly resolves over the course of 6 months to 2 years. Patients with a history of Guillain–Barré syndrome may be graded 1–5 . . .

Grade 1	Able to run
Grade 2	Able to walk 5 m but not to run
Grade 3	Able to walk 5 m with assistance
Grade 4	Chair- or bed-bound
Grade 5	Intubated and ventilated

Only 10% of patients remain at grade 4 or 5 one year after the initial syndrome began. Even complete initial paralysis may be compatible with subsequent complete recovery.

The most sinister complication is **respiratory impairment** (50% of patients) that may progress to failure (in 33% of patients). Other significant complications include **autonomic instability** (urinary retention, sweating, tachycardia, dysrhythmia, fluctuating blood pressure, orthostatic hypotension), pain, secondary respiratory tract infection (due to suboptimal ventilation), papilloedema, DVT and pressure ulcers.

Q. What is the treatment?

A.

The treatment depends on whether neuromuscular respiratory impairment/failure is present. **Regular measurement of FVC** and arterial blood gases should be performed. In the presence of an FVC of <1.5 L, a $PaCO_2$ of >6 kPa or a PaO_2 of <10 kPa, strong consideration of transfer to intensive care and intubation with **IPPV** should be made. If respiratory impairment is not a feature, then management should take the form of . . .

- **Monitoring for autonomic instability**: ECG, frequent measurement of BP and HR
- **CSF analysis**: to reveal rising protein levels, which peak at around 6 weeks
- **IV immunoglobulin**: for 5 days has been shown to speed recovery (superior to plasmapheresis)
- Good nursing care: to avoid DVT and pressure sores

NB There is no evidence that steroids are beneficial in Guillain–Barré syndrome.

OSCE station 41

A 19-year-old student presents to A&E complaining of a 12-h history of gradual-onset, **worsening severe headache**. She has been previously fit and well, apart from a 2-day history of earache. She has no history of migraine or other recurrent severe headache. There is no history of head trauma. She has **vomited** once at home. She is up-to-date with her childhood vaccinations. You are asked to examine her . . .

On examination you find an extremely poorly-looking girl. She is pale and is **shielding her eyes from the light in the cubicle**. Though you turn the light off she continues to narrow her eyes to the faint ambient light from outside. Her BM is 4.5. Her temperature is **38.9°C**. She has **no evidence of rash**. She is **tachycardic**, 115/min. Her blood pressure is 115/76. Her heart sounds are normal with no murmurs. Her chest is clear. GIT examination is unremarkable. GCS 15, AMTS 10. There is no focal abnormality on examination of her PNS. The only discernible abnormality on CNS examination is some **bilateral blurring of the optic discs** on fundoscopy. You also feel that there is some **reproducible nuchal rigidity**. Both Kernig's and Brudzinski's tests are positive.

*Q. You are immediately told by the examiner that this is **not** a case of bacterial meningitis (in fact, it is and he/she is just being mean). What is the differential diagnosis of such a presentation when meningitis is ruled out?*
A.
The differential diagnosis of acute bacterial meningitis is wide. **Other infectious causes of meningitis** must be considered: **viruses** (e.g. enteroviruses like echovirus and Coxsackie virus), **TB**, **fungi** (e.g. *Cryptococcus*), *Rickettsiae* (e.g. Rocky Mountain spotted fever), and *Spirochaetes* (e.g. syphilis). **Subarachnoid haemorrhage, brain abscess, brain tumour** and **iatrogenic causes** (e.g. medications, operations and spinal anaesthesia) may all cause a similar clinical picture.

Q. Describe your initial management of this patient.
A.
As with every answer to immediate management you would be expected to answer this along the principles of ABC. Once you had ensured that the airway was patent and being maintained, that the chest was clear with a rea-

sonable respiratory rate and SpO_2 (+/– supplementary O_2), and that heart rate and BP were satisfactory and heart sounds were normal, you would then be free to move on to the specifics of acute management of (likely bacterial) acute meningitis.

Intravenous access should be secured immediately and **blood taken for all routine tests** (U+E, FBC, bicarbonate, glucose and clotting screen) and **blood cultures**. If not already given, the patient should receive **intravenous penicillin or ceftriaxone** (or alternative third-generation cephalosporin). In patients allergic to penicillins, consider intravenous erythromycin and chloramphenicol (if in hospital, discuss with resident microbiologist). Any of the recognized complications of acute bacterial meningitis should be treated as they occur (e.g. seizures should be treated with benzodiazepines, raised ICP should be treated with steroids and mannitol).

Ultimate diagnosis of the aetiology of the meningitis is based on examination of the CSF. However, **lumbar puncture (LP) should rarely be undertaken without first having a head CT** performed to rule out raised ICP. Performing lumbar puncture in a patient with raised ICP can be rapidly fatal due to brainstem herniation through the foramen magnum. Some groups say that CT head should only be performed if there are focal neurological signs, papilloedema, reduced conscious level or frequent seizures. We feel that unless the presentation is extremely benign, CT head should be performed in all cases of ?meningitis, as not only does it allow raised ICP to be identified, but it also allows a number of other pathologies that present like bacterial meningitis to be excluded, e.g. subarachnoid haemorrhage (still need LP to exclude), infarction, tumour and brain abscess. Unfortunately, a normal head CT is not 100% accurate in identifying all cases of raised ICP, and cerebral herniation and death still occur on LP in patients with normal CT scans.

Lumbar puncture should be performed and CSF should be sent for **Gram stain, microscopy, culture, sensitivity, WCC, protein measurement and glucose measurement**. Broad-spectrum antibiotics should be continued until results are available from microbiology that may better direct therapy.

Public health services should be notified in any case of bacterial meningitis. They will give advice on treatment and will assist in contact tracing. **Prophylaxis** should be given to all contacts (rifampicin or ciprofloxacin).

OSCEs

The patient in the above question has a CT scan that shows 'no evidence of raised intracranial pressure (no midline shift, no dilatation of the ventricles, no papilloedema)'. You perform a lumbar puncture. Initial results show the following . . .

Appearance:	Cloudy
Cells per mm³:	1005
Predominant cell type:	Small cells with multilobular nuclei

Glucose:	20% of blood glucose
Protein:	1.2 g/L

Q. *Describe how you would use a sample of CSF to differentiate between bacterial, viral, tuberculous and fungal causes of meningitis.*

A.

By remembering the following table . . .

		CSF in . . .			
Characteristic	*Normal CSF*	*bacterial meningitis*	*TB meningitis*	*viral meningitis*	*fungal meningitis*
Appearance	Clear, colourless, does not clot in tube	Turbid	Clear	Clear	Clear
Cells/mm³	0–5	5–2000	5–1000	5–500	5–500
Main cell type	Mononuclear	Neutrophil	Lymphocyte	Lymphocyte	Lymphocyte
Glucose	>50% of blood glucose	Very low (<30% blood glucose)	Low	Normal	Normal or mildly decreased
Protein	<0.4 g/L	High (often >1)	Very high (>>1)	Normal or mildly raised	High (often >1)
Smear	No organisms	Organisms	May see occasional organism	No organisms	No organisms; may see fungal hyphae with correct stain
Lactic acid (mmol/L)	0.8–2.8	>35	>35	<35	<35
Opening pressure (mmH₂O)	70–200	>200	Within normal range	Within normal range	Within normal range
Other tests		Bacterial antigen	Ziehl–Nielsen, fluorescence, PCR	PCR	Special stains

Based on the results of the CSF, you decide that the likely cause of the patient's clinical state is bacterial meningitis.

Q. Describe how you would use clinical information to decide which bacterium is most likely to be the culprit.
A.
Several clinical variables give clues as to the most likely infecting bacterium in cases of meningitis. These are . . .
1. **Age of patient**
   - **0–4 weeks**
   Group B *Streptococcus*; *Escherichia coli*; *Listeria monocytogenes*; *Klebsiella pneumoniae*; *Enterococcus* spp; *Salmonella* spp
   - **4–12 weeks**
   Streptococcus agalactiae; *E. coli*; *L. monocytogenes*; *Haemophilus influenzae*; *Streptococcus pneumoniae*; *Neisseria meningitidis*
   - **months–18 years**
   S. pneumoniae; *N. meningitidis*; *H. influenzae*
   - **18–50 years**
   S. pneumoniae; *N. meningitidis*
   - **>50 years**
   S. pneumoniae; *N. meningitidis*; *L. monocytogenes*; aerobic Gram-negative bacilli
2. **Immunocompromized state**
   S. pneumoniae; *N. meningitidis*; *L. monocytogenes*; aerobic Gram-negative bacilli (including *Pseudomonas aeruginosa*)
3. **Basilar skull fracture/chronic otitis/sinusitis**
   S. pneumoniae; *H. influenzae*; Group A β-haemolytic streptococci
4. **Head trauma/post-neurosurgery**
   Staphylococcus aureus; *Staphylococcus epidermidis*; aerobic Gram-negative bacilli (including *P. aeruginosa*)
5. **CSF shunt (in patients with hydrocephalus)**
   Staph. aureus; *Staph. epidermidis*; aerobic Gram-negative bacilli (including *P. aeruginosa*); diphtheriods; *Propionibacterium acnes*

The most likely cause of this patient's meningitis given her age, her history of earache and the overall clinical picture is *S. pneumoniae*.

Q. Describe the proper procedure for elucidating Kernig's and Brudzinski's signs. What is the significance of the result in this patient?
A.
Kernig's sign (named after Russian physician Vladimir

Kernig, 1840–1917) is elicited by lying the patient flat on their back. Flex one leg to 90° at both hip and knee. Keeping the hip flexed, extend the leg at the knee. Discomfort behind the knee is to be expected in normal subjects. However, **pain at the back of the neck and resistance to extension of the knee** suggests Kernig's sign. For the sign to be positive, the pain and resistance has to be present on testing *both* legs. It suggests meningeal irritation.

Brudzinski's sign (named after Polish physician Josef von Brudzinski, 1874–1917) is elicited by passively flexing the neck of the patient. If this manoeuvre causes **reflex flexion of the hips and knees**, then Brudzinski's sign is positive. It suggests meningeal inflammation.

This patient has both a positive Kernig's and Brudzinski's sign, meaning that there is almost certainly a meningitic process occurring. The absence of these signs, however, does not rule out meningitis: only 50% of patient with meningitis demonstrate positivity for these signs.

OSCE station 42

Q. The patient has joint problems. Examine their hands.
A.
The hand examination routine in rheumatology . . .
- Ask the patient if they have any joint pain first
- Place the hands on a pillow on the patient's lap with the dorsal surface upwards
- Inspect the hands commenting on any typical deformities which might suggest rheumatoid arthritis
  - Ulnar deviation
  - Swan neck deformity
  - Boutonniere deformity
  - 'Z' thumb deformity
  - Tendon rupture
- Inspect for the Bouchard's (PIPJs) and Heberden's nodes (DIPJs) of osteoarthritis
- Inspect the nails closely for the pitting and oncholysis of psoriasis (remember it is possible to have psoriatic arthropathy with limited or absent skin lesions)
- Remember to look closely for nail fold vasculitis and steroid-induced skin atrophy and purpura
- Comment on any wasting of the interrossii (guttering between the metacarpals)
- Ask the patient to turn the hands palm upwards and look for palmar erythema
- Then examine very carefully for active synovitis, by looking at the patient's face for tenderness whilst

gently palpating the dorsal aspects of the metacarpophalangeal joints
- Check the motor and sensory function of the hands (possible carpal tunnel syndrome and mononeuritis multiplex)
- Ask the patient to perform some motor tasks to assess hand function (e.g. grip a key or pen, fasten a shirt button)
- Finally check around the elbows for rheumatoid nodules

Q. How is the diagnosis of rheumatoid arthritis made?
A.

On the clinical picture . . .
- The onset of a symmetrical inflammatory (morning stiffness for >1 h) arthritis most commonly affecting the metacarpo-phalangeal joints
- The findings of typical peri-articular erosions, soft tissue swelling, and deformity on radiography
- The presence of rheumatoid factor (in 70%)

Rheumatoid arthritis is much loved in medical examinations because the disease is multisystemic and the patients have stable physical signs. A **symmetrical** deforming polyarthritis occurs involving the MCPJs, wrists, elbows, shoulders, cervical spine, knees, ankles and MTPJs. An erosive synovitis occurs with 'boggy' soft tissue swelling and tenderness. It **tends not to involve the axial skeleton**, sacroiliac joints and the hips.

Q. What is the epidemiology of rheumatoid arthritis?
A.

Remember mnemonic **3344** . . .

3	1–<u>3</u>% of the population
3	<u>3</u>:1 female:male ratio
4	HLA DR<u>4</u>
4	<u>4</u>0 years or over is age of typical onset

Q. What are the radiographic findings in rheumatoid arthritis?
A.
- Soft tissue swelling
- Peri-articular erosions
- Cartilage thinning
- Subluxations/ deformity

Q. What are the (extra-articular) complications of rheumatoid arthritis?
A.
- **Skin complications**

- Vasculitis
- Nail fold infarcts
- Sensory neuropathy
- Steroid changes (skin atrophy and purpura)
- Nodules (in 30%): any site is possible, e.g. skin, lung, bone (patients will be positive for rheumatoid factor)
- Drug reactions
- **Haematological complications**
  - **Anaemia:**
    Anaemia of chronic disease
    Haemolytic anaemia
    Drug side effects
       Blood loss due to NSAID usage
       Marrow suppression with DMARTs
    Associated (autoimmune) pernicious anaemia
  - **Felty's syndrome:**
    Neutropenia
    Splenomegaly
    RA
    Occasionally with leg ulcers, pigmentation and lymphadenopathy
  - **Thrombocytosis**; reflects the degree of disease activity
- **Pulmonary complications**
  - Effusions (most common feature)
  - Rheumatoid nodules (which may cavitate)
  - Caplan's syndrome (nodular fibrosis with coal dust exposure)
  - Fibrosing alveolitis
  - Obliterative bronchiolitis
- **Ophthalmic complications**
  - Anterior uveitis
  - Episcleritis
  - Scleritis
  - Scleromalacia
  - Scleromalacia perforans
  - Sjögren's syndrome:
    Keratoconjunctivitis sicca
    Xerostomia
    RA
- **Neurological complications**
  - Peripheral nerve entrapment (carpal tunnel syndrome)
  - Polyneuropathy
  - Atlanto-axial subluxation
- **Cardiological complications**
  - Pericarditis (pericardial effusions and tamponade)
  - Nodules in the myocardium
- **Others**

- Amyloidosis
- Lymphadenopathy in proximity to an inflamed joint
- Weight loss
- Depression
- Medication side effects

Q. What modes of presentation of rheumatoid arthritis do you know?

A.

- **Insidious onset** of small joint pain, swelling and morning stiffness with remissions and relapses; the most common presentation (70%)
- **Pallindromic RA**: moves between different affected large joints with resolution between attacks; 50% convert to the more typical form especially if rheumatoid factor positive
- **Systemic onset**: extra-articular features predominate
- **Rapid progression RA**: deformity and disability occurring over a few years; high occurrence of extra-articular features and resistance to usual treatments occur
- **Transient RA**: usually seronegative disease which resolves following a bout of synovitis; good prognosis

Q. What do you know about rheumatoid factor in rheumatoid arthritis?

A.

- Rheumatoid factor is IgM, G or A directed against the Fc portion of IgG
- It occurs in **4%** of the normal population, but in 70% of those with RA. This rises to 100% if there are extra-articular features, e.g. nodules, Felty's syndrome, pulmonary involvement, etc.
- It may also be variably positive in various other conditions (where there is excessive immune system activity) . . .
  - **Infections:**
    Syphilis
    Bacterial endocarditis
    TB
  - **Autoimmune illnesses:**
    Fibrosing alveolitis
    Sarcoidosis
    Chronic autoimmune hepatitis
    SLE
    Systemic sclerosis
    Polyarteritis nodosa
- It supports the diagnosis of RA when taken with the clinical picture, and predicts more severe disease when present

Other possibilities for rheumatology OSCE stations

- Other joint examinations
- Joint radiographs
- Spot diagnoses plus assorted supplementary questions (especially tophaceous gout and ankylosing spondylitis)
- History/ counselling stations
  - Explain RA
  - Discuss available treatments
  - Full history (emphasis on functional difficulties, social situation plus aids and appliances)
- Assorted management questions, e.g.
  - Risks of NSAIDS
  - Side effects of DMARTS

Other possible rheumatology diagnoses

- RA (the most likely case)
- Osteoarthritis
- Ankylosing spondylitis [see EMQ 18 (5), p. 131]
- Psoriatic arthritis [see EMQ 23 (4), p. 155]
- Scleroderma (systemic sclerosis) [see OSCE 28, p. 277]
- Tophaceous gout [see EMQ 23 (5), p. 155]
- Dermatomyositis [see EMQ 15 (5), p. 123]
- SLE [see EMQ 6 (5), p. 77]
- Vasculitis [see EMQ 15 (4), p. 122]

Other hand examination spot diagnosis OSCE stations

- **Acromegaly** ('spade like', thick greasy skin plus typical habitus)
- **Thyroid disease** (fine tremor, tachycardia, clubbing)
- **Marfan's disease** (arachnodactyly)
- **Raynaud's disease** (white finger, digital infarcts, ?features of scleroderma)
- **Stigmata of bacterial endocarditis**
- **Clubbing**
- **Chronic liver disease** stigmata (palmar eythema, flap, leukonychia)
- **Peripheral neuropathy** (media, ulnar nerve and radial nerve palsies)
- **Dermatological problems**, e.g. psoriasis, nail dystrophy

---

OSCE station 43

A 61-year-old man presents to A&E complaining of a **1-h** history of **worsening severe tearing interscapular back**

pain accompanied by **heavy central chest pain**. It came on whilst he was painting the living room and at first he thought that he had merely pulled a muscle, hence the delay in presentation. He has **never suffered with any chest pain in the past**, although he does have a history of musculoskeletal back pain and **hypertension**, currently being treated by 2.5 mg bendrofluazide daily. In the last 10 min he has begun to complain of **tingling and numbness affecting his left arm**.

On examination, the patient has a heart rate of **121/min, regular**, and a blood pressure of **185/119** in the right arm. He is fidgeting around the bed unable to get comfortable due to the pain. He is peripherally cold and cyanosed, and has a **capillary refill time of 3 s**. He seems to be becoming **more confused** the longer he remains in the cubicle, and you note a degree of agitation beginning to appear. His heart and breath sounds appear normal, and his respiratory rate is 30. You note **absence of femoral, popliteal, posterior tibial and pedal pulses bilaterally**. Grossly, you note a **decrease in sensation and power in the left arm** compared to the right.

Q. What would be the four most important initial investigations to perform?
A.
1. **ECG**: this is vitally important to check for myocardial ischaemia/infarction in a patient who presents in such a way
2. **Right and left arm blood pressure**: potentially shows great difference between right and left arms depending on the location and spread of an aortic dissection. A difference of 20 mmHg systolic is considered significant
3. **Chest X-Ray**: expected to show widening of the mediastinum and blurring of the normal mediastinal anatomy, including obscuration of the aortic knuckle
4. **Transoesophageal echocardiography (TOE)**: preferable to CT/MRI scan in the unstable patient, this diagnostic technique can confirm or rule out the diagnosis, and also give an idea of the extent of the dissection. However, due to restricted emergency access to skilled TOE technicians, patients often receive a CT scan

Q. How are dissecting thoracic aortic aneurysms classified?
A.
There are two main ways in which dissecting thoracic aneurysms are classified . . .
1. **DeBakey classification**

- *DeBakey I*: dissection originates in ascending part of aorta, and involves the arch and the descending aorta
- *DeBakey II*: dissection originates in and is confined to the ascending aorta
- *DeBakey III*: dissection originates in the first part of the descending aorta distal to the origin of the left subclavian artery, and migrates distally
2. **Stanford classification**
- *Stanford A*: dissection affects the ascending aorta, whether its origin is proximal or distal
- *Stanford B*: dissection does not affect the ascending aorta

Q. What are the complications of dissecting aneurysms, excluding death?
A.
Retrograde dissection, whereby the stripping of the intimal lining of the vessel from the media progresses backward toward the aortic valve. Should the dissecting process reach the valve, torrential aortic regurgitation ensues along with acute cardiac failure. The coronary ostia also become occluded, leading to acute severe myocardial ischaemia. The most devastating consequence of retrograde dissection is however when it progresses to the aortic root and free rupture occurs into the pericardial sac, leading to acute tamponade and usually rapid death.

    Anterograde dissection may also occur. If the dissection begins in the ascending aorta, then it may involve the brachiocephalic vessels and lead to acute stroke. If the dissection originates in the descending aorta, the dissection can come to involve the renal, mesenteric, spinal and even femoral and iliac vessels, leading to ARF, mesenteric ischaemia, neurological symptoms, or ischaemia of the lower limbs.

Q. What are the main causes of dissecting aneurysms?
A.
The main causes of dissection can be remembered using the mnemonic **PATC$_3$H** . . .
  P   Pregnancy
  A   Aortic coarctation
  T   Trauma
  C   Connective tissue disorders, specifically Marfan's and Ehlers–Danlos syndrome
       Congenital cardiac disease, specifically Turner's and Noonan's syndrome
       Cocaine and other stimulant drugs of abuse
  H   Hypertension, being *by far the most common*

What the above conditions have in common is **hyperdynamic blood flow** and a **damaged/deranged medial arterial layer**. In this situation, a small tear in the intimal lining of the artery allows the turbulent blood flow access to the defective media, and a false lumen arises, cleaving the intima from the media for a variable distance.

Q. What is the treatment of dissecting aneurysms?
A.

There is much debate about the best manner in which to treat dissections, including postulations that some dissections should be treated surgically whilst others should be managed conservatively by physicians. In general, the **results of treatment are poor** (mortality is 1–2% per hour for the first 24–48 h). It is currently thought that *all type A dissections should be treated surgically*, whilst *only certain subgroups of patients with type B dissections should be treated surgically* (those patients with dissections that are leaking, ruptured or compromising blood flow to a vital organ; also patients with Marfan's or in whom medical treatment is failing to control BP should have their distal dissection treated surgically). Medical treatment is usually directed towards **aggressively lowering the inevitable hypertension** with a combination of **sodium nitroprusside and a β-blocker, such as labetalol**. Surgical treatment involves **resection of the diseased portion of the aorta**, with distal and proximal closure of the aorta and replacement of the resected part with an appropriate graft material, such as Dacron®. Where possible, surgical treatment should be delayed until the patient is medically stable.

OSCE station 44

Q. Examine this patient's gastrointestinal system for evidence of liver dysfunction.
A.

The patient appears **thin** with obvious **muscle wasting** (malnutrition/chronic liver synthetic dysfunction) and **jaundiced** from the end of the bed. There is evidence of **clubbing** and **scratch marks**. There is a **liver flap**, **Dupuytren's contracture** and **palmar erythema**. The skin is **thin, bruised** and there are **scratch marks**. The **conjunctiva appear yellow (and pale?)**. There is evidence of **parotid gland enlargement**. There are numerous large **spider naevi** on the face and upper chest (compress with a digit and watch them refill from the centre outwards). There is **gynaecomastia** (palpate for subareolar glandular development).

The abdomen appears **distended uniformly (ascites)**. There are dilated collateral veins over the abdominal wall with blood flowing away from the umbilicus (**caput medusae**). There is a **fluid thrill and evidence of shifting dullness**. The **liver and spleen are (or are not) enlarged** (comment on the size and surface of the liver). There is **testicular atrophy**. There is pitting **oedema** of the ankles.

The patient may be **agitated, restless and confused**, consistent with hepatic encephalopathy? (Unlikely in an examination.)

The patient has signs consistent with chronic liver disease.

Q. What are the possible complications of liver failure?
A.

- Bleeding tendency
  - Reduced hepatic synthesis of coagulation factors
  - Vitamin K deficiency: a fat-soluble vitamin (ADEK) requires bile acids to help adsorption
  - Thrombocytopenia due to consumption by large spleen (hyperspenism)
  - Impaired platelet function due to abnormal liver function
  - Disseminated intravascular coagulation
- Hepatic encephalopathy
- Infections
- Hypoglycaemia (impaired gluconeogenesis)
- Portal hypertension and variceal haemorrhage
- Ascites
- Hepatorenal syndrome
  - In essence, nitric oxide accumulates in liver failure, which is a vasodilator producing hypotension reducing renal blood flow and precipitating renal failure. The prognosis is poor
- Hepatocellular carcinoma
  - Chronic viral hepatitis
  - Haemachromatosis

Q. What is cirrhosis, and what are the possible causes?
A.

Cirrhosis occurs where there is damage to liver cells with nodular regeneration of tissue associated with fibrosis. Fibrosis eventually dominates the picture with declining liver function. The nodular regeneration is either micronodular (<3 mm; mainly alcohol) or macronodular (often hepatitis B).

Although hepatomegaly may be present early in the condition, cirrhosis is eventually characterized (variably) by a small non-functioning liver, persistent jaundice, ascites, a bleeding tendency and encephalopathy. There is usually a continued insult (e.g. alcohol, autoimmunity or chronic viral hepatitis infection) perpetuating the liver damage.

The picture is one of chronic liver disease. The causes could include . . .
- **Alcoholic liver damage**
- **Infections**
  - Hepatitis B (D), C
- Autoimmune
  - Chronic autoimmune hepatitis
  - Primary biliary cirrhosis
- Drugs
  - Carbon tetrachloride
  - Methotrexate
  - Isoniazid
  - Rifampicin
  - Amiodadrone
  - Many others
- Blood (stasis)
  - Right ventricular failure
  - Budd Chiari syndrome: hepatic vein occlusion/ thrombosis due to 'bush tea', chemotherapy, radiotherapy or thrombophilic predisposition
- Bile (stasis)
  - Common bile duct stricture or stone
  - Congenital biliary atresia
- Metabolic
  - α_1-antitrypsin deficiency (cirrhosis and emphysema)
  - Haemochromatosis
  - Wilson's disease (always exclude this treatable condition in young patients with liver disease or apparent Parkinson's disease)
- Miscellaneous
  - Cystic fibrosis
  - Sickle cell disease
  - Osler–Weber–Rendu syndrome
  - Idiopathic

Q. What is the prognosis in cirrhosis?
A.
The **Child–Pugh grading** scores cirrhosis based on the following point system . . .

Score	1	2	3
Bilirubin*	<34	34–50	>50
Albumin (g/L)	>35	28–35	<28
INR (seconds prolonged)	<4	4–6	>6
Encephalopathy	None	Mild	Severe
Ascites	None	Mild	Severe

- Child's grade A = <7, B = 7–9, C = >9
- Grade C has an expected survival of less than 12 months
- *for sclerosing cholangitis or primary biliary cirrhosis the bilirubin grading is; <68, 68–170 and >170

Q. This patient is jaundiced, what questions would you like to ask?
- Alcohol intake?
- Travel?
  - Hepatitis A, B from blood products and sexual transmission
- Blood transfusions?
  - Especially in less developed countries
  - All blood in developed countries are now screened for hepatitis B and C virus, and HIV
- Haemophilia?
  - Hepatitis C
- Sexual history?
  - Particularly recent unprotected intercourse/ homosexual sex
- IV drug abuse?
  - Especially needle sharing
- Medications?
  - Many drugs can cause liver damage!
  - Paracetamol overdose
  - Ask for recent changes to medications
- Family history (Gilbert's syndrome)?
- Previous episodes (Gilbert's syndrome)?
- Past medical history?
  - Gallstones
  - Inflammatory bowel disease (sclerosing cholangitis)

- Haematological conditions, e.g. sickle cell disease
- Pregnancy?
  - A cause of an acute cholestatic jaundice and fulminant hepatic failure
- Abdominal pain?
  - Gallstones
  - Pancreatic malignancy (late feature)
  - Sepsis
- Colour of urine and stools?
  - Pale stools and dark urine in obstructive jaundice
- General systemic review?
  - Weight loss
  - Fevers
  - Vomiting

Q. What are the possible causes of jaundice?

If you get a question such as this, which appears to warrant an extremely long answer, it is best to respond initially by giving the general headings, to avoid being overwhelmed. For example, in response to 'Tell me some causes of weak legs' you could start with: 'The possible causes may be divided into muscular weakness, neuromuscular junction problems (myasthenia gravis, Eaton Lambert), motor neuropathy, anterior horn cell damage (motor neurone disease), spinal cord pathology, or cerebral hemisphere pathology (stroke) etc . . .'.

A.

Jaundice may be classified into . . .

- **Haemolytic jaundice (prehepatic)**
  The increased red cell breakdown in the various haemolytic anaemias leads to an excess of unconjugated bilirubin as liver enzyme (glucuronosyl transferase) systems are overloaded. The unconjugated ('raw') bilirubin is water insoluble and does not appear in the urine (i.e. acholuric; urine is not dark). However, the liver does 'process' more bilirubin than usual, which leads to greater production of urobilinogen in the terminal ileum following the reduction of bilirubin. This urobilinogen appears in the urine.
  Suspect a haemolytic jaundice if . . .
- Liver function tests are normal
- Unconjugated hyperbilirubinaemia
- Elevated urinary urobilinogen
- There is evidence of increase RBC destruction:
  Splenomegaly
  Abnormal RBC shapes (spherocytes, fragments, sickle cells)

- Evidence of increased RBC production (to compensate):
  Immature RBCs in the circulation (reticulocytes)
  Expansion of the marrow production (erythroid hyperplasia)
  RBC production in non-marrrow sites (extramedullary haematopoiesis), e.g. liver (hepatomegaly) and spleen (splenomegaly)
- **The congenital hyperbilirubinaemias**
  Unconjugated
  - **Gilbert's syndrome:**
    Reduced glcuronosyl transferase
    Periodic jaundice that is mild (bilirubin <100 μmol/L) and otherwise normal LFTS
    Jaundice may be precipitated by 24-h fast, infections or IV nicotinic acid infusion
    Common and does not require any intervention
  - **Criggler Najjar:**
    Rare
    Absent (recessive type) or virtually absent (dominant type) glucoronosyl transferase
    Liver transplantation is required
  Conjugated
  - **Dubin Johnson:**
    Recessive inheritance
    Black liver due to melanin deposition
    Good prognosis
  - **Rotor syndrome:**
    Dominant inheritance
    Good prognosis
- **Liver disease causing cholestasis (see above list)**
- **Common bile duct obstruction**
  - Stones
  - Stricture
  - Tumour (pancreatic, ampulla of Vata, bile duct)

Q. How would you investigate this patient who is jaundiced?

A.

A young person with jaundice is likely to have an **infective**, **immunological** or **toxic** (drugs and alcohol) related cause for their jaundice.

An older patient is more likely to have **malignancy** (liver primary or secondary, biliary tract, peri-portal tract lymphadenopathy, or carcinoma of the head of pancreas) or **gallstones** as the cause.

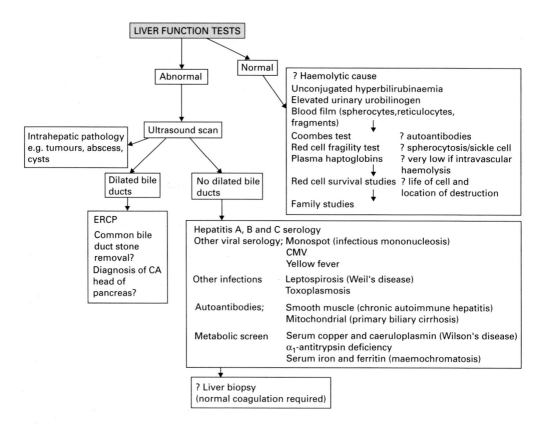

Q. *Assess this patient for possible porto-systemic encephalopathy (PSE)?*

A.

- End of the bed **general observations**
  - Agitated
  - Vomiting
  - Fetor hepaticus
  - Seizures/ abnormal jerking movements
- Assessment of consciousness: perform the **Glasgow Coma Scale**
- **Abbreviated Mental Test Score** 1–10 (current year, date of birth, address, where are they now, name two people in the room, World War II, name the Prime Minister, name the Queen, count from 20 to 1, remember '42 West Street' and ask in 2 min).
- **Myoclonus** (asterixis)
  - Arms outstretched, wrists extended, fingers spread and eyes closed
  - Look for repeated, jerking, forward flap of the palms
- **Constructional apraxia**
  - Assess ability to construct five-pointed star (practice doing this yourself!) . . .

or join numbers . . .

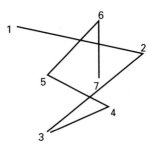

Q. What factors can precipitate encephalopathy in patients with liver failure?

A.

Note that hepatic encephalopathy may complicate acute or chronic hepatic failure. Many toxins have been implicated but ammonia is generally thought to be the most important agent. Failure of normal hepatic 'detoxification' of these compounds leads to brain dysfunction.

Encephalopathy may be precipitated in a patient with hepatic dysfunction by . . .
- **Infection** (spontaneous bacterial peritonitis)
- **More toxins**
  - Alcohol
  - Drugs
  - High protein diet
  - GIT haemorrhage
  - Constipation
- **Electrolyte imbalance**
  - Hyponatraemia (frequent in liver failure)
  - Diuretics
  - Ascites (especially following paracentesis)
- **Surgery**

Q. What is the management of PSE?

A.

The management centres on removing the offending agent or cause, placing the patient on a low protein diet, maintaining good electrolyte balance and treating infections.
- **Give antibiotics** to sterilize the bowel in all cases (metronidazole and rifamixin)
- **Evacuate bowels** (lactulose) to limit ammonia absorption
- **Correct electrolyte imbalances**
- **Stop offending drugs**
- **Diet**: high calorie but restricted protein (for 48 h)

Q. What are the possible causes of acute fulminant hepatic failure?

A.

This may be defined as *acute liver failure* within 8 weeks in a patient with a previously healthy liver.
- Infections
  - All the hepatitis viruses (even hepatitis A)
- Drugs
  - Paracetamol
  - Steroids
  - Halothane

- Sodium valproate
- Isoniazid
- Aspirin (Reye's syndrome in children)
- Toxins
  - Carbon tetrachloride (an industrial solvent)
  - *Amanita phylloides* (death cap mushroom)
- Pregnancy
- Wilson's disease

OSCE station 45

You are asked to examine a 66-year-old female who has been brought into A&E by her concerned husband and daughter who have become unable to cope with her new, yet very **violent mood-swings** over the past fortnight. The patient herself admits that her mood is 'out-of-control' at times, but she doesn't really see the problem, and is most displeased about being in hospital. Her daughter mentions to you quietly that her mother is usually a placid woman, but over the last 10 days or so, has transformed into 'a monster', hitting out at her father and other relatives, over-reacting to minor stressors and **not sleeping**, pacing through the house all night. She has also noticed her mother talking to people who are not there and occasionally **seeing 'bugs'** that are also not physically present. She also states that she has **gained a significant amount of weight** over the last 2 weeks or so, and was wondering if it was this that had caused her mood to alter. She apologizes profusely, but states that her mother's behaviour at home has become so abhorrent over the last 48 h that herself and her father did not know what else to do.

Of note in her past medical history, the patient has asthma, controlled by salbutamol and beclomethasone metered dose inhalers. She also takes 'a baby aspirin', 2.5 mg bendrofluazide o.d. and hormone replacement therapy. She is also currently on a **reducing dose of 60 mg prednisolone o.d.** secondary to 'a particularly nasty chest infection' she suffered 'about a month' ago. She has not yet had her dose reduced because she has had problems getting an appointment to see her GP. She is allergic to penicillin. She is a lifelong smoker with a 50-pack-year history.

On examination, you note a flushed, large, balding woman, who is irritable and restless. Her heart rate is 82, regular. Her blood pressure is **178/99**. The character and volume of the pulse are normal. Her JVP is normal.

Examination of her eyes, mouth and face is unremark-able. Her trachea is undisplaced. She is too obese to pal-pate an apex beat. Heart sounds are normal, as are breath sounds. The abdomen is soft and non-tender. There is no focal neurological abnormality. There are numerous bruises over the patient's extremities and abdomen.

ECG shows sinus rhythm and nil else. Urine dipstick reveals glucose and nil else. Routine blood tests reveal . . .

Na$^+$	143 mmol/L
K$^+$	3.1 mmol/L
Ur	5.2 mmol/L
Cr	87 μmol/L
Hb	12.9 g/dL
WCC	10.8×10^9/L
MCV	90 fL
Platelets	302×10^9/L
INR	1.2
Glucose	14.1 mmol/L

Q. What is the likely cause of this woman's acute symptoms?

A.

It is likely that this woman has developed an **acute psychosis** secondary to **excessive inappropriate thera-py with prednisolone**, an exogenous corticosteroid meant to control her asthma during a presumed lower respiratory tract infection. She has been taking what was initially meant to be a reducing dose for too long, and she has also been taking an inappropriately high dose given her clinical situation and age. Be aware that patients will commonly take the incorrect dose of prednisolone be-cause the manner in which the drug is produced (in 2.5- or 5-mg tablets) means that patients have to take multi-ple tablets in a single dose. An appropriate dose for a mild asthmatic with a lower respiratory tract infection would be 40 mg, reduced quickly after a course of 1 week (e.g. by 5–10 mg/day). This lady has been taking 60 mg for approximately 4 weeks, and not only has developed an acute psychosis, but also has developed some of the features of Cushing's syndrome: plethora, weight-gain, hair-thinning, hypertension and easy bruising.

Q. What other signs and symptoms would you expect in patients with a similar medical problem, not necessarily of the same aetiology?

A.

Other symptoms of Cushing's syndrome include . . .

- Depression
- Menstrual disturbance
- Poor libido
- Thinning of the skin
- Hirsuties
- Acne
- Muscular weakness
- Polyuria
- Polydipsia

Signs include . . .
- Purple abdominal striae
- Osteoporosis
- Moon face
- Water retention
- Buffalo hump (due to a supraclavicular fat pad) kyphosis
- Predisposition to infection
- Poor wound healing
- Hyperglycaemia

Q. Does the patient in the above question have Cushing's syndrome, Cushing's reflex or Cushing's disease?

A.

Cushing's syndrome describes the aforementioned col-lection of signs and symptoms that result due to the pres-ence of excessive corticosteroid (in the form of cortisol) within the blood from any cause. This is the condition that the patient in the question should be described as suffering from.

   Cushing's disease describes the clinical situation of an **ACTH secreting adenoma of the pituitary** leading to Cushing's syndrome.

   Cushing's reflex (also known as the Cushing effect or phenomenon) describes the clinical situation of hyper-tension and bradycardia (the *opposite* of shock) that oc-curs in patients with acutely raised intracranial pressure (usually ICP>150% systolic BP).

   All three of the above were first described by the American neurosurgeon Harvey W. Cushing (1869–1939).

Q. What are the potential causes of Cushing's syndrome?

A.

These should be divided depending on whether ACTH is the cause of the syndrome . . .

ACTH-independent	ACTH-dependent
Adenoma of the adrenal gland	Adenoma of the pituitary gland— Cushing's disease
Carcinoma of the adrenal gland	Ectopic production of ACTH (e.g. bronchial carcinoma)
Iatrogenic/ exogenous glucocorticoid administration	Iatrogenic ACTH administration

An important clinical discriminator is that patients with ACTH-dependent Cushing's will suffer from similar skin, scar and buccal hyperpigmentation as patients with Addison's due to the high circulating levels of ACTH. Patients with ACTH-independent Cushing's will not suffer from hyperpigmentation.

Q. How would you go about making the diagnosis?
A.

The diagnosis of Cushing's syndrome is made based on the results of the **dexamethasone suppression test**, as well as other supportive clinical parameters. The dexamethasone suppression test takes three forms, which are often employed one after the other until the cause of the Cushing's syndrome is finally elucidated . . .

1. **The overnight dexamethasone suppression test**
    *   Used as an out-patient **screening tool** for Cushing's syndrome
    *   Patient given 1 mg dexamethasone at night
    *   Blood taken for plasma cortisol levels at +12 hours
    *   Negative result: plasma cortisol <100 nmol/L
    *   Positive result: plasma cortisol >100 nmol/L → go on to . . .

2. **The low dose dexamethasone suppression test**
    *   Used to **definitively diagnose Cushing's syndrome**
    *   Patient given 0.5 mg dexamethasone every 6 h for a total of 8 doses from 09.00 hours on day 0
    *   Blood taken for plasma cortisol levels at 09.00 hours on day 0 and day +2
    *   Negative result: plasma cortisol suppressed to <50 nmol/L in normal individuals
    *   Positive result: plasma cortisol not suppressed in Cushing's syndrome (i.e. remains above 50 nmol/L) → go on to . . .

3. **The high dose dexamethasone suppression test**
    *   Used to differentiate **whether Cushing's syndrome is due to pituitary disease or adrenal disease/ ectopic ACTH production**
    *   Patient given 2 mg dexamethasone every 6 h for a total of 8 doses from 09.00 hours on day 0
    *   Blood taken for plasma cortisol at 09.00 hours on day 0 and day +2
    *   Pituitary-dependant disease will be suppressed by the high dose of dexamethasone given: cortisol result on day 2 will be <50% that seen on day 0
    *   Adrenal-dependent disease or ectopic ACTH secretion will not be suppressed, even by the high doses of dexamethasone given: cortisol result on day 2 will be ≥50% that seen on day 0, although it will commonly be even higher than this

Supplementary tests in Cushing's syndrome that may aid diagnosis include . . .
*   **Random cortisol**: much debated, value now thought to be very low
*   **Increased urinary free cortisol on 24-h collection**: a good test, but commonly limited by practical failure of collection
*   **Circadian variation in serum cortisol**: test patient without warning and once they have settled as an in-patient; take serum cortisol levels at 09.00 and 00.00 hours (midnight). Normal patients show large drops in cortisol at night-time, but those with Cushing's will show markedly raised midnight cortisol levels
*   **Routine bloods**: hypokalaemia, hypochloraemia, hyperglycaemia, hypercholesterolaemia
*   **Arterial blood gas**: metabolic alkalosis
*   **CT** adrenals to look for neoplasm
*   **MRI** pituitary to look for mass
*   A full **search for malignancy** should be launched if ectopic ACTH production is suspected, beginning with a chest radiograph

Q. How would you treat this woman?
A.

The treatment of Cushing's syndrome very much depends on the cause. If it is left untreated, however, regardless of the cause, then the prognosis is poor, with death occurring due to hypertension, cardiac failure or infection due to immunosuppression. In this patient, **withdrawal of the exogenous steroid should take place on** an **accelerated basis**. Whenever exogenous steroids are withdrawn, consideration should be given to the possibility of **acute adrenal insufficiency**, which may occur after just a few days of high-dose steroid therapy (>60 mg/day prednisolone or equivalent) or two weeks of lower dose therapy (<60 mg/day prednisolone or equivalent). Significant interpersonal variability exists in tolerating withdrawal, though it is likely, given the dose and length of treatment in this patient that adrenal insufficiency would result if steroids were abruptly withdrawn. Hence, she should be treated by accelerated withdrawal of prednisolone, and by **phenothiazine medications** to combat the psychosis (e.g. haloperidol, thorazine). Steroid psychosis can be expected to fully resolve in 90% of cases, whilst **10% go on to experience continuing psychiatric disturbance**.

Patients with other causes for their Cushing's syndrome can be treated in a variety of ways . . .
- **Pituitary adenoma**
  - External beam radiotherapy to the pituitary
  - Trans-sphenoidal surgical removal of adenoma
  - Medical therapy to counter excess ACTH (e.g. bromocriptine)
  - Bilateral adrenalectomy
- **Adrenal adenoma:**
  - Unilateral surgical removal
  - 3–12 months of glucocorticoid replacement
- **Adrenal carcinoma**
  - If no evidence of metastases, surgically remove
  - Follow up with adrenolytic medications (e.g. op'DDD) and radiotherapy
- **Ectopic ACTH secretion**
  - Remove the source neoplasm if possible
  - If not, treat symptoms with metyrapone, ketoconazole or adrenolytics

NB Before any surgery or radiotherapy, cortisol oversecretion should be controlled with the 11-hydroxylase blocker metyrapone.

OSCE station 46

Q. Take a history from this patient who has chronic liver disease and diabetes.

A.

The patient has primary haemochromatosis

So-called 'bronzed diabetes' idiopathic haemochromatosis is an autosomal **recessive** (chromosome 6) condition in which iron is deposited in various organs causing fibrosis and dysfunction. The main brunt of the disease falls upon the endocrine glands (pancreas, pituitary and adrenals) and the liver (cirrhosis). Women are less severely affected due to iron loss through menstruation. Alcoholism exacerbates the pathological process.

The chief features are . . .
- **Liver**
  - Gradual fibrosis leading to cirrhosis
  - Hepatocellular carcinoma (30% of those with cirrhosis)
- **Skin: bronze pigmentation**
- **Endocrine**
  - Piuitary hypogonadism (small testicles) and libido failure
  - Adrenals:
    Addison's disease
    Pancreas — type I diabetes
- **Cardiac**
  - Cardiomyopathy/conduction system abnormalities
- **Joints**
  - Calcium pyrophosphate deposition causing pseudogout and calcification of cartilage (chondrocalcinosis).

Q. How is the diagnosis confirmed?
A.
- The diagnosis replies upon finding evidence of iron overload, e.g. elevated ferritin, reduced total iron binding capacity
- Liver biopsy will again show evidence of iron overload with either fibrosis or established cirrhosis
- Liver function tests classically remain normal despite advanced cirrhosis

Q. How are these patients managed?
A.
Management involves . . .
- **Repeated venesection** until the MCV starts to reduce, indicating iron depletion
- **Avoidance of alcohol**
- **Hormone replacement**: insulin, testosterone and steroid replacement as required (for the general endocrine failure)
- **Iron chelation therapy**, e.g. using desferrioxamine, is

rarely required and is reserved for those who cannot tolerate the venesections
- **First-degree relative can be easily screened** as heterozygotes will have elevated ferritin levels

---

OSCE station 47

Q. *Perform spirometry on this patient.*
A.
- Introduce yourself and explain the procedure to the patient
- The patient should ideally stand to get the best readings, but if elderly or infirm can remain seated
- Ask the patient has to breathe in maximally, and then exhale at maximum velocity into the spirometer and keep going until he can exhale no further ('until your lungs are empty')
- Perform three tests
- Ideally a bronchodilator (e.g. 5 mg of nebulized salbutamol) should be administered and the spirometry performed again after 15 min. 'Reversibility' in FEV1 > 20% differentiates COPD (<20%) from asthma (>20%)

Q. *What is the value of spirometry?*
A.
The time/ volume expired curve produced allows assessment of . . .

FEV1	Volume of air expelled in the first second
FVC	Forced vital capacity (total functional lung volume)
FEV1/FVC ratio	Typically around 80% irrespective of age, height and sex.

It therefore can help differentiate . . .
- **Obstructive defects**: which reduce air flow (FEV1) more than lung volume (FVC)
- **Restrictive defects**: which reduce lung volume (FVC) move than airflow (FEV1)
- Reversibility testing allows **COPD to be differentiated from asthma**

Q. *Interpret the following spirometry results.*
1.

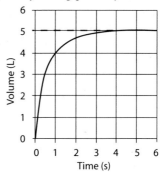

A.

FEV1	=4 L
FVC	=5 L
FEV1/FVC	**=0.8 (normal)**

2.

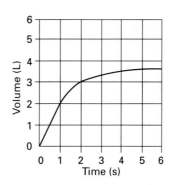

A.

FEV1	=1.8 L
FVC	=3.5 L
FEV1/FVC	**=0.5 (obstructive, e.g. COPD)**

3.

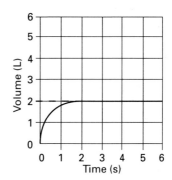

A.

FEV1	=1.8 L
FVC	=2 L
FEV1/FVC	**=0.9 (restrictive, e.g. pulmonary fibrosis)**

OSCE station 48

You are faced in your OSCE with a man in his 20s. You are asked to examine the peripheral nervous system in his legs.

On inspection from the end of the bed you note that the patient has **wasting** of the muscle bulk of his left leg. You note that he does not move it normally. You also note, on inspecting his back, that he has a **circular scar** just lateral to the left side of his lumbar spine region that does not look like it was made by a surgeon. You ask the patient what it is. He says he was shot there 2 years ago. Examination of the PNS in his legs reveals the following . . .

	Left leg	*Right leg*
Tone	Increased	Normal
Power	1/5 (fasciculations)	5/5
Reflexes	Generalized hyperreflexia	Normal
Co-ordination	Not assessable due to weakness	Normal
Sensation	Loss of vibration and proprioception sense; intact pain and temperature sense	Loss of pain and temperature sense; intact vibration and proprioception sense
Plantars	Up-going	Down-going

Q. What is the significance of the neurological findings? What is the name of this syndrome?

A.

The patient is demonstrating unilateral (left-sided) hypertonia, hyperreflexia, weakness (damage to corticospinal tract) and loss of vibration and proprioceptive sensation (dorsal columns), with contralateral loss of pain and temperature sensation (spinothalamic tracts). This picture is characteristic of **Brown–Sequard syndrome**, a situation where there is effectively **hemisection** of the spinal cord, either by trauma (as in this situation), infection, neoplasia, MS or neurodegenerative disease. The crossed neurological findings are a consequence of the differing patterns of decussation of the fibres carrying sensory modalities distally to proximally; the spinothalamic tracts cross to the contralateral side of the cord almost as soon as they enter the dorsal root, whereas the dorsal column fibres remain ipsilateral until their decussation in the brainstem.

OSCE station 49

Q. Take a history from this patient with chronic liver disease.

A.

The history is of **insidious onset of pruritis**. On examination there is a middle-aged **female** patient who is **jaundiced** with scratch marks (itching is the first and main symptom), **spider naevi and xanthelasmata**. There is enlargement of the liver and possibly the spleen if there is portal hypertension.

Primary biliary cirrhosis (PBC)

Progressive **autoimmune** damage occurs to the intrahepatic biliary tree. On histology, **granulomas** are present in the liver. **Anti-mitochondrial antibodies are raised** in around 95%. **Alkaline phosphatase is elevated early**, even before symptoms occur.

There is **hypercholestrolaemia** and an **elevated IgM** occurs. Progression occurs to cirrhosis and eventual liver failure

Q. What are the conditions are associated with PBC?
A.

Like all autoimmune illnesses there are various associated autoimmune conditions; e.g. Sjögren's disease, renal tubular acidosis, RA, dermatomyositis, systemic sclerosis and coeliac disease.

Q. What are the available treatments for this condition?
A.

- **Ursodeoxycholic acid**: improves the liver biochemistry and pruritus, but no effect on survival
- **Cholchizine** improves liver biochemistry, but again has no effect on survival
- Cyclosporin and steroids have been used with **minimal benefit**
- Symtomatic treatments for . . .
  - Pruritus: cholestyramine, rifampicin and naloxone
  - Malabsorbtion of fat-soluble vitamins A, D, E and K
  - Calcium supplements
  - Hyperlipidaemia
- Liver transplantation

OSCE station 50

You arrive at an OSCE station, and the examiner says to you that he would like you to put in a femoral long line by the Seldinger technique.

The vast majority of techniques for accessing the central veins (e.g. femoral, internal jugular and subclavian) employ what is known as the Seldinger technique. This will be fully described below for femoral venous cannulation, then the differences explained for the other sites of central venous access.
- **Introduce** yourself to the patient
- **Explain** what you are about to do — *'I am going to put a big drip into the vein in your groin, so that we can give you all the fluid and medications that you require'* — often an explanation is not required as these patients are very poorly, although you should always attempt to give one
- Attempt to **gain consent**, even though this may also not always be possible due to the reasons outlined above
- Get all your **equipment** ready; for this procedure you will need . . .
  - Sterile gloves
  - Sterile gown
  - Surgical towels
  - Antiseptic solution (e.g. Betadine ®)
  - Dressing kit (cotton-wool, gauze, etc.)
  - A long-line kit, consisting of:
    Long, wide-bore needle
    10-mL syringe
    Guidewire
    Dilator
    Scalpel blade
    Long-line itself
  - Suture
  - Adhesive, clear dressing
  - 10 mL normal saline or water for injection
  - 10-mL syringe
- Place the patient in a supine position
- Palpate the femoral arterial pulsation: the **vein is just medial** to this
- Thoroughly **clean** the area around the proposed site of venepuncture
- **Cover** in sterile surgical towels, leaving a 10 cm² window over the proposed site of venepuncture
- **Wash** your hands

- Empty all the kit onto a sterile trolley, keeping it sterile
- Don sterile surgical gown and sterile gloves
- If patient is awake, use **local anaesthetic**
- Whilst palpating the femoral pulse with the non-dominant hand, take the wide-bore needle and syringe and insert it just medial to the femoral pulsation, 15° cephalad and posteriorly
- Once through the skin, advance the needle slowly whilst exerting **negative pressure** on the syringe
- As the vein is punctured, dark venous blood will fill the syringe; beware the syringe filling itself without negative pressure, or bright cherry-red blood, as these may be signs of femoral artery puncture
- Hold the base of the needle firmly with the non-dominant hand: do not allow this to move from its position
- Remove the syringe from the needle
- Observe the bleeding from the needle in the patient's femoral vein: it should be a **venous ooze** rather than an arterial pulse
- If you are happy the needle is in the correct place, take the wire in the dominant hand and thread it through the base of the needle and into the vein
- Once the wire is approximately three-quarters of the way into the vein, remove the needle back over the wire, **constantly maintaining your grip on the base of the wire**
- Once the wire is visible at the patient's skin, move your grip on the wire to where wire and skin meet, slipping the needle entirely off the back of the wire at the same time
- Whilst maintaining your hold on the wire, make a **nick** in the patient's skin where wire and skin meet with the scalpel blade
- Maintaining a grip on the wire at all times, slip the **dilator** over the base of the wire and down to the skin surface, and with gentle pressure insert the dilator into the soft tissues for about **2 cm**
- Remove the dilator back over the wire, keeping a firm grip on the wire at all times
- You may also need to exert some pressure on the skin where the dilator has just been; this process commonly causes a great deal of bleeding
- Keeping a firm grip on the wire at all times, insert the **long-line** over the wire as far as it will go, whilst feeding the wire up the line
- As the wire emerges from the base of the long-line, take a hold on it and advance the apparatus *en-masse*, up into the vein

- Holding the long-line in place, gently remove the wire
- Either cap off the long-line, or connect it to an infusion (consider taking blood prior to this)
- Suture the line to the skin
- Apply adhesive dressing
- Remove drapes
- **Clean** patient up
- **Thank** patient
- **Document** the procedure in the notes
- Consider the need for radiological confirmation of site of catheter

It is the **hollow needle in → wire in → hollow needle out → dilator in → dilator out → cannula in → wire out** that is the technique described by Seldinger.

This exact procedure can be repeated to access the internal jugular or subclavian veins, using a different catheter (commonly a triple-lumen central venous catheter) and different anatomical landmarks . . .

Internal jugular venous access
- Patient needs to be **supine, at least 15° head-down to assist filling of central veins** (even more important in shocked and hypovolaemic patients) and also to **prevent entraining of air and air embolism** upon venepuncture
- Turn patient's head away from the venepuncture site
- Sterile technique
- **Local anaesthetic** if awake
- Palpate carotid artery with non-dominant hand
- Puncture internal jugular vein by inserting needle just lateral to the fingers on the carotid artery, at the mid-point of a line joining the mastoid process to the ipsilateral medial head of the clavicle. Insert the needle at 30° to the horizontal, and aim towards the nipple
- Follow the Seldinger technique described above, **monitoring the ECG** whilst inserting the guidewire (the guidewire may irritate the heart from the inside, leading to arrhythmia)
- **Document** procedure
- A **chest radiograph** is mandatory post-procedure, both to check position and to ensure that a pneumothorax has not been caused

Subclavian venous access
- Patient again needs to be supine, at least 15° **head-down**, for the same reasons described above
- Sterile technique

- **Local anaesthetic** if awake
- Palpate the clavicle, and feel for the slight cephalad bend in the bone at the junction of its medial and middle one-thirds
- Puncture the subclavian vein by inserting the needle 1 cm below the junction of the middle and medial thirds of the clavicle, and heading medially and behind the clavicle, slightly upwards towards the sternal notch, almost parallel with the frontal plane until the vein is punctured
- Follow the Seldinger technique described above, **monitoring the ECG** whilst inserting the guidewire
- **Document** the procedure
- Again, a **chest radiograph** post-procedure is mandatory

Following guidelines from the National Institute of Clinical Excellence (NICE), it is felt that (where available) **ultrasound guidance should be used to assist placement of central venous catheters**. If you do hit the artery, abandon the procedure and exert direct pressure on it until it stops bleeding. Do not go on to attempt a similar procedure on the contralateral side, without consulting a senior.

Always bear in mind that whilst attempting to secure central venous access, there are multiple potential complications, and these are summarized in the table below . . .

Complications of femoral venous access	*Complications of subclavian/internal jugular venous access*
Arterial injury	Pneumothorax
Nerve damage	Haemothorax
Infection	Chylothrox
Deep venous thrombosis	Central venous thrombosis
Arteriovenous fistula formation	Arterial injury
	Nerve damage
	Arteriovenous fistula formation
	Air embolism
	Infection

House Officer Skills for the OSCE

Increasingly, medical schools are introducing stations into the OSCE setting where they test the skills commonly used by the house-officer. These have taken the form of four general stations . . .

1. The drug chart
2. The observation chart
3. The fluid chart
4. The pronunciation of death/ death certification

The drug chart

During this station, you will be asked to label a drug chart correctly, and then write the patient up for a number of different drugs on differing regimes. It is very important to be able to understand the common abbreviations used in writing up medications, and the main ones are summarized below . . .

i.v.	Intravenously
i.m.	Intramuscularly
i.t.	Intrathecally
s.c.	Subcutaneously
p.o.	Abbreviation of Latin *per os* = by mouth
p.r.	Abbreviation of Latin *per rectum* = by rectum
p.v.	Abbreviation of Latin *per vaginum* = by vagina
SR	Slow release
MR	Modified release
stat	Abbreviation of Latin *statim* = at once, immediately
o.d.	Abbreviation of Latin *omni die* = every day, once daily
o.m.	Abbreviation of Latin *omni mane* = every morning
o.n.	Abbreviation of Latin *omni nocte* = every night
mane	Mornings
nocte	Night times
b.d.	Abbreviation of Latin *bis die* = twice daily
t.d.s.	Abbreviation of Latin *ter die sumendus* = to be taken three times daily
q.d.s.	Abbreviation of Latin *quater die sumendus* = to be taken four times daily
q.i.d.	Abbreviation of Latin *quater in die* = four times a day
q3h/q10h	Every 3 h/ every 10 h
p.r.n.	Abbreviation of Latin *pro re nata* = as required

Use **abbreviations** where appropriate on drug charts. Fill in **all boxes** asking for demographic details. Use the **generic names** for medications, **not the manufacturers name**. Write **clearly** and spell correctly. Be familiar with how to use the **British National Formulary** (BNF), as candidates have been asked to do so in the past. If you make a mistake, do not try to change it: instead, **score through the whole box** and start on a new line. **Minimize ambiguity** at all times. Be familiar with the layout of drug charts: even though they vary from place to place, the information required on all of them is essentially the same. Always give a **start *and* a finish date for antibiotic prescriptions**. Stop medications with a firm line through the **entire** box that it was written in.

A typical drug chart is shown overleaf . . .

DRUG PRESCRIPTION AND ADMINISTRATION RECORD

Date Chart Commenced		Ward	Consultant		Weight	Height	Hospital Site
Number Of Drug Chart / Total Number of Charts Currently in Use					Unit No.		DOB
					Surname		
					Forename(s)		
					Use Addressograph Label		

ONCE-ONLY and PRE-MEDICATION

Drug Allergies / Sensitivities		
Signature	Bleep	Date

Date to give	1. Drug		Route	Signature / Name	Date given	Given by
Time to give	Dose	Direction		Bleep	Time given	Pharm
Date to give	2. Drug		Route	Signature / Name	Date given	Given by
Time to give	Dose	Direction		Bleep	Time given	Pharm
Date to give	3. Drug		Route	Signature / Name	Date given	Given by
Time to give	Dose	Direction		Bleep	Time given	Pharm
Date to give	4. Drug		Route	Signature / Name	Date given	Given by
Time to give	Dose	Direction		Bleep	Time given	Pharm

REGULAR PRESCRIPTIONS

	Drug Allergies/Sensitivities		

Unit Number	Date of Birth			
Surname	Forename	Signature	Bleep	Date

Circle times to be given. Use extra boxes for other times.			Indicate day and month below. Year…													

1. Drug		0600														
Dose	Route	1000														
Start	Finish	1200														
Special Directions		1400														
Sig./Name		1800														
Bleep		2200														

2. Drug		0600														
Dose	Route	1000														
Start	Finish	1200														
Special Directions		1400														
Sig./Name		1800														
Bleep		2200														

3. Drug		0600														
Dose	Route	1000														
Start	Finish	1200														
Special Directions		1400														
Sig./Name		1800														
Bleep		2200														

4. Drug		0600														
Dose	Route	1000														
Start	Finish	1200														
Special Directions		1400														
Sig./Name		1800														
Bleep		2200														

AS REQUIRED PRESCRIPTIONS

Drug Allergies/Sensitivities		

Unit Number	Date of Birth
Surname	Forename

Signature	Bleep	Date

---

1. Drug		Dose		Date/Time							
Route	Frequency and max 24° dose										
				Dose							
Start	Stop	Signature/Name	Bleep								
				Given by							

2. Drug		Dose		Date/Time							
Route	Frequency and max 24° dose										
				Dose							
Start	Stop	Signature/Name	Bleep								
				Given by							

3. Drug		Dose		Date/Time							
Route	Frequency and max 24° dose										
				Dose							
Start	Stop	Signature/Name	Bleep								
				Given by							

4. Drug		Dose		Date/Time							
Route	Frequency and max 24° dose										
				Dose							
Start	Stop	Signature/Name	Bleep								
				Given by							

5. Drug		Dose		Date/Time							
Route	Frequency and max 24° dose										
				Dose							
Start	Stop	Signature/Name	Bleep								
				Given by							

Now, to practice what you will be asked to do in the OSCE, either take a photocopy of the charts, or write on them in the book, and prescribe the following for the patient detailed . . .

Your patient is a 64-year-old woman Mrs Betty Smith, born on 14 February 1940, and you are working on ward 63 at the Royal London hospital for a Mr Jones, vascular surgeon. You are writing this chart on the 16 May 2004. Mrs Smith weighs 68 kg and stands 1.43 m tall. Her unit number is 786768. This is chart 1 of 1 currently in use. She has a well-documented drug allergy to Septrin. Your bleep number is 4312, and your name is Campbell. The time is 11.00 hours. Mrs Smith needs the following medications . . .

* 40 mg furosemide intravenous stat
* Dihydrocodeine 30 mg, two tablets as required, maximum 6-hourly
* Regular 40 mg furosemide b.d. orally
* Aspirin 75 mg o.d. orally
* Paracetamol 500 mg tablets orally or rectally, up to 1 g at a time, q.d.s. as required
* Bisoprolol orally 5 mg once daily
* Zocor 10 mg by mouth at night
* Diazepam orally 5 mg at night as required, maximum once at night

* Cyclizine 50 mg as required by mouth, intravenously or intramuscularly, maximum three times per day
* Oramorph 10 mg/ 5 ml, 10 mg as required, at most every 2 h

The answers are at the end of this chapter.

The observations chart

Another exercise that you will commonly be asked to perform is the filling out of an observations chart. Be aware that the information an 'obs' chart can carry varies, but, at the very least, you can expect it to contain such information as . . .

* Temperature (°C)
* Heart rate (beats/ min)
* Blood pressure (mmHg)
* Respiratory rate (b.p.m.)
* Oxygen saturations (%)
* Blood glucose

Intensive care unit and high dependency unit observation charts will commonly carry much more information, but you would be highly unlikely to encounter such a chart in you undergraduate finals OSCE. An example observations chart is shown overleaf . . .

4-HOURLY OBSERVATIONS CHART

Surname	Forename(s)	DOB	Unit Number	Date	Ward

Time

Temperature (°C)

| 39.5 |
| 38.5 |
| 37.5 |
| 36.5 |
| 35.5 |

Heart Rate (bpm)/ Blood Pressure(mmHg)

| 220 |
| 200 |
| 180 |
| 160 |
| 140 |
| 120 |
| 100 |
| 80 |
| 60 |
| 40 |
| 20 |
| 0 |

| RR (/min) |
| SpO₂ (%) |
| BM |

In order to practice for what you will be asked to do in the OSCE, either photocopy the chart or complete it *in situ* with the following details. The patient's demographic details are the **same** as in the question on completion of the drug chart.

Mrs Smith returns from theatre late at night following a vascular surgery procedure. Her obs from that moment on for the remainder of her stay in hospital are shown in the table below. Fill out the obs chart.

| Day | Sunday 14 May | | | | | |
Time	02.00	06.00	10.00	14.00	18.00	22.00
T	36.2	36.5	36.2	37.1	37.0	37.1
HR	81	83	88	98	99	140
BP	130/90	135/81	139/70	119/68	115/65	98/63
RR	15	14	16	16	17	22
SpO$_2$	98	98	97	95	99	96
BM	5.6	5.1		6.2	4.9	

| Day | Monday 15 May | | | | | |
Time	02.00	06.00	10.00	14.00	18.00	22.00
T	37.3	37.1	36.8	38.1	38.5	37.6
HR	145	139	99	90	88	75
BP	95/59	110/75	109/71	119/68	125/76	134/68
RR	23	22	18	18	18	17
SpO$_2$	97	98	97	96	98	96
BM		4.8	6.7		5.1	

| Day | Tuesday 16 May | | | | | |
Time	02.00	06.00	10.00	14.00	18.00	22.00
T	37.2	37.8	36.8	37.2	37.5	37.3
HR	70	79	78	73	81	75
BP	131/76	127/71	119/69	126/80	134/78	130/73
RR	19	16	15	17	15	18
SpO$_2$	96	94	96	97	96	95
BM		5.9			5.1	

The above observations give the typical postoperative findings of increasing heart rate with decreasing blood pressure (postoperative bleed/ inadequate fluid intake), along with a bout of postoperative fever, a common finding due to either lower respiratory tract or urinary tract infection in the first few days after surgery. The other common pattern of observations that you may be given is an increasing blood pressure with a decreasing heart rate, i.e. the Cushing reflex.

The fluid chart

You will commonly be asked to prescribe daily maintainence fluids to a patient as part of an OSCE station.

This necessitates that you know a little about fluid balance, and sodium and potassium homeostasis within the body. It also means that you need to know a little about what intravenous infusion prescription charts look like. An example, slimmed down chart is shown below . . .

BLOOD/ I.V. INFUSION FLUID AND ADDITIVE CHART				Unit No.							
				Surname							
Consultant			Ward		Forename(s)						
Date	Type of I.V. fluid	Vol	Time to be infused	Additive Name and dose	Sig	Dispensed	Batch/ bottle no.	Time started	Sig Witness	Time stopped	Vol infused

Briefly, an otherwise fit person who is nil by mouth will require approximately **3 L of intravenous fluid per day** to fulfil their bodily needs at rest. In addition to this (and in the short term) patients also require **60–150 mmol of sodium and 60 mmol of potassium per day**, unless they are losing sodium- or potassium-rich body fluids, in which case they would require more of the relevant lost electrolyte, and more fluid. Always base fluid replacement above this 3 L/day on the quantity that is lost: get nursing staff to start an intake–output chart to keep an eye on urinary losses of fluid/ vomitus/ diarrhoea and replace fluid accordingly.

Pearls of wisdom with fluids include . . .
- **1 L of normal saline (0.9%) contains the full adult daily requirement of sodium** (150 mmol each of sodium and chloride)
- **1 L of dextrose saline (4% dextrose, 0.18% sodium chloride) contains one-third of the adult daily requirement of sodium** (30 mmol each of sodium and chloride)
- Avoid normal (0.9%) saline in patients with ascites or liver failure: it will make these conditions worse. Instead give 5% dextrose
- Avoid 5% dextrose in hyponatraemia: use normal saline instead, and fluid restrict to <3 L/day
- Patients with pyrexia require **10% more intravenous fluids for every degree that their temperature is above 37°C**
- Go slow with fluids in the elderly, even if they appear

dehydrated: it is too easy to compound the problems they already have by tipping them into cardiac failure with over-zealous usage of fluids
- **Stick to the fluids you know**: rarely be tempted to use hypertonic solutions, as these can be very dangerous indeed in the wrong hands
- Always start fluid replacement with **crystalloids**, and

move on to colloids later if no success. As a rule, only use blood if the haemoglobin is <8.5 g/dL, or has dropped by >2–3 g/dL
- Always bear in mind the electrolyte composition of various body fluids: if you know that these are being lost, you will be able to replace the electrolytes appropriately. These are shown in the table below . . .

Fluid	*Sodium (mmol)*	*Chloride (mmol)*	*Potassium (mmol)*	*Bicarbonate (mmol)*	*Daily production*
Sweat	45	40	5	Negligible	Variable
Gastric juice	80	100	10	Negligible	1.5–2 L
Bile	145	100	5	30	500 ml
Pancreatic secretions	150	75	5	100	500 ml
Ileal secretions	145	100	5	30	3 L
Diarrhoea (measure!)	50	45	35	50	Variable

If you are asked to write up a day's worth of maintenance fluids for a patient, you essentially have two choices. Either . . .
1. **1 L normal (0.9%) saline over 8 h, followed by 2×1 L 5% dextrose over 8 h each, or . . .**
2. **3×1 L dextrose/saline (4%/0.18%) over 8 h each**

Regardless of which of the above two you choose, you will need to add **20 mmol potassium chloride (KCl) to each bag** to ensure daily potassium requirements are met. Practice writing up a full day's worth of maintenance fluids on the above chart for a patient who is nil by mouth, but who is having no abnormal daily losses (see end of chapter for model answer).

The other thing that you may potentially be asked to write up on a fluid chart is **insulin for a sliding scale**. No matter the rate of the sliding scale, the infusion that is used is always of the same strength: **50 international units of human Actrapid insulin in 50 ml normal saline**, to be given as per sliding scale. You should practice writing this up on the fluid chart also (see end of chapter for model answer).

The pronunciation of death/death certification

These stations are becoming increasingly common in OSCEs, as when performed inadequately by the ill-

prepared house-officer, they can be the source of a great deal of trouble. If you are asked to certify that a patient is dead, you must . . .
- Ensure privacy
- Uncover the patient if they have been covered by a nurse
- **Identify** the patient (wristband, ankle bracelet, personal belongings)
- Loudly **shout the patient's name** whilst **shaking them lightly** by the shoulders, in an attempt to rouse them
- Exert a **painful stimulus** on the patient in an attempt to rouse them, either by rolling a pen over the nail cuticle or by gently rubbing a knuckle over the sternum
- Palpate the **carotid pulse**: note no pulsation for 3 min
- **Auscultate the heart**: note no heart sounds for 3 min
- **Auscultate the lungs**: note no breath sounds for 3 min; also look out for lack of excursion of the chest wall
- Attempt to elicit the **pupillary light reflex**: note fixed and dilated pupils
- If you are at all unsure, perform an ECG (no electrical activity) or perform fundoscopy (cattle-trucking of the blood in the retinal veins, caused by blood separating into blotches)
- **Annotate the notes** to show all the things you have checked for, stating 'pronounced dead', then note the date, the exact time, your name, your bleep number and signature (important to allow bereavement liason officers and/or the coroner to contact you)

- Note the presence of a pacemaker or radioactive implants (important for person doing cremation form)
- Inform relatives: annotate notes once relatives informed
- Inform GP: annotate notes once GP informed
- Ask your senior (preferably your consultant) what the cause of death was, and write this in the notes. If a cause of death cannot be given, you may need to inform the coroner

Filling in a death certificate is an especially difficult skill, and one which you will no doubt get wrong a few times when you are a house officer. Attempt to limit your mistakes, as queries from the registrar of births and deaths have the potential to delay the funeral. There are again multiple steps to the completion of a death certificate . . .

- **Ensure that you knew the patient**: if you feel you did not and that someone on your firm/ a different firm knew the patient better than you, consider calling them and asking them to complete the certification
- Fill in the many **demographic details** of the patient: surname, forename(s), age, date of birth, consultant, etc.
- In section 1 of the certification, you need to give **details of the condition(s) that caused the patient's death**
  - In 1a you must state the condition that **directly caused the patient's death**. These conditions must be **recognized pathological states**, e.g. MI, septicaemia. They must not be too vague. There are a number of unacceptable things to put in section 1a, including organ failure, brain failure, asphyxia, cachexia, coma, exhaustion, hepatic failure, renal failure, shock, etc. All of these are 'modes' of death, not causes of death and will be rejected. You *must* be more specific. If you are struggling, discuss this with a senior. It may be that you will flag up the need for an autopsy
  - Sections 1b and 1c allow details of **diseases underlying 1a to be detailed**, e.g. if 1a was MI, 1b might be ischaemic heart disease, and 1c might be familial hypercholesterolaemia
- Section 2 allows detailing of **diseases not directly linked to 1a, but which may have contributed to the demise of the patient**, e.g. if 1a is MI, 1b is ischaemic heart disease, 1c is familial hypercholesterolaemia, then 2 might be DM.
- Ensure that you sign your name, print your name, and detail your relevant contact details
- Fill in the stub with the relevant details that are already on the main body of the certifcate
- Ensure that whenever you get the chance, watch another doctor filling out the death certificate and ask questions as to why they arrived at the conclusions that they did

Example: a 28-year-old female who has a 10-year history of alcoholism and biopsy-proven grade 4 liver fibrosis is admitted to hospital with haematemesis. She deteriorates, developing group B streptococcal septicaemia and multi-organ failure, and eventually dies after a 7-day stay on intensive care. A suitable death certification would be . . .

1a *Septicaemia*
1b *Multi-organ failure*
1c *Upper gastrointestinal bleed*
2   *Alcoholic cirrhosis*

MED A
24 000000

BIRTHS AND DEATHS REGISTRATION ACT 1953
(Form prescribed by the Registration of Births and Death Regulations 1987)

MEDICAL CERTIFICATE OF CAUSE OF DEATH

For use only by a Registered Medical Practitioner WHO HAS BEEN IN ATTENDANCE during the deceased's last illness, and to be delivered by him forthwith to the Registrar of Births and Deaths.

	Register to enter No. of Death Entry

Name of deceased ....

Date of death as stated to me .... day of .... Age as stated to me ....

Place of death .... day of ....

Last seen alive by me ....

1 The certified cause of death takes account of information obtained from post-mortem.
2 Information from post-mortem may be available later.
3 Post-mortem not being held.
4 I have reported this death to the Coroner for further action.

Please ring appropriate digit(s) and letter

a Seen after death by me.
b Seen after death by another medical practitioner but not by me.
c Not seen after death by a medical practitioner.

CAUSE OF DEATH

The condition thought to be the 'Underlying Cause of Death' should appear in the lowest completed line of Part I.

These particulars not to be entered in death register

Approximate interval between onset and death

I (a) Disease or condition directly leading to death†

(b) Other disease or condition, if any, leading to I(a).

(c) Other disease or condition, if any, leading to I(b).

II Other significant conditions CONTRIBUTING TO THE DEATH but not related to the disease or condition causing it.

The death might have been due to or contributed to by the employment followed at some time by the deceased.

Please tick where applicable

†This does not mean the mode of dying, such as heart failure, asphyxia, asthenia, etc; it means the disease, injury, or complication which caused death.

I hereby certify that I was in medical attendance during the above named deceased's last illness, and that the particulars and cause of death above written are true to the best of my knowledge and belief.

Signature ....

Qualifications as registered by General Medical Council

Residence ....

Date ....

For deaths in hospital: Please give the name of the consultant responsible for the above-named as a patient

---

MED A
24 000000

(Form prescribed by the Registration of Births and Deaths Regulations 1987)

NOTICE TO INFORMANT

I hereby give notice that I have this day signed a medical certificate of cause of death of

....

Signature ....

Date ....

This notice is to be delivered by the informant to the registrar of births and deaths for the sub-district in which the death occurred.

The certifying medical practitioner must give this notice to the person who is qualified and liable to act as informant for the registration of death (see list overleaf). Where the informant intends giving information for the registration outside of the area where the death occurred, this notice may be handed to the informant's agent.

DUTIES OF INFORMANT

Failure to deliver this notice to the registrar renders the informant liable to prosecution. The death cannot be registered until the medical certificate has reached the registrar.

When the death is registered the informant must be prepared to give to the registrar the following particulars relating to the deceased:

1. The date and place of death.
2. The full name and surname (and the maiden surname if the deceased was a woman who had married).
3. The date and place of birth.
4. The occupation (and if the deceased was a married woman or a widow the name and occupation of her husband).
5. The usual address.
6. Whether the deceased was in receipt of a pension or allowance from public funds.
7. If the deceased was married, the date of birth of the surviving widow or widower.

THE DECEASED'S MEDICAL CARD SHOULD BE DELIVERED TO THE REGISTRAR

MED A
24 000000

COUNTERFOIL

For use of Medical Practitioner, who should complete in all cases.

Name of deceased

Date of death

Age

Place of death

Last seen alive by me

Post-mortem/*
Coroner   1   2   3   4

Whether seen after death*   a   b   c

Cause of death:—
I (a)
  (b)
  (c)
II

Employment?   *Please tick where applicable*

B. Further information offered?

Signature

Date

*Ring appropriate digit(s) and letter.

PERSONS QUALIFIED AND LIABLE TO ACT AS INFORMANTS

The following persons are designated by the Births and Deaths Registration Act 1953 as qualified to give information concerning a death; in order of preference they are:

DEATHS IN HOUSES AND PUBLIC INSTITUTIONS

(1) A relative of the deceased, present at the death.

(2) A relative of the deceased, in attendance during the last illness.

(3) A relative of the deceased, residing or being in the sub-district where the death occurred.

(4) A person present at the death.

(5) The occupier* if he knew of the happening of the death.

(6) Any inmate if he knew of the happening of the death.

(7) The person causing the disposal of the body.

DEATHS NOT IN HOUSES OR DEAD BODIES FOUND

(1) Any relative of the deceased having knowledge of any of the particulars required to be registered.

(2) Any person present at the death.

(3) Any person who found the body.

(4) Any person in charge of the body.

(5) The person causing the disposal of the body.

*"Occupier" in relation to a public institution includes the governor, keeper, master, matron, superintendent, or other chief resident officer.

Complete where applicable

A

I have reported this death to the Coroner for further action.

Initials of certifying medical practitioner. _____

The death should be referred to the coroner if:

- the cause of death is unknown
- the deceased was not seen by the certifying doctor *either* after death *or* within the 14 days before death
- the death was violent or unnatural or was suspicious
- the death may be due to an accident (whenever it occurred)
- the death may be due to self-neglect or neglect by others

B

I may be in a position later to give, on application by the Registrar General, additional information as to the cause of death for the purpose of more precise statistical classification.

Initials of certifying medical practitioner. _____

- the death may be due to an industrial disease or related to the deceased's employment
- the death may be due to an abortion
- the death occurred during an operation or before recovery from the effects of an anaesthetic
- the death may be a suicide
- the death occurred during or shortly after detention in police or prison custody

LIST OF SOME OF THE CATEGORIES OF DEATH WHICH MAY BE OF INDUSTRIAL ORIGIN

MALIGNANT DISEASES — Causes include

(a) Skin
 – radiation and sunlight
 – pitch or tar
 – mineral oils

(b) Nasal
 – wood or leather work
 – nickel

(c) Lung
 – asbestos
 – chromates
 – nickel
 – radiation

(d) Pleura and peritoneum
 – asbestos

(e) Urinary tract
 – benzidine
 – dyestuff manufacture
 – rubber manufacture
 – PVC manufacture

(f) Liver
 – radiation

(g) Bone
 – radiation

(h) Lymphatics and haematopoietic
 – benzene

POISONING

(a) Metals — e.g. arsenic, cadmium, lead

(b) Chemicals — e.g. chlorine, benzene

(c) Solvents — e.g. trichlorethylene

INFECTIOUS DISEASES — Causes include

(a) Anthrax
 – imported bone, bonemeal hide or fur

(b) Brucellosis
 – farming or veterinary

(c) Tuberculosis
 – contact at work

(d) Leptospirosis
 – farming, sewer or under-ground workers

(e) Tetanus
 – farming or gardening

(f) Rabies
 – animal handling

(g) Viral hepatitis
 – contact at work

CHRONIC LUNG DISEASES

(a) Occupational asthma
 – sensitising agent at work

(b) Allergic alveolitis
 – farming

(c) Pneumoconiosis
 – mining and quarrying
 – potteries
 – asbestos

(d) Chronic bronchitis and emphysema
 – underground coal mining

NOTE:—The Practitioner, on signing the certificate, should complete, sign and date the Notice to the Informant, which should be detached and handed to the informant. Where the informant intends giving information for the registration outside of the area where the death occurred, the notice may be handed to the informant's agent. The Practitioner should then, without delay, deliver the certificate itself to the Registrar of Births and Deaths for the sub-district in which the death occurred. Envelopes for enclosing the certificates are supplied by the Registrar.

Answers

DRUG PRESCRIPTION AND ADMINISTRATION RECORD

Date Chart Commenced 16th May 2004	Ward 63	Consultant Mr Jones		Weight 68kg	Height 1.43m	Hospital Site Royal London

Number Of Drug Chart / Total Numberof Charts Currently in Use	Unit No. 786768	DOB 14/02/40
	Surname Smith	
1/1	Forename(s) Betty	
	Use Addressograph Label	

# ONCE-ONLY and # PRE-MEDICATION	Drug Allergies / Sensitivities Septrin		
	Signature Campbell	Bleep 4312	Date 16/5

Date to give 16/5/4	1. Drug Furosemide		Route Iv	Signature / Name Campbell	Date given	Given by
Time to give 11:00	Dose 40mg	Direction stat		Bleep 4312	Time given	Pharm

Date to give	2. Drug		Route	Signature / Name	Date given	Given by
Time to give	Dose	Direction		Bleep	Time given	Pharm

Date to give	3. Drug		Route	Signature / Name	Date given	Given by
Time to give	Dose	Direction		Bleep	Time given	Pharm

Date to give	4. Drug		Route	Signature / Name	Date given	Given by
Time to give	Dose	Direction		Bleep	Time given	Pharm

REGULAR PRESCRIPTIONS

Drug Allergies/Sensitivities
Septrin

Unit Number 786768	Date of Birth 14/02/40
Surname Smith	Forename Betty

Signature	Bleep	Date
Campbell	4312	16/5

Circle times to be given. Use extra boxes for other times.

Indicate day and month below.   Year…

16 5															

1. Drug Furosemide		0600																
Dose 40mg	Route PO	(1000)																
Start 16/5	Finish	1200																
Special Directions		(1400)																
Sig./Name Campbell		1800																
Bleep 4312		2200																

2. Drug Aspirin		0600																
Dose 75mg	Route PO	(1000)																
Start 16/5	Finish	1200																
Special Directions		1400																
Sig./Name Campbell		1800																
Bleep 4312		2200																

3. Drug Bisoprolol		0600																
Dose 5mg	Route PO	(1000)																
Start 16/5	Finish	1200																
Special Directions		1400																
Sig./Name Campbell		1800																
Bleep 4312		2200																

4. Drug Simvastatin		0600																
Dose 10mg	Route PO	1000																
Start 16/5	Finish	1200																
Special Directions		1400																
Sig./Name Campbell		1800																
Bleep 4312		(2200)																

AS REQUIRED PRESCRIPTIONS		Drug Allergies/Sensitivities Septrin		
Unit Number 786768	Date of Birth			
Surname Smith	Forename Betty	Signature Campbell	Bleep 4312	Date 16/5

1. Drug Dihydrocodeine	Dose 30mg	Date/Time
Route PO	Frequency and max 24° dose ii, max QDS	Dose
Start 16/5	Stop	Signature/Name Campbell	Bleep 4312	Given by

2. Drug Paracetamol	Dose 500mg	Date/Time
Route PO/PR	Frequency and max 24° dose ii, max QDS	Dose
Start 16/5	Stop	Signature/Name Campbell	Bleep 4312	Given by

3. Drug Diazepam	Dose 5mg	Date/Time
Route PO	Frequency and max 24° dose Max ON	Dose
Start 16/5	Stop	Signature/Name Campbell	Bleep 4312	Given by

4. Drug Cyclizine	Dose 50mg	Date/Time
Route po/iv/im	Frequency and max 24° dose Max TDS	Dose
Start 16/5	Stop	Signature/Name Campbell	Bleep 4312	Given by

5. Drug Morphine 10mg/5ml	Dose 10mg	Date/Time
Route PO	Frequency and max 24°dose Max q2hrs	Dose
Start 16/5	Stop	Signature/Name Campbell	Bleep 4312	Given by

4-HOURLY OBSERVATIONS CHART

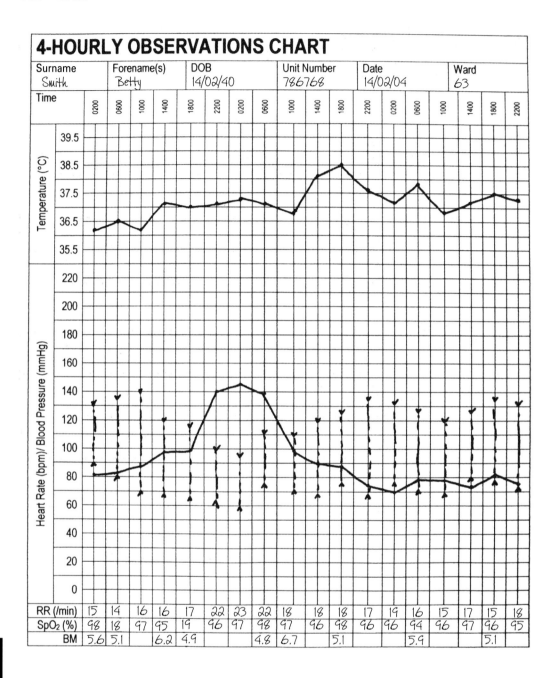

Surname	Forename(s)	DOB	Unit Number	Date	Ward
Smith	Betty	14/02/40	786768	14/02/04	63

Time	0200	0600	1000	1400	1800	2200	0200	0600	1000	1400	1800	2200	0200	0600	1000	1400	1800	2200
RR (/min)	15	14	16	16	17	22	23	22	18	18	18	17	19	16	15	17	15	18
SpO₂ (%)	98	18	97	95	19	96	97	98	97	96	98	96	96	94	96	97	96	95
BM	5.6	5.1		6.2	4.9			4.8	6.7		5.1			5.9			5.1	

Temperature (°C): 39.5, 38.5, 37.5, 36.5, 35.5

Heart Rate (bpm)/ Blood Pressure (mmHg): 220, 200, 180, 160, 140, 120, 100, 80, 60, 40, 20, 0

BLOOD/ I.V. INFUSION FLUID AND ADDITIVE CHART

Unit No. 786768
Surname Smith

Consultant Jones	Ward 63	Forename(s) Betty

Date	Type of I.V. fluid	Vol	Time to be infused	Additive Name and dose	Sig	Dispensed	Batch/ bottle no.	Time started	Sig Witness	Time stopped	Vol infused
16/5	0.9% saline	1L	8 hours	20mmol KCl	AC						
16/5	5% dextrose	1L	8 hours	20mmol KCl	AC						
16/5	5% dextrose	1L	8 hours	20mmol KCl	AC						

… or alternatively…

16/5	dextrose/ saline	1L	8 hours	20mmol KCl	AC						
16/5	dextrose/ saline	1L	8 hours	20mmol KCl	AC						
16/5	dextrose/ saline	1L	8 hours	20mmol KCl	AC						

For sliding scale…

16/5	0.9% saline	500 ml	As per sliding scale	50 I.U. Actrapid	AC						

Index